AIDS

THE UNNECESSARY EPIDEMIC

America Under Siege

The frightening story telling how the AIDS and
Gay Lobbies have been able to prevent physicians
from monitoring or controlling this epidemic.

Dr. Stanley Monteith, M.D.

Cover Design by Peggy Anderson
AndArt, Capitola, CA and
Marsha Smith — the Forum
Santa Cruz, CA

Published by

Covenant House Books
P.O. Box 4690
Sevierville, TN 37864-4690

Printed in the United States of America
ISBN 0-925591-17-3

ABOUT THE AUTHOR
AND THIS BOOK

Dr. Monteith is a nationally known orthopedist who has practiced surgery in California for thirty years. For many years, he has been the senior delegate from Santa Cruz County to the California Medical Association. For five years, he battled within the structure of organized medicine in an effort to have HIV (the virus responsible for AIDS) disease considered an infectious disease so that it could be monitored and controlled in the same manner as other diseases.

As the years progressed, the author increasingly came to realize that there were powerful forces which were aligned to prevent the implementation of a logical, compassionate approach to the epidemic.

The book takes the reader behind the political machinations within organized medicine and the U. S. Public Health Service. It takes the reader into the Centers for Disease Control and into the White House itself. The story tells how even the President of the United States, Ronald Reagan, was unable to implement a logical public health policy in regards to this epidemic.

The frightening conclusion of the story offers a solution and a challenge to every reader, for if the American people do not awaken to the very real danger that faces our nation, we may soon see the same breakdown in the structure of our society that is, today, occurring across the continent of Africa.

DEDICATION

To my wife, Barbara, who has patiently worked beside me during the two years it took to research and write this book. With me, she has read and reread the manuscript to correct it and make it more readable. She has labored lovingly, and without her support and encouragement this story would never have been told.

ACKNOWLEDGMENTS

I would like to acknowledge the permission of St. Martin's Press to quote from Randy Shilts' book, *And The Band Played On;* the *American Journal of Medicine* for permission to quote from Doctor William Darrow; the *New American Magazine* for permission to reprint from their articles; the *McClatchy News Service* for the description of the gay march in San Francisco in 1986; to *AIDS Policy and The Law* (A Burnaff publication) for permission to quote from their articles, and the *Los Angeles Times* and the *New York Times*.

Many of the information sources are listed but many are not. I have read the AMA News, the CDC AIDS Weekly, the MMWR and literally thousands of articles to verify the information quoted.

I would acknowledge the help of my wife, Barbara and my secretaries, Judy and Shirley in the preparation of the manuscript. I would also like to thank Dr. J. Ricker Polsdorfer for his help in reading journals.

Many of the ideas presented are not my own. They are the thoughts of various people who are discussed in this book. No one else is responsible for any misstatements or misinformation which I may have inadvertently included. Any blame for the contents of this book is mine.

The events which I have recorded here, I have personally witnessed and they are all true. For over four years, I have lived a nightmare, knowing what was happening in our nation, but being unable to effectively disseminate that information to my fellow physicians and to the nation. This book is written in an effort to educate the public about our peril, for AIDS is an unnecessary epidemic and today our nation is under siege.

— Stanley K. Monteith, M.D.

TABLE OF CONTENTS

INTRODUCTION

Once to every man and nation, comes the moment to decide.
In the strife of truth with falsehood for the good or evil side...
Then it is the brave man chooses, while the coward stands aside.
Til the multitudes make virtue of the faith they had denied.
Though the cause of evil prosper, yet 'tis truth alone is strong.
Though her portion be the scaffold and upon the throne be wrong.
Yet that scaffold sways the future and behind the dim unknown
Standeth God within the shadow, keeping watch above His own.

James Russell Lowell (1819-1891)
From his poem "The Present Crisis"

The truth of this poem is eternal and is as apropos today as we face the AIDS crisis as it was when James Russell Lowell wrote of the crisis which our nation faced during the era of slavery. Now is the time to decide — for our nation and for every citizen. There is a "strife of truth with falsehood" and each one of us must choose "for the good or evil side."

In the past, there have been a few brave men and women who have taken a stand, but their efforts have been tragically inadequate. I write this book in the hope of motivating its readers to become involved and to follow through with a logical, intelligent and humanitarian approach to the epidemic that faces our nation.

To be able to better understand the story I am about to tell, you will need to know the various personalities involved. I should point out that I do not know the motivation of any of the people I have listed. Many times, well-meaning people will take unexplainable positions until they come to realize that they are wrong. I certainly hope that many of those who are listed who have opposed a logical approach to the epidemic will one day see the error of their position — while there is still time.

MAYOR ART AGNOS: Former Assemblyman from San Francisco. In 1985, he authored AB403 which effectively blocked doctors from doing routine HIV testing in California. Later, Agnos became the Mayor of San Francisco.

DOCTOR FRED ARMSTRONG: President of the California Medical Association — 1987-88.

DOCTOR AXELROD: The physician in charge of the Department of Public Health for the State of New York...a persistent opponent of routine HIV testing.

GARY BAUER: Chief Advisor to President Reagan on domestic policy issues.

WILLIAM BENNETT: Secretary of Education during the Reagan Administration, subsequently to be the "drug czar" under President Bush.

TED BLANCHARD: Administrative Aide to State Senator John Doolittle of California.

DOCTOR WARREN BOSDICK: Pathologist, former President of the CMA, former Dean of the UC-Irvine Medical School.

ASSEMBLYMAN WILLIE BROWN: The Democratic Speaker of the California State Assembly and a leading spokesman for the AIDS Lobby.

COLONEL DONALD BURKE: A research virologist at Walter Reed Hospital. He was the physician in charge of the HIV testing program for the United States Army.

DOCTOR PAUL CAMERON: A research psychologist who heads the Family Research Institute in Washington, D. C.

DOCTOR CORLIN: Los Angeles physician, Speaker of the House of Delegates of the California Medical Association.

DOCTOR THERESA CRENSHAW: A member of the Presidential AIDS Commission, frequent speaker on the AIDS issue and director of a sex therapy clinic in Southern California.

DOCTOR LARIMORE CUMMINS: A gastroenterologist from Santa Cruz, California — Chairman of the Santa Cruz Medical Society AIDS Task Force. He was instrumental in writing Proposition 102.

DOCTOR JAMES CURRAN: Chief of the Venereal Disease Division of the Centers for Disease Control. In that position, he is primarily involved in monitoring the AIDS epidemic for the CDC in Atlanta, Georgia.

CONGRESSMAN WILLIAM DANNEMEYER: Outspoken conservative Republican Congressman from Orange County, California.

DOCTOR LORRAINE DAY: Associate Professor of Orthopedic Surgery at the University of California in San Francisco, Chief of Orthopedic Surgery at San Francisco General Hospital (until February of 1990).

BRUCE DECKER: A gay activist, appointed by Governor Deukmejian as his representative on the California AIDS Commission; advisor to Senator Pete Wilson and the coordinator for the Committee to Defeat Proposition 102.

SENATOR JOHN DOOLITTLE: Conservative Republican State Senator in California, leader of the Senate Republican caucus.

GOVERNOR GEORGE DEUKMEJIAN: The Republican Governor of the State of California (through 1990).

DOCTOR ANTHONY FAUCI: The Director of AIDS Research at the National Institute of Allergy and Infectious Disease, (NIAID), a division of the National Institute of Health of the U. S. Public Health Service.

DOCTOR DON FRANCIS: West coast representative of the Centers for Disease Control, an outstanding clinical epidemiologist, but firmly opposed to Proposition 102 and routine HIV testing.

DOCTOR ROBERT GALLO: Internationally acclaimed scientist. Father of retrovirology, employed at the National Cancer Institute; discoverer of the HTLV-I, HTLV-II retroviruses and co-discoverer of the HIV virus.

PAUL GANN: An elderly political activist in the State of California who was infected with the HIV virus. He mobilized his statewide organization in support of Proposition 102.

DOCTOR STEPHEN JOSEPH: Health officer in charge of the Department of Public Health for the City of New York.

DOCTOR KOLODNY: A sex therapist and author who worked with Masters and Johnson on their book, *Crisis*.

LYNDON LAROUCHE: A radical left wing revolutionary who submitted Propositions 64 and 69 in the State of California.

DOCTOR ARNOLD LEFF: A former public health official now practicing internal medicine in Santa Cruz, California. He represented the Santa Cruz County Medical Society in testimony before the State Legislature and the AMA Convention in Chicago in 1987.

COUNCILMAN LISA: A liberal Democrat, New York City Councilman who headed the City Council's Health Commission.

DOCTOR LAWRENCE McNAMEE: A radiologist from Whittier, California who headed "California Physicians For A Logical AIDS Response," a physicians' organization supporting Proposition 102.

CAROL LEIGH: The national representative of "COYOTE," the prostitutes' union.

DOCTOR JONATHAN MANN: In charge of the "Global AIDS Project" of the World Health Organization.

DOCTOR JAMES MASON: Formerly Director of the Centers for Disease Control, later to become Assistant Secretary of Health in the Department of Health and Human Services (HHS).

DOCTOR LUC MONTAGNIER: Chief of Cancer Research at the Pasteur Institute in Paris, co-discoverer of the HIV virus.

DOCTOR WILLIAM O'CONNOR: A family practitioner who has written and lectured on the epidemic and has recommended quarantine of those infected.

DOCTOR DAVID PENCE: A former anti-war activist, who gave a speech on the AIDS epidemic which has been published and widely quoted.

MRS. PENNY PULLEN: A legislator in the State of Illinois. She was primarily responsible for the AIDS legislation in that state, including premarital testing.

LT. COL. ROBERT REDFIELD: Chief Medical Officer in charge of the AIDS Ward at Walter Reed Hospital and one of the original researchers on the epidemic. He was the first physician to recognize the progressive nature of HIV disease.

ED ROWE: A conservative minister who heads the National Association for AIDS Prevention, one of the two organizations in America working effectively to treat the HIV epidemic as if it were an infectious disease.

DOCTOR MERVYN SILVERMAN: Former Public Health Officer from San Francisco, influential leader of several public health organizations and a firm opponent of the widespread use of routine HIV testing. Currently President of the American Foundation for AIDS Research (AMFAR).

SHEPHERD SMITH: Founder of "Americans For A Sound AIDS Policy," a Washington, D.C. based group coordinating citizens who want to face the epidemic medically.

CONGRESSMAN HENRY WAXMAN: Liberal Democratic Congressman from Southern California and an opponent of using testing and contact tracing to control the epidemic.

DOCTOR LAURENS WHITE: Oncologist from San Francisco — Chairman of the Council of the California Medical Association in 1986. President-Elect of the CMA 1987-88, and ultimately President of the California Medical Association — 1988-89.

FOREWORD

For of all sad words of tongue or pen,
The saddest are these: it might have been.

— Maude Muller, 1856

When historians of the future record the events surrounding the AIDS epidemic, they may well record the tragedy of "what might have been." For there was no reason for this epidemic to strike our nation in the 1980's.

With health facilities readily available all across America, with public health officers in every major county in this land and with our ability to track and control the spread of disease in the 1980's and 1990's, there was no reason for a major, new epidemic to threaten the stability of our nation.

When historians of the future record the history of this epidemic, they will record a story of malice and mistakes, illusion and delusion, deceit and deception, of dying and death. They will record how the liberal media, highly placed government officials and the U. S. Public Health Service worked in collusion to deceive the American public and convince them that every effort was being made to monitor and control the spread of the disease when, in truth, exactly the opposite was the case.

In 1986, the Centers for Disease Control announced that there were between a million and a million and a half people infected with the virus. In 1987, 1988 and again in 1989, the Centers for Disease Control announced there were probably between a million to a million and a half people infected. By 1990, the CDC estimated that there were probably only about one million people infected with the HIV virus. However, the truth of the matter is that the CDC has steadfastly refused to monitor this epidemic.

Congressional investigators have challenged the Centers for Disease Control figures and said that they were grossly underestimating the incidence of the disease in the heterosexual community.

The Hudson Institute, an independent research foundation founded by Herman Kahn in Indianapolis, Indiana, estimated that there were already 2-1/2 million Americans infected with the virus by mid-1989 and that there might be 14 million Americans infected with the virus by the turn of the century (the year 2002) if our nation did not start using accepted public health techniques to control the disease.

The financial impact of this epidemic will certainly destroy the Social Security System and Medicare, the private health and life insurance industry and the national welfare system. The expenses incurred in dealing with this epidemic will eventually bankrupt and disrupt our nation.

Yet, faced with an epidemic of this magnitude, the U. S. Public Health Service and its agency, the Centers for Disease Control, have consistently refused to recommend the control measures which have been accepted by public health authorities for decades to bring epidemics under control.

If this indeed is the case, you may ask, "Why have I never been told?" and "Why is nothing being done?" As I will document in this story, there has been an intentional cover-up by certain government agencies and the liberal media in America.

There is a Gay Media Task Force that reviews television scripts for all three major networks. No program is shown in this nation without their concurrence. When NBC dared to show an episode of "Midnight Caller" in December of 1988 that had not been cleared by homosexual leaders, there were violent demonstrations in San Francisco.

When CBS commentator, Andy Rooney of "60 Minutes" made remarks which were offensive to homosexual leaders, he was accused by homosexuals of making racial slurs against blacks and initially suspended for three months by his employer.

Members of the "Brotherhood of Promiscuity" work in all governmental agencies, the media, our schools and our communities. Any homosexual who refuses to acquiesce to the homosexual agenda is threatened and attacked.

In California, in 1988, every major newspaper in the state distorted the truth and opposed Proposition 102, a State Initiative written by doctors that would have allowed physicians to begin to stop the epidemic. I, personally, polled 100 California newspapers after the election. Only 3 of the small newspapers that replied supported the initiative. Virtually all other newspapers in California lied to the public about Proposition 102 and opposed a sound, logical, medical approach to the epidemic.

Public health officials have come and told me, privately, that they knew what needed to be done — but they had been threatened and were afraid to speak out.

Physicians across the nation who have been courageous enough to challenge the conspiracy of silence have repeatedly had their lives threatened. I have been threatened. Several major demonstrations have been staged in an effort to intimidate me. A letter that I wrote to a friend was stolen from my office (or from the mail) and circulated to every major newspaper in the State of California in an effort to discredit me. This pattern of harassment is understandable when you consider the ultimate consequences of this epidemic and the motives of some of those intent upon blocking effective measures from being used to stop the spread of this disease.

Even the President of the United States, Ronald Reagan, was unable to influence public health policies in this nation during his tenure in office. The President was booed in Washington, D. C. on May 31, 1987 when he spoke out, advocating the use of accepted public health techniques to bring the epidemic under control. Directives which were sent from the White House to public health agencies were ignored. When the President contacted Republican governors across this nation in 1987 trying to convince them that they must start taking steps to bring the epidemic under control, the Surgeon General of the United States, C. Everett Koop, and others, went to those states to convince local authorities that they should not carry out the President's recommendation.

You have probably read in your local newspapers the statistics which are regularly released by the Centers for Disease Control on the incidence of AIDS in America. Those statistics are published for only one reason — to give the American public the impression that the CDC is monitoring the epidemic. Nothing could be further from the truth.

First of all, the disease is not AIDS. The disease is HIV disease. AIDS is simply the terminal stage of the disease. HIV disease is a chronic, progressive retroviral infection which has an average ten-year latency period. That means that the average time period from contracting the disease to developing the terminal stage (which is referred to as "AIDS") is ten years.

Thus 25% of the people who contract the disease will have progressed to AIDS in five years, 50% in ten years, 75% in fifteen years and it is assumed that somewhere between 95% and 100% of the people will have progressed to the terminal stage in twenty years.

The published AIDS statistics tell us the average incidence of the epidemic ten years ago. When you read in your newspaper that there are 130,000 reported cases of AIDS in America it means that in 1980—ten years ago—there were approximately 260,000 people already infected. AIDS statistics which are published in the 1990's tell us that in the 1980's only 4% of the HIV-infected individuals were heterosexual and that the preponderance of the infection was in homosexuals and intravenous drug users. Those statistics give us absolutely **no** information as to the incidence or the pattern of the epidemic in our nation today.

Then why are the statistics published? Simply to reassure the public and give the impression that public health authorities are monitoring the epidemic.

We have only a very few statistics available on the incidence and pattern of HIV disease in our population today.

The Army statistics on recruits show that about 30% of the infected applicants are women.

Masters and Johnson, the sex therapists, released the result of their research in March of 1988 in a book entitled, *Crisis*. They documented that 5% of promiscuous heterosexual men (those with over 5 sexual partners a year) and 7% of promiscuous women in Los Angeles, Chicago and New York City, were already infected with the disease by the end of 1987. If a woman in New York City had 12 sexual partners a year, 14% were infected.

The results of their extensively documented study were viciously attacked by the Surgeon General and officials of the CDC because the "AIDS statistics didn't confirm their studies." Yet CDC statistics published in their weekly bulletin, the MMWR, had already shown the spread of disease into the heterosexual population.

Anonymous testing has been done on our college campuses. We know that on some of our college campuses, almost 1% of the students already carry the virus — but — since the testing was done anonymously, no measures can be taken to identify those who are infected in order to break the chain of transmission and death.

We know that in hospitals such as Bellevue Hospital in New York City in 1988, 2% of the women who delivered children were infected with the virus—but the testing was done anonymously so that there was no way to identify those who were infected so physicians could break the chain of transmission and, ultimately, the chain of death.

Testing in hospitals across our nation is carried out by the CDC by analyzing anonymous blood specimens from newborn children. By 1989, it was recognized that only 1/3 of the children born to HIV-infected mothers were infected with the virus at the time of birth; however, many children are infected secondarily by nursing. Anonymous testing of newborn children was specifically designed so that no one could know which mothers were infected. As a result, no measures could be taken to protect newborn infants from being infected unnecessarily because **we are intentionally not trying to identify the mothers who are infected.**

This is the first epidemic in all recorded history where physicians have been told not to try to identify those who are infected in the general population!

We do know that in 1987, at the Bronx-Lebanon Hospital in New York City, 17% of the people coming in off the street to the emergency room were infected with the HIV virus. By 1988, the percentage of infected people walking in off the street was 23%. We do know that in New York City, 30% of male prisoners being admitted to the prisons between the ages of 30 and 39 carry the virus.

It is estimated today that there are as many as 400,000 people in New York City who are already infected and will die. Even the CDC admits that by 1993, there will be 445,000 people with AIDS in America, but no one ever mentions the fact that for every patient with AIDS, there will be 20 or 30 who carry the virus and will ultimately progress to AIDS and die.

The problem is that every effort is being made to block the widespread use of HIV testing to identify those who are infected. Without identifying those who are infected, how can physicians begin to stop the chain of transmission?

Doctors are consistently told by the Center for Disease Control that they should test only patients in risk groups (i.e., bisexuals, homosexuals, IV drug users and sexual partners of IV drug users), yet numerous studies have shown that the majority of those infected are not in risk groups. By testing only high risk individuals, we guarantee that the disease will continue spreading in the heterosexual community.

Despite the fact that health care workers commonly come in contact with blood and body secretions in their work and these products are known to transmit the disease, hospitals are told that HCW's should **not** be tested for their protection **or** for the protection of their families. The CDC has acknowledged that the incidence of infection in health care workers is 1 seroconversion for every 200 needle sticks with an HIV infected needle. Health care workers, however, are assured that they are in very little danger and that 1 seroconversion in 200 needle sticks is **low risk.**

On the other hand, CDC officials acknowledge that having unprotected anal sex with someone who is infected will lead to infection of their sexual partner in 1 in 200 exposures. Unprotected anal sex, however, is referred to as "high risk sex." The question might be asked, "Why is an infection rate of 1 in 200 exposures considered **low risk** for health care workers while an infection rate of 1 in 200 exposures with unprotected anal intercourse is considered **high risk** activity?"

By early 1990, there were over 6,000 health care workers dead or dying in the terminal stages of HIV disease (which we refer to as AIDS). Yet the Centers for Disease Control tells us that health care workers are not in danger and they insist that most of the infected HCW's are either homosexuals or IV drug users.

In 1983, only 1.7% of all AIDS cases were in health care workers. By 1985, 3% of all AIDS cases were in health care workers. By August 1987, 5.7% of all AIDS cases were in health care workers. In August 1987, the Centers for Disease Control assured health care workers that they had little to worry about, but at that same time the CDC issued a directive stating that all HCW's should start treating every patient who came into the hospital as if they were infected. HCW's were told to use **universal precautions** and that they should all be wearing gloves and/ or gowns or gloves and masks depending upon the type of exposure that they had to body secretions.

Although the CDC publicly states that there are only 18 to 25 cases of HIV disease in HCW's, private discussions with highly placed CDC officials suggest that there are between one and two hundred cases that they know of, but these cases cannot be confirmed because the CDC objects to routine testing of HCW's so they are unable to determine when the infections occurred. Most of these cases in HCW's have been picked up accidentally at blood banks since the CDC persists in recommending that HCW's should not be routinely tested.

In the Federal Register, OSHA (Occupational Safety and Health Administration) notes that there are close to 200 cases of HIV infection reported in HCW's without any known risk factors, yet the CDC consistently recommends against routine testing of HCW's to find the true incidence of the disease.

Health care workers are told that **they should never know which patients are infected** because knowing which patients are infected would be dangerous!

Health care workers are told that physicians **should not try** to identify hospital patients who are infected because if HCW's knew who was infected, it would only increase their risk. Why is this? Because, on rare occasions, there would be patients who were infected but whose blood test had not yet turned positive. This might be only a fraction of a percent of the infected cases or perhaps 1 in every 1,000 to 1 in every 100,000 patients admitted to a hospital (depending on the incidence of infection in the population). However, HCW's are assured that knowing who is infected would cause health care workers to be careless with people who **they thought were uninfected** and, therefore, would be hazardous to their health.

Is this line of reasoning madness or something far more sinister?

Health care workers are told that there is absolutely no danger of acquiring the disease from saliva. On the other hand, HCW's are told that they should not perform mouth to mouth resuscitation on patients and that resuscitator bags are to be available on all wards. Dentists and dental workers are told that they are in danger from working in peoples' mouths and that they should use universal precautions on all cases.

Laboratory workers are told that there is little danger of contracting the disease — although there are a number of reported instances where laboratory workers have become infected — even those who used universal precautions. Indeed, there was one instance in which a laboratory worker obviously contracted the disease by the respiratory route. Despite this fact, public health officials have consistently assured the public that there is no way that this disease can be spread by respiratory means.

The public has been assured over and over that there is no danger from casual spread of the disease. All mention of the few confirmed cases of casual transmission have been suppressed. Casual transmission occurs very infrequently and then usually only in families with long exposure, but it does occur.

I will recount, later in my story, the evidence that I have personally researched.

What needs to be done? We need to tell the public the truth about the magnitude and the dangers of this epidemic. We need to start treating HIV disease like a disease rather than a civil rights issue.

We need to deal with HIV disease just as we deal with other primarily sexually transmitted diseases.

(1) We need to identify those who are infected and find out who they may have acquired the disease from and to whom they may have transmitted it. Thus we can break the chain of transmission of this disease as physicians have done with all other sexually transmitted diseases.

(2) Every case should be reported to the public health officers so we can determine the true incidence of the disease.

(3) 75% of our population goes to a hospital or a doctor every year. Doctors should routinely perform the blood test on all office patients and *all* hospital patients. Had we done that in 1985, the epidemic would have been under control by the end of 1986. However, physicians were blocked from using the test in 1985 and physicians are actively discouraged from doing routine HIV testing today. As a result, the dying and the death continues.

(4) We should test all school students above the age of 12.

(5) We should move rapidly against street prostitutes and houses of prostitution since we are dealing with a fatal, sexually transmitted disease.

(6) We should shut down gay bathhouses, sex clubs and pornographic stores.

(7) In our schools, we have consistently given our children the wrong message. We should stress moral values, sexual responsibility and chastity instead of reassuring our children of the safety of condoms. We should tell our children of the danger from deep, passionate kissing.

(8) We should move rapidly to effectively stop the use of illicit drugs and provide drug treatment centers for drug users instead of bleach and clean needles and a program of "Just Say No To Drugs." In countries with a mandatory life sentence (or death penalty) for selling drugs, there is very little drug trafficking.

Tragically, instead of doing what was necessary to control this epidemic, every possible barrier has been placed in the way of physicians to discourage them from addressing this disease. I know, because I have been in the front lines of this battle for four years.

If someone wanted to destroy our nation, is there a better way to accomplish that goal than to allow this almost universally fatal disease, with an average latency period of 10 years, to silently spread across our land?

If a foreign nation were to attack our shores and kill 10,000 Americans, it would be considered an act of war. Yet, millions of Americans have already been unnecessarily infected in this epidemic and they will almost all die. The tragedy is that this epidemic should never have occurred.

> For of all sad words of tongue or pen,
> The saddest are these: It might have been.

When historians of the future record the events surrounding the AIDS epidemic, they may well record the tragedy of "what might have been" had responsible public health officials been allowed to deal with this epidemic as they have traditionally dealt with all previous epidemics.

BOOK ONE

CHAPTER ONE

The bitter truth was that AIDS did not just happen to America —
it was allowed to happen by an array of institutions, all of which failed
to perform their appropriate task to safeguard the public
health...There was no excuse in this country and in this time for the
spread of a deadly, new epidemic.

— Randy Shilts, *And The Band Played On—People, Politics and
The AIDS Epidemic*

There was a festive atmosphere in Montreal on that afternoon of June
3, 1989. The air was cool and crisp as thousands of people milled about
the registration hall and the veranda outside the Palais Des
Congres...the great convention hall located on the edge of downtown
Montreal.

There were visitors from all over the world: Europe, Asia, Africa and
South America who had gathered for the 5th International Conference
on AIDS, to learn of the latest research and treatment in controlling the
HIV epidemic. Thousands of strangers passed one another or simply sat
about on benches in the sunshine looking at the schedule which held the
summary of the hundreds of speeches, seminars and poster displays that
would be presented during the next four days.

There was also an air of anticipation, for in the distance you could hear
the chants of demonstrators and the blast of the electronic microphone
as young men clad in black T-shirts were being readied for the coming
confrontation.

Almost all the young men wore either black or pink arm bands. They
were affiliated with the New York based organization, ACT UP (Aids
Coalition To Unleash Power). From the beginning of the epidemic, this
group and similar groups had used threats, confrontation and intimidation to direct the course of our nation's response to "the plague."

On this day and the four following days, I watched the demonstrators
and came to recognize just how effective they could be. These groups
have held our public health policy hostage. They have utilized the horror
of the epidemic to gain their political and social objectives. Their
domination of our nation's response to this epidemic has led to the
unnecessary spread of the disease not only in the homosexual population, but throughout the drug-using population and now into the hetero-

sexual population.

The actions of these groups, along with the coordinated programs of the AIDS Lobby[1] and the liberal media, have been effective since April of 1982 in blocking effective public health measures from being used to control the epidemic.

Soon the young men were beginning to parade around in a circle adjacent to the large cement patio on the side of the convention hall. Their signs had obviously been prepared in advance of the meeting. Some of the signs bore the slogan: SILENCE EQUALS DEATH, the same slogan that was imprinted on the front of their black T-shirts beneath the scarlet triangles (A's) they wore on their chests. Many of the signs were dual colored — the top half in yellow, bearing the slogan: WE ARE SICK OF, and the lower half in red having various slogans such as: YOUR NEGLECT, YOUR POLITICS, AIDS HYSTERIA, HOMOPHOBIA, YOUR NEGLIGENCE.

There were other signs that said: RELEASE THE DRUGS, STOP THE PROFITEERING, AIDS TREATMENT NOW, ILLNESS IS DEATH, WE'VE GOT IT, SILENCE EQUALS MY DEATH, STOP AIDS, and AIDS ACTION NOW.

The marchers chanted the slogans as they paraded about in a circle. One of their leaders would call out a slogan and soon the chorus would be taken up by the growing numbers of black-shirted men. Some of the group passed out fliers, some passed out a document entitled "The Manifesto of Montreal," others distributed a large, colored poster that bore a picture of the classic three monkeys — SEE NO EVIL, HEAR NO EVIL, SPEAK NO EVIL — with the caption beneath: SILENCE EQUALS DEATH.

The sound of the chants, the sound of the blowhorn and the sense of anger and hostility that they represented, could be heard and felt by the thousands of people milling about, waiting to enter the great conference hall where over twelve thousand people would soon gather for the opening ceremonies.

There were physicians and administrators from 106 countries in attendance. There were public health officers, university professors, treating physicians, members of the press and just plain citizens who were concerned about the spread of this epidemic.

These were the people who were willing to put out the thousands of dollars necessary to attend such a convention. These were the citizens of the world who were intimately involved with the international effort to try to stop the spread of the virus.

Out in front of the Palais Des Congres, the young men in their black shirts continued to march, shouting ever more angrily and demanding that their programs for control of the epidemic be continued. And they did have a program, a program which was primarily responsible for the fact that this epidemic was continuing to spread across our land.

At 4:00 p.m., the registrants were allowed to ascend to the great conference hall.

Paid employees of the Canadian convention center, wearing their bright red sport jackets, stood beside the escalators and stairways moving that great mass of humanity quickly and efficiently up the escalators into the conference hall.

The opening ceremony was to start at 4:30 with the introductory remarks to be made by Mr. Robert Bourassa, Prime Minister of Quebec. Then there was to be a talk by the permanent representative of Barbados to the United Nations, followed by Dr. Jonathan Mann, head of the Global Program on AIDS of the World Health Organization. The program was to be concluded with remarks by Brian Mulroney, the Prime Minister of Canada and Kenneth Kaunda, the President of the Republic of Zambia.

As we sat in that great conference hall, decked with flags, with three giant television screens suspended across the front of the auditorium, we patiently waited for the event to begin. Behind the stage was a giant sign in blue — the word SIDA in white letters on one side and AIDS on the other. The term SIDA is French for AIDS.

Between SIDA and AIDS was a large circle which was reminiscent of the world. Around the periphery on one side of the circle were the characteristic sequential projections that one associates with a picture of the HIV virus. The theme that it symbolized — AIDS was encircling our world.

It seemed that there was an endless supply of people moving about the auditorium and into chairs, waiting for the program to begin.

And then it happened. You could almost hear the quiet come over the audience as the black-shirted young men carrying their signs marched triumphantly towards the podium. There must have been between 100 and 200 of them on the stage, moving their signs up and down and chanting in unison, "STOP AIDS NOW" — "STOP AIDS NOW" — "STOP AIDS NOW" or "RELEASE THE DRUGS" — "RELEASE THE DRUGS" — "RELEASE THE DRUGS," or "AIDS TREAT-

MENT NOW, AIDS ACTION NOW," or "STOP AIDS NOW" or "STOP THE PROFITS!!!"

Then one of their leaders moved to the microphone. I was surprised to see that the microphone was turned on. As he started speaking, a hush fell over the audience.

"Today, after five years in office, Prime Minister Brian Mulroney has promised that he would stand up and say the 'A' word, or in French, the 'S' word...We find that it is unprecedented that the Mulroney government does not have a policy in respect to AIDS. It is not just AIDS activists who have said that the conservative government has no policy. Last month, the Secretary of Health of the conservative government said that the government had no AIDS policy. People have died in Toronto because medicines available in Buffalo, New York are not available in Canada. People are dying unnecessarily. Our government has victimized its people to appease the homophobic segment of society......"

Then the leader of the ACT UP demonstrators called for a moment of silence to show support for those courageous young Chinese demonstrators who had died in Beijing the night before, as if somehow the demonstrations in Montreal by those dressed in black could be equated with the sacrifice of those thousands of Chinese who had been killed or wounded in Tiananmen Square the previous night.

The audience obediently fell silent.

Then there were calls from the demonstrators for a reading of The Manifesto. "Read the demands, read the Manifesto!" they shouted.

I looked about the auditorium. Everywhere I looked, I saw men hugging men in the aisles. I saw other young men in black shirts who were not on the podium moving about the aisles with their black or pink arm bands on. Many of them were not wearing name tags which meant that they had not paid the $500.00 that I had paid to attend the convention.

How were they able to get in without paying? How soon would the directors of the convention bring in guards to evict the demonstrators? Certainly, something would be done soon to bring order back to the conference...or so I thought at that moment.

Today, as I look back at my experiences over the past four years in dealing with the epidemic, it is amazing how often I have been wrong. For I always expect that there will be a logical response to a given situation. Tragically, that seldom occurs.

The spokesman on the podium began speaking into the public address system again, reading the list of demands from "The Manifesto of Montreal."

"All government and all international and national health organizations must treat HIV disease positively and aggressively as a chronic manageable condition. Insuring access and availability of treatment must be part of the social and moral obligation of governments to their citizens.

"Governments must recognize that HIV disease is not highly infectious. Casual contact presents **no** threats of infection and **irrational fears of transmission must be fought.**

"An International Code of Rights must preserve the humanity of people with HIV disease."

He then presented the following list which he said "This code must include":

A. Antidiscrimination laws to legislate and protect the jobs, housing and access of services of people with HIV disease.

B. Active involvement of the affected communities of people with HIV disease in any decision making that may affect them.

C. Guaranteed access to approved experimental drugs and treatments and quality medical care.

D. The right to **anonymous** and absolutely **confidential** HIV antibody testing.

E. Pre — and post — test **counseling** will be available.

F. The right to medically appropriate housing.

G. No restriction on the international movement or immigration of people with HIV disease.

H. Full legal recognition of lesbian and gay relationships.

I. No **mandatory** testing under any circumstances.

J. No quarantine under any circumstances.

K. Protection of the reproductive rights of women with HIV disease including their right freely to choose the birth and spacing of their children and have the information and means to do it.

L. Special attention to the unique problems and needs of intravenous drug users including provision of substance abuse treatment on demand.

M. Special attention to the unique problems and needs of prisoners with HIV disease and guarantees that they receive the same standard of care and treatment as the general population.

N. The right to communicate and all services concerning HIV disease in all languages (written, signed or spoken) of his/her choice, through an interpreter if necessary.

O. The provision of reasonable accommodations, services and facilities for disabled people.

P. Catastrophic/immunity rights, the guaranteed right of people faced with a life-threatening illness to choose treatments they deem beneficial for themselves.

I listened as the speaker read the demands. Yes, it was all there. The whole homosexual agenda.

(1) ANONYMOUS TESTING so that public health officials could not know who was infected. In that way, irresponsible homosexuals and heterosexuals could continue spreading the disease without fear of being identified and accused of infecting others...as had occurred so often in the past and still continues to this very day.

(2) CONFIDENTIAL HIV TESTING which had been used in California to threaten physicians with prison and fines of $10,000.00 for doing testing if, under any circumstances, they released information on a patient's antibody status.

(3) The PRETEST COUNSELING PROGRAM which had been used so effectively to discourage doctors from doing routine HIV testing to bring the epidemic under control.

(4) NO MANDATORY TESTING. By blocking mandatory testing, they had been able to prevent routine premarital testing and unsuspecting men and women were marrying infected partners all across our nation. Sooner or later, the marital partners would become infected and die. The AIDS Lobby had been able to prevent prenatal testing as well which had led to the unnecessary infection of infants by breast feeding from their HIV infected mothers.

(5) NO QUARANTINE UNDER ANY CIRCUMSTANCES. But what about infected prostitutes who knowingly continue spreading the disease or homosexuals who knowingly continue spreading the disease within the gay community?

(6) There is no **casual spread** of infection. The homosexuals demanded that government agencies accept that position to allay the fears of the public.

I wondered how many people had already contracted the disease unnecessarily and how many more would die in this epidemic which had

been allowed to happen...allowed to happen because of the effectiveness of the organized efforts of the AIDS and Gay Lobbies in keeping
physicians from addressing the epidemic.

The speaker droned on:

> "International educational programs outlining comprehensive sex
> information supportive of all sexual orientations in culturally sensi-
> tive ways and describing safe sex and needle use practices and other
> means of preventing HIV transmission must be made available."

Yes, there it was. They wanted sex education down at the lowest level
— sex education starting in kindergarten — though it would have
nothing but harmful effects on the minds of young children. They were
demanding that teachers present gay and lesbian relationships as normal
alternative lifestyles and sexual promiscuity as a normal means of self
expression. And condoms. Condoms were their solution to the AIDS
epidemic. That was the lie circulated by organized medicine, public
health officers, gay activists, the AIDS Lobby and the mass media.

The speaker went on:

> "The unequal social position of women affecting their access to
> information about HIV transmission must be recognized as well as
> their right to programs redressing this inequality including respect for
> a woman's right to control her own body."

That was simply a call for abortion "rights," for the gay activists had
made common cause with the National Organization For Women
(NOW) and Planned Parenthood. The entire spectrum of the political
left had joined together. The National Organization For Women was
supporting the homosexuals' demands while the gay activists were
supporting the position of the pro-abortion forces.

The speaker continued:

> "It must be recognized that in most parts of the world, poverty is a
> critical co-factor of HIV disease. Therefore, conversion of military
> spending worldwide to medical health and basic social services is
> essential."

Yes, the American government should no longer spend money for
armaments to defend our freedoms. Rather, America should send its
money to the rest of the world to build up the living standard of the
underdeveloped countries.

The message presented might just as easily have come from **Pravda**
or the **People's Daily World,** the official Communist publication in
America.

The demonstration ended after fifteen minutes. The sign carriers and the black-shirted youth quickly moved into the seats at the front of the auditorium which were reserved for VIPs. There they sat with their signs raised overhead while their leaders shouted into a portable loudspeaker.

A man appeared at the podium and spoke into the public address system. It was obvious that he represented the committee which had organized the convention.

"We had an agreement. We agreed to let you demonstrate for fifteen minutes. We even turned on the microphones so that you could address the convention. But you promised that you would leave at the end of that time; you promised that you wouldn't disrupt the rest of the meeting. Won't you keep your agreement?"

You could hear the shouts from the front of the auditorium. The signs went up and down, the portable loudspeaker blared and you could hear the chanting, "STOP AIDS NOW, STOP AIDS NOW" and "STOP THE PROFITS, STOP THE PROFITS," and "SILENCE IS DEATH, SILENCE IS DEATH." The demonstration kept on as the speaker left the podium. His parting words to the demonstrators were: "Please keep your agreement — Won't you please keep your agreement?"

I smiled sadly. Did he really think that these young men would keep their agreement, that they would keep their promises? The one thing they understood was force.

Undisciplined children will push an authority figure as far as they can. And if the authority figure does not have the courage to take a stand, they will push further.

That is exactly what the undisciplined boys were doing. The immature young men who had embraced the homosexual lifestyle had never grown up. They were now acting out their juvenile aggressions and demonstrating that they could bring the 5th International Conference on AIDS to its knees.

I left my seat and went forward to see what was happening. There, clad in a dress made from an American flag with the blue background and stars making up the skirt and red and white stripes making up the top of the low cut blouse, stood a fat, large and unattractive woman. She had very red hair and was wearing a red feathered hat perched on top of her head. Her bosoms were bursting from the top of her blouse. She wore excessive make-up, too much rouge and pinned to her chest was a large button which proclaimed, "PROSTITUTES USE CONDOMS — DO YOU?"

I immediately recognized her as Carol Leigh of COYOTE, the

prostitutes' union (Call Off Your Old Tired Ethics). I had seen her many times on television programs. She paraded up and down the aisles, smiling broadly and chatting with passers-by, adding a sense of frivolity to the demonstration. Television cameramen moved up and down the aisles with their assistants following close behind carrying their video recorders.

All the best seats in the center of the auditorium had now been seized by the demonstrators. A few of the red-coated monitors stood beside velveted ropes which cordoned off the front of the auditorium where the demonstrators were yelling, shouting and chanting in unison.

The disruption lasted for almost one hour while the twelve thousand registrants, who had each paid $500.00 to attend the conference, sat and waited. Finally, the leaders of the demonstrators ascertained that they were in complete control of the meeting. At that point, they told their supporters to sit down and be quiet so the meeting could begin.

The scheduled speakers began giving their presentations from the podium. Occasionally there were hoots and screams from the demonstrators. Time passed and the speeches continued. Finally, two red-coated members of the Royal Canadian Mounted Police, wearing their wide-brimmed hats, entered the back of the auditorium followed by a train of dignitaries, including Prime Minister Brian Mulroney of Canada and President Kenneth Kaunda of Zambia. They were escorted to the front of the auditorium amidst catcalls from the demonstrators.

When the Prime Minister was finally introduced, it was to the disparaging cries of the demonstrators. As he attempted to speak, he was frequently interrupted.

To his credit, he handled himself with poise. He delivered his speech, seemingly oblivious to the mass of black-shirted young men shaking their fists and chanting whenever their leaders gave the signal. Fortunately, the loudspeaker system worked and we were able to hear most of what was said over the crude and rude chanting from the front of the auditorium.

I kept wondering when they were going to bring in the police or riot squad and evict the demonstrators. Before long it became obvious that no one had any intention of trying to stop the disruption of the conference. Although there were almost 13,000 people who attended that conference, people who had come from all over the world because of their grave concern about this epidemic, a small, well-organized group was able to force their will, views and opinions on that convention.

What became obvious that evening and during the days that followed was that no one had the courage to stand up against the demonstrators. Of all the 13,000 people who were there, there were only a few of us who dared to challenge their effort to dominate that convention.

In the next few days, I was to see a clear picture of everything that was wrong with the handling of this epidemic. I would see good men reiterate philosophies which they obviously knew were incorrect. Everyone seemed to be in agreement on how the epidemic was to be handled and no one wanted to openly challenge the demonstrators.

As I observed the charade, I vividly recalled Hans Christian Anderson's children's story of the king who wore no clothing. Only one small boy had the courage to stand up and say, "The king is as naked as the day that he was born."

*** *** ***

The following day was Monday and it was on Monday morning when Dr. Stephen Joseph, the City Health Commissioner of New York City, was to be one of the primary speakers. Doctor Joseph is the man who was primarily responsible for the failure of public health policy in the City of New York and the unnecessary spread of the disease through the homosexual and drug-using population there.

By 1989, over 60% of the hundreds of thousands of drug users in that city were infected and will ultimately die. Doctor Joseph had consistently refused to close the gay bathhouses during the early part of the epidemic in order to stop the spread of the disease throughout the gay population. Why? Because of the agitation of gay leaders.

He had left the houses of prostitution open. He had consistently refused to suggest that HIV disease be considered a communicable, sexually transmitted disease for public health purposes so that contact tracing could be carried out in an effort to identify those who were infected. As far as I was concerned, Dr. Stephen Joseph had failed dismally in his responsibility as the Chief Public Health Officer of the City of New York.

As Dr. Joseph mounted the podium on Monday morning, you could hear the cries and screams from the assembled gay demonstrators to his left. Fifty of them were standing up with their arms raised overhead, each hand holding a wrist watch to signify that "time was running out." They chanted in unison, "RETIRE — RETIRE — RETIRE" and

"SHAME — SHAME — SHAME," screaming at the top of their lungs. It was only when the convention engineers turned up the public address system that we were able to hear Dr. Joseph's words.

Doctor Joseph appeared to be a man in his 40's with dark hair and a full beard streaked with gray. His face was sad as he spoke of his concern for the epidemic which had spread extensively throughout his city. As he spoke, the demonstrators continued to heckle, yell and scream, trying to disrupt his speech. I couldn't help but have a feeling of empathy for him.

In his city, newborn infants had been anonymously tested to determine the incidence of HIV disease in child-bearing women. But mothers were never told that they were infected because the testing was always anonymous. That meant that they would nurse their children and many newborns would become infected. That meant that the women would go home and pass on the disease to their sexual partners...because they were never told of their infection.

As I listened to Dr. Joseph, I wondered how many hundreds of children had already contracted the disease unnecessarily and how many more would contract the disease because **he** had consistently refused to insist that standard public health techniques be used to control the epidemic.

Doctor Joseph spoke on. My feeling of anger at his failure and my sympathy for those thousands of people who would suffer and die because of his failure was mixed with a feeling of admiration for this man who stood — as I had stood in the past — against the wrath, fury and anger of the demonstrators.

As the speaker concluded his remarks, he nodded to the crowd and returned to his seat. The audience broke into applause. The clapping was constant and went on longer than applause for any of the speakers who had preceded him. A number of people in the audience jumped to their feet and I found myself among them — applauding enthusiastically for this man who had failed so miserably.

You could see the close-up picture of his face projected on the television screens; a sad, resigned, public health official, who, at this point, must have known that all his efforts to placate the gay and AIDS activists had failed — and he had failed.

After that meeting, Dr. Joseph was interviewed and came out strongly in favor of beginning to do contact tracing in New York City to try to bring the epidemic under control. At long last, Dr. Joseph was willing to begin approaching HIV disease as a communicable disease instead of a civil rights issue. But, by then, it was too late.

There were hundreds of thousands of people in New York City already infected with the virus and there was no way to identify them all. There was no way to take care of them. Hundreds of thousands of people would die in New York City, **because of an array of public institutions all of which had failed to carry out their appropriate task to safeguard the public health.**

✳✳✳

Another speaker that morning was a very handsome Eurasian. His name was Mechai Viravaidya. He was founder of the Population and Community Development Association of Thailand. In years past he had received awards from Planned Parenthood and many other organizations for his efforts at promoting birth control. He was a poised and accomplished speaker who expressed his deep concern over the rapid spread of HIV infection in the intravenous drug users of Bangkok. He pointed out that the infection rate had gone from almost 0 to 40% in a little over one year and the infection rate among prostitutes in Bangkok was now in the neighborhood of 40%. He was sincerely concerned about the ravages of the infection in his land and he had a program which he was championing, not only for Thailand, but for the entire world.

He stood on the podium blowing up a condom, sealing it at one end and allowing it to bounce across the stage. He pointed out that his daughter had never played with any other sort of a balloon besides a condom. She started playing with condoms at the age of six and now, at thirteen years of age, was busy passing out condoms to all her friends at school. He projected on the overhead screen, pictures of a giant condom balloon that he was taking from city to city in Thailand to popularize the idea of wearing prophylactics to stop the spread of HIV disease.

Condoms were being distributed in classrooms; condoms were being distributed in universities; condoms were being distributed in clinics and by public health officials.

His concept of condoms as a solution to the problem was being embraced by people throughout the countryside of Thailand. Condoms were the answer. What we needed were more condoms and better condoms with wider distribution of condoms and wider acceptance of condoms.

His theme was that children should play with condoms in school;

mothers should give condoms to their children and intravenous drug users and prostitutes should exchange condoms between one another.

His talk was well received and was broadcast by television all across America. The message was loud and clear. Condoms would solve the problems of the epidemic.

A giant condom balloon flew over the Palais Des Congres in Montreal. Condoms were passed out freely from various exhibits. Speakers spoke in glowing terms of the success of condom distribution. There were pictures of condoms on bananas and condoms on cucumbers. There was an art exhibit and here we saw pictures of two hands touching — but on the index finger of each hand there was a condom. There were other pictures that were labeled, "Aids Art," with pictures of condoms on all sorts of various vertical objects — pencils, pens and carrots.

In the days that followed, speakers spoke at various seminars on the importance of distributing condoms to stop the AIDS epidemic. There was only one problem — and it was that problem that bothered me as I sat and listened to the talks and watched the smiling salesmen handing out condoms from their booths in the exhibit section of the convention center. That problem was that no one ever stopped and asked if condoms really worked efficiently to stop the spread of HIV disease.

After all, in a nation as dedicated to scientific studies as is America, a nation where drugs are kept off the market for years even after they have been released in other countries (until those drugs have been proven definitely effective by double-blind studies), in a nation where every effort is made to keep air pollution to a minimum and OSHA will not allow workers to work around any chemical that may be in the least bit hazardous, there were only a very few controlled studies to demonstrate the effectiveness of condoms in stopping the spread of the virus from an infected individual to one who was not infected.

We know that in the era before "the pill" was available to prevent conception, if couples used condoms on a regular basis during sexual intercourse, the condoms failed at the rate of about 10% a year or about 1% per month. The source of concern with these figures is that women are only fertile for a period of two or three days a month and the sperm is certainly far less capable of perforating a condom than an HIV virus would be.

There was a study which was reported at the 3rd International Conference on AIDS in 1987 by Doctor Fishel of Miami, which reported a 16% failure of condoms to prevent HIV infection — when one partner was infected and the other partner was not — over an 18 month period. Once again, the failure rate was about 1% a month.

At the meeting in Montreal in June of 1989, a study was reported out of Africa that, once again, showed about a 1% a month failure rate with the use of condoms when one partner was infected and the other was not.

Another controlled study from Nairobi was presented, with prostitutes who ordinarily (but not always) used condoms. One group used Nonoxynol-9, a virocidal, spermicidal cream and the other control group used a placebo instead of Nonoxynol-9. The group of prostitutes using Nonoxynol-9 cream and condoms **actually had a higher rate of HIV infection** than the group that did not use Nonoxynol-9. Yet, Nonoxynol-9 was being pushed by the Centers for Disease Control and other public health officials across our nation as "protection" against HIV infection.

In view of the presumed failure rate of condoms of 1% a month, is it really safe to recommend that our young people use condoms to protect themselves from HIV disease? How effective are condoms?

Much of the campaign to control HIV infection is coordinated through the National Research Council which is funded through the Rockefeller Foundation, the Russell Sage Foundation and the U. S. Public Health Service. In their report, "AIDS, Sexual Behavior and Intravenous Drug Use" published in 1989,[2] the council issued the following statement to the insiders — those within the hierarchy of the public health establishment:

"Little is known about the effectiveness of condoms...in actual use. Condom failure rates for contraception are known to vary with some sets of users experiencing high failure rates...The committee recommends that the public health service begin a research program to begin determining the extent to which the use of condoms and spermicides reduces the risk of HIV transmission."

There it is...the very words of those who are directing the condom campaign in America in 1989. They don't know if condoms are really effective. They are experimenting with the lives of your children.

The fact is, there is no proof as to how efficiently condoms work. A gigantic experiment is being carried out on our young people and on young people all across the world — hoping against hope that the use of condoms may somehow slow down the spread of HIV disease. Now I am not suggesting that if you are going to be promiscuous that you shouldn't use a condom. The difficulty is the message that we give our youth with condom distribution and condom education and condom advertising. It is the message that if you use a condom you are safe (or safer), whereas, all the scientific evidence suggests a 1% failure rate per month in a virtually 100% fatal disease.

Every young person in our schools, indeed, every person in America — should sign a disclaimer statement acknowledging that they do not mind our public health agencies experimenting with their lives, utilizing an entirely unproven approach to stopping the epidemic.

Condoms are not "safe sex." Condoms are not "safer sex." Condoms are "suicidal sex" in the era of AIDS.

When addressing young people, I will often tell them — "If you want to have premarital sex, if you want to play in the lottery of death — be sure to use a condom. But remember, you are playing Russian Roulette in the lottery of death, a lottery in which there are no winners, only losers. If you are going to play, use a condom. But understand that there is a 1% per month failure rate if your partner is infected and there is no second chance. Once you lose, you can only look forward to the fact that you will **never** be able to have a normal, intimate marriage relationship. You will never be able to raise a family. What you can look forward to is a slow, prolonged, painful and perhaps demented death. Is it really worth the risk?"

When presented in that manner, most young people will say "no." The message of the condom, however, is exactly the opposite. The message of "the condom" is the message that the gay activists and the AIDS Lobby were pushing at the 5th International Conference on AIDS and that same message is being presented all across our land today.

✳✳✳

Just outside the registration hall in Montreal, under the full jurisdiction of the organizing committee of the convention, there was a table that sold T-shirts. On the front of some T-shirts, there was a picture of two men embracing and kissing with the caption underneath, "READ MY LIPS." There were other T-shirts with two women kissing passionately with the same identical caption. There were T-shirts that said, "SILENCE IS DEATH." Other fliers and posters were handed out on the grounds of the Palais Des Congres by members of ACT UP (AIDS Coalition to Unleash Power).

✳✳✳

Along the streets adjacent to the convention center, there were young prostitutes passing out fliers from ACT UP, the homosexual organization. The young girls wore buttons stating — "I'M A SAFE SLUT" or "I'M A PRO" or "PROSTITUTES USE CONDOMS — DO YOU?"

The pink form they distributed asked:

"Why are prostitutes being scapegoated in this conference? Identifying prostitutes as if they were vectors of infection is not only bad science, but a criminal misrepresentation of the facts..."

All throughout Africa, prostitutes are spreading the disease. In New Jersey, in 1987, 57% of the prostitutes tested by the Centers for Disease Control were already infected with the virus, yet nothing was done to stop the spread of the disease. Today, the epidemic is exploding in New Jersey, New York City, Maryland and Washington, D. C. Yet, in Montreal, prostitutes were proclaiming that "identifying prostitutes as if they were vectors of infection is not only bad science but a criminal misrepresentation of the facts."

In 1989, I wrote to the police forces in all the major cities of America where HIV disease is rampant to see what was being done to stop the spread of this sexually transmitted disease. In the majority of those cities, nothing was being done to stop infected prostitutes from continuing to spread the disease.

As I read the flier being passed out by the young prostitutes that day, I reflected that the world had gone mad and those who seemed to be in control were the maddest.

✳✳✳

The red-headed prostitute, Carol Leigh of COYOTE, was busy demonstrating with the black-shirted activists from ACT UP. She paced up and down, wearing her American flag dress — that low cut dress which forced her breasts out over the top of the red and white stripes. On that day her red-dyed hair cascaded down onto her shoulders. She used an electric blowhorn and proclaimed the rights of prostitutes to continue plying their trade and teaching their customers about safe sex and the use of condoms.

✳✳✳

In the small seminars that were held after 11:00 every day, between Monday and Thursday, almost all the speakers followed the same line. Physicians should **not** report HIV-infected patients to public health officers and should **not** do contact tracing as they do with all other diseases. Physicians should **not** do routine testing on patients in their offices or those being admitted to the hospital. Physicians should **not** do routine premarital testing or prenatal testing. Physicians should **not** try to identify patients in the general community who are infected.

There were numerous homosexual speakers who were lauded and applauded for their statements.

At most of the conferences we were told that we could not do testing without written **consent** from the patients, without **pre-** and **post-test counseling,** without preserving **confidentiality,** there was no **casual transmission** of the infection and physicians should always encourage **condom** use.

Of course, there were a few voices of reason. By June of 1989 it was obvious to public health officials all over the nation that the public health strategy which had been embraced in the past had failed. The epidemic was frankly out of control on the eastern seaboard and it was obvious it would soon be out of control in other parts of the country where the infection had already made deep inroads. For this reason, a few responsible public health officials had decided to embrace a new strategy.

Now you must understand that there have been a whole series of new words introduced into our vocabulary as a result of this epidemic. **Homophobe** is a term used to refer to anyone who is concerned about homosexuals teaching in our schools or for political leaders who do not proclaim homosexuality as a normal alternative lifestyle.

Anyone who is concerned about AIDS and its spread into the heterosexual population is labeled as "AIDS-phobic." People infected with AIDS are referred to as "PWA's" or "People With AIDS."

But now there were to be other new terms that would be introduced into our vocabulary. You see, the Gay and AIDS Lobbies objected to the term "contact tracing" — the time-proven method used by public health officers to identify those who had transmitted an infectious disease to another person. And so a new phrase had been developed. It was "partner notification." Partner notification was really contact tracing but public health officials had to use this new term so they would not inflame or antagonize the homosexual activists and the AIDS Lobby.

In 1989 another new phrase was introduced. Those of us who have been involved in the struggle for years wanted to do routine HIV blood testing to identify those who were infected and to begin controlling the epidemic but all efforts to encourage routine HIV testing had been opposed and effectively blocked by the left-wing establishment. So a new phrase was introduced by responsible public health officers... **"early diagnosis."** Of course **"early diagnosis"** was simply **"routine testing"** of people in an effort to find out who was infected. It was hoped that the new phrase would not promote the same angry and vindictive response that the term "routine testing" had evoked.

And so it was that on Sunday morning, June 3, before the conference had actually begun and before the demonstrators had seized the podium at the Palais Des Congres to denounce Prime Minister Brian Mulroney, I attended a preconvention meeting on counseling and testing that had been sponsored by the American Medical Association. The concluding speaker was Dr. James Mason, then the Assistant Secretary of Health in the Department of Health and Human Services.

Doctor Mason is a career bureaucrat. He has tried to play the political game and survive as a public health officer in a government dominated by the radical left, where liberal politicians can harass and hound responsible and concerned physicians to the point where they are forced out of office. For a number of years, before moving to the Department of HHS, Doctor Mason had been Director of the Centers for Disease Control and had taken a middle-of-the-road position in order not to offend the liberals and homosexuals in government.

Since the liberal Democrats hold power in both the Senate and the House of Representatives, any spokesman from the public health department has to accede to their demands and avoid any semblance of anti-gay bias or opposition to the gay program for America — both as far as promotion of the gay lifestyle and following the gay program to deal with the AIDS epidemic.

Later in my story, I will tell you of my first encounter with Doctor Mason and his testimony before a congressional committee. I shall have to admit that I had a very low impression of his integrity and sincerity at that time but, looking back on that episode, I rather feel that I was unkind in my judgment. One must realize that it is very difficult to be courageous when one is a government employee and sometimes, in government, being able to survive is an accomplishment and an end in itself. Courageous men are fired or destroyed. Whistle-blowers are drummed out of government. That is why no one in government breaks the code of silence and tells the public the truth about this epidemic.

And so it was, on the morning of June 3, 1989, Dr. Mason addressed a group of perhaps 150 attendees at the preconference-conference at the Bonaventure Hilton Hotel in downtown Montreal.

Doctor Mason is of medium height with a round face, graying hair and wears rimless glasses. He speaks well and clearly. During the course of his talk, he announced that the theme of the 5th International Conference in Montreal was to be the encouragement of "early diagnosis" in an effort to stop the spread of disease. His words and his sentiments were well stated and I was initially filled with hope and encouragement as the audience warmly applauded his remarks. Then came the time for questions from the audience.

One of the AIDS activists from San Francisco sprang to his feet — a physician who has often attacked me at the meetings of the House of Delegates of the California Medical Association —

"You're not suggesting we do routine testing?" he demanded. "You are not suggesting that we do testing without **consent** and **confidentiality** and pre- and post-test **counseling?**" he reiterated in an angry tone of voice. "Certainly, you are not suggesting that we simply do **routine** testing?"

It was at that point that I saw why we, as a nation, are losing the battle. Doctor James Mason, former Director of the CDC, and at that time, the Assistant Secretary of Health in the Department of Health and Human Services, began backing away from his statements on "early diagnosis." He assured the speaker that he had no intention of suggesting that physicians should do testing without consent and confidentiality and pre- and post-test counseling. He agreed that those steps were vitally important to combat the epidemic. Nothing more was said about the importance of **early diagnosis to stop** the ravages of the disease and protect both the infected and uninfected from this horrible, progressive, fatal illness. Once again, I saw how good men would retreat under attack from a well organized minority whose political allies held the reins of power in Washington, D. C.

Later during the convention, Dr. Mason was asked how he stood on mandatory contact tracing of partners of HIV infected persons.

Now, all across America, public health departments carry out mandatory contact tracing on all other serious diseases to stop their spread; however, the Gay and AIDS Lobbies have consistently opposed mandatory contact tracing for HIV disease. How did Mason respond?

"Love, concern and consideration should be the motivation in partner notification, not the force of law."

Yes—Dr. Mason understands the rules of the game. Never offend the Gay or AIDS Lobbies. That's how you survive in government service.

⁂

Each day, Monday through Thursday, between 11 a.m. and 5:30 p.m., dozens of separate 1-1/2 hour seminars were presented on varied subjects with 5 or 6 speakers presenting their views. At one of these sessions, a woman who was a public health official from Wisconsin got up and spoke about the importance of beginning to report HIV disease to public health departments as physicians do with all other diseases. Immediately, gay activists were at the microphones shouting and condemning her. One young man shouted:

"You want my name on a list. You want to quarantine me. You want to lock me up!"

Almost every person at the microphones was either a gay activist or a liberal activist and the speaker from Wisconsin was badgered with the same question over and over, putting her into a totally defensive position. Nobody from the audience would speak up on her behalf. Finally, the moderator interrupted the questions and went on to the next speaker.

At this point, another woman from the public health service got up and suggested that public health officials should begin keeping files and records on those who were infected just like they do with all other serious diseases.

The response to her remarks was similar. The black-shirted, gay activists and the liberal activists were at the microphones angrily denouncing the idea that public health officers should keep any lists of the names of people who were infected. The threats of quarantine and discrimination were raised, with a very pointed suggestion that the only reason anybody wanted to treat HIV disease as we do other diseases was so that government and homophobes could eventually discriminate against those who were infected.

Sitting in the back of the room, I could see the woman on the podium beginning to wilt under the vicious verbal attacks from the audience. I walked to the microphone in the rear of the room and when my turn came, I started out with a simple statement:

"First of all, I would like to thank you for suggesting that we should begin to address HIV disease as an epidemic.

"Secondly, I have a question. By this time there have probably been more than one hundred thousand cases of AIDS and HIV disease reported, in confidence, to public health officers all across our nation. Do you know of even one instance where reporting of a case of AIDS or HIV disease to a public health officer, in confidence, has ever led to release of that information and discrimination against that patient?"

The room went wild. Gay activists from all sides of the room began yelling and screaming and waving their arms. Of course, I had anticipated this reaction, but I could not imagine sitting in the room and allowing them to viciously, verbally attack the quiet, young woman at the speaker's podium. The woman at the podium could not answer my question because **there are no cases of discrimination resulting from public health officers releasing the names of infected patients.**

One gay activist in the room began shouting out the name of Roy Cohn. "How about Roy Cohn," he screamed, "How about Roy Cohn?"

I looked at him, "The public health officer didn't release Roy Cohn's name — that was the coroner. He was dead."

The yelling and hurling of insults continued. At the microphone, I raised my voice and said, "Once again, let me congratulate you for beginning to address this epidemic as an epidemic."

There was a warm round of applause from the audience, because, you see, most of the people in the audience knew and understood that we were treating HIV disease as a civil rights issue and not as an epidemic. Yet no one else had the courage to stand and make that statement publicly.

As I moved to my seat, the chairman of the session called for order and the next speaker. At this point, a small man, wearing a red jumper-jacket, his braided hair hanging down to his mid-back, rushed to the microphone and demanded an opportunity to speak.

"You let that big doctor speak, now I want an opportunity to speak," he shouted, angrily, "You let that fat-ass doctor get up and talk and I want an opportunity to counter what he said."

Someone from the audience spoke up, "This is a professional meeting — why don't you act professionally?"

The man at the microphone shouted angrily, "I'm a doctor too and I can tell you that we (meaning the gay activists) have saved an awful lot of lives."

That was the response that anybody could expect if they stood up and talked about addressing HIV disease as a disease. I spoke out several other times at the conference and almost every time I was greeted with rounds of applause from those in the audience and screams and shouts from the gay and AIDS activists.

The tragedy was that there were only two physicians out of the thousands of physicians in attendance who had the courage to stand and challenge the AIDS Lobby and Gay Lobby's control of the 5th International Conference on AIDS in Montreal.

✳✳✳

There was only one talk in the entire meeting which I felt dealt with the real problem that we face today. The talk was given by Doctor S. I. Okware, who is the Director of the Ugandan AIDS Control Program in Entebbe, Uganda. This frail, thin, black man presented his country's approach to the AIDS epidemic.

Doctor Okware spoke in somewhat halting English and it was difficult to understand him. He talked about his nation, ravaged with disease, with one of the highest rates of HIV infection anywhere in Africa. Certainly, a large segment of the reproductive population of his nation was already infected and were going to die as a result of this epidemic. And how were they handling the epidemic in Uganda?

They had mobilized the community. They had gone to the media and into the schools and insisted that they present an educational program based on moral precepts. They had gone into the churches and insisted that their ministers inform their parishioners about the epidemic and about the moral implications of the disease. They had gone to all government employees and insisted that they be educated about the epidemic and its moral implications.

Any government official who wanted a promotion had to take a test to make sure that he understood the epidemic. They were using education all across Uganda — but a far different type of education from what was being used in America, Western Europe or most of Africa.

After his talk, I went to the podium and asked Doctor Okware if I had understood him correctly.

"What are you having your ministers tell the people?" I asked.

"The ministers are to preach morality."

"But what about condoms. Aren't you passing out condoms?"

He looked at me quizzically:

"Condoms?" he queried. We don't pass out condoms. The President of my country has said that we will not pass out condoms. Our President says that if we pass out condoms, we give our young people the wrong message. Condoms tell our youth that promiscuity is all right. Our program in Uganda is to encourage morality and our program is working. It used to be that our sexually transmitted disease clinics would have 10 or 15 cases of STD's a day. Now we have perhaps 1 case a week, if that. We are cutting back on the transmission of HIV disease and venereal disease in our country."

I looked at this black man from Africa who was talking about **morality.**

America, for years, has been the center of Christianity. America is a nation sending Christian missionaries to Africa, but in America, the nation which today is financing most of the Christian evangelism throughout the world, almost no one in a position of power ever talks about concepts of Christian morality.

America's answer to the epidemic was "condoms." We were telling our young people that sexual promiscuity is perfectly acceptable as long as they use condoms. After years of intensive education, our sexually transmitted disease clinics all across America are crowded with clients. The epidemic continues to spread, teenage pregnancy continues unabated and syphilis rates continue to rise year after year after year.

Yet here was a man from Africa talking about morality as the answer to the epidemic. Our former Surgeon General, Dr. C. Everett Koop, would never publicly mention morality, nor would any of the medical leaders or public health leaders of our nation. Had our nation deteriorated so far spiritually and morally that we would have to look to doctors from Africa for leadership? That was a question that would haunt my thoughts during the rest of that convention.

America has lost its position of moral leadership; America has lost its vision; America has turned its back on its heritage of freedom under God. Americans have forgotten the admonition of our greatest libertarian, the man who wrote the Declaration of Independence. His words have long since been forgotten, although they are still chiseled in the granite of the Jefferson Monument in Washington, D. C.:

"God who gave us life gave us liberty. Can the liberties of a nation be secure when we have removed a conviction that these liberties are the gift of God? Indeed, I tremble for my country when I reflect that God is just, that His justice cannot sleep forever."

In a nation where we inscribe "In God We Trust" on our money; where the Congress opens every day with a prayer; where above the seat of the Chief Justice of the Supreme Court are inscribed the Ten Commandments, in that nation, Americans cannot mention God in school because we are told that we would be violating the principle of "the separation of church and state."

Faced with a moral crisis and a sexually transmitted epidemic, our leaders and public health officials across our nation, our Surgeon General and our Centers for Disease Control — and organized medicine — are all advocating the use of **condoms.**

I looked at the slightly built, black physician in front of me and grasped his hand.

"Thank you and God bless you," I said.

✳✳✳

One of the more interesting exhibits appeared in the poster section of the convention. Here, the Centers for Disease Control had a very elaborate series of posters to demonstrate **why mandatory premarital HIV blood testing was unnecessary.** They pointed out that:

1. There would be 4,778,00 men and women who would be married in 1990. Of these 4,778,000 people, 9,697 would marry a partner who was HIV positive. At $40.00 each for an HIV test (over 10 times what the U. S. Army pays for each HIV test) it would cost $191,121,000.00 to identify those 9,697 people who carry the virus or over $200,000 for each person whose life might be saved.

2. In addition, there would be 48 people who would be incorrectly told they had the disease (i.e., have a false-positive blood test) who would have their lives ruined. The poster exhibit went on to point out that;

3. The Centers for Disease Control only receives $211,889,000.00 a year for all its activities. Thus, the expenditure of $191,121,000.00 was wasteful just to identify those 9,697 people who were infected and who were entering into a life long sexual relationship with their uninfected partners.

The purpose of this exhibit was obviously to convince those attending the conference that mandatory premarital blood testing was a poor expenditure of money. The poster exhibit presented the following conclusions:

1. The cost of identifying infected people getting married is high compared with other preventative programs.

2. We don't know what happens when people find out that the person they are intending to marry is infected.

3. If premarital testing is carried out in one state, then people will

simply journey to another state to get married so they won't have to waste money for the HIV blood test.

What is basically wrong with this scenario?

1. By CDC figures, it is costing a little over $200,000.00 to identify one person who has a positive HIV test based upon the premise that they will have to test 5000 people at $40.00 per test to find one person who tests positive. On the other hand, what will be the cost to take care of the marriage partner who will become infected by their undiagnosed husband/wife because the CDC opposes premarital blood testing? The cost for caring for **one** patient will be $50,000.00 to $70,000.00 per year. They may well live for three years with current treatment. With new medical programs, perhaps they will live four to five years.

Yet, the CDC opposes doing the testing. Thus, by the CDC's own figures, 9,697 uninfected people will marry infected partners in 1990 and the vast majority of them will become infected via sexual relations...unnecessarily.

2. How much does it cost to take care of one child who is going to be conceived as a product of these marriages? Taking care of a child is three or four times more expensive than taking care of an adult. It will ordinarily cost $150,000.00 to $200,000.00 yearly to take care of an infected child if they remain in the hospital.

3. If the U. S. Public Health Service was really intent upon addressing the epidemic, they would suggest getting the HIV test done in the same manner as the Army does. The test could be drawn at the local public health clinics or at a doctor's office when the routine premarital examination is performed. The blood test could then be sent to one of the public laboratories used by the Army and all the testing could be done for less than $4.00 per test.

That would mean that instead of spending $191,121,000.00 for the nationwide premarital testing, it would really cost only a little over twenty million dollars to test the entire group or a total of about twenty thousand dollars for each life we could expect to save. In addition, the government does not put out the money. The money is put out by those getting married. Wouldn't most individuals honestly really rather put out $4.00 to protect the life of someone they love and prevent them from becoming infected unnecessarily?

4. The idea that someone is simply going to journey to another state would **not be valid if laws were introduced in every state. Furthermore, people should be** educated as to the importance of having

premarital HIV testing rather than being purposely frightened with all the possible social and economic implications of the blood test, most of which are simply fear tactics circulated by the Gay Lobby and the AIDS Lobby.

5. The specter of false-positive HIV tests is invalid if the proper sequence of testing is done and a confirmatory test is drawn. At the most, there might be 3 or 4 false-positives among the 4 million marriage applicants tested and the 9,697 lives saved.

6. The next point that the CDC ignores is the question, "What is a human life really worth in dollars and cents?" I'm certain that no one in Atlanta really wants to answer that question.

Recently there has been a great deal of concern about asbestos insulation used in public buildings and schools across America. Currently, Congress has passed the "Asbestos Hazard Emergency Response Act" which requires the EPA to contact school districts to monitor and label asbestos contaminated buildings. It is estimated that our nation will spend 100 to 150 billion dollars to remove asbestos from school buildings and other buildings in the coming decade — to protect the public health. What is the danger to school children? In an article in the prestigious New England Journal of Medicine, June 29, 1989, it was estimated that the danger of death to school children in America from cancer and disease as a result of asbestos insulation was between .37 and .02 per million school children per year. Thus, the danger is somewhere between 1 in 3 million children to 1 in 20 million children who may die from the complication of asbestos insulation yearly.

But as many as 9,697 people will contract HIV infection in 1990 from their infected marriage partners because the CDC has determined that premarital blood testing is "just too expensive."

How many infected children will be born with the virus or contract the virus from breast feeding?

But we can spend 100 to 150 billion dollars to take asbestos insulation out of our school buildings to prevent unnecessary deaths and "preserve the public health."

This CDC poster exhibit was simply another example of the sophistry that has been used so effectively by certain groups within the CDC. Even more interesting is the response that I got when I went to the Centers for Disease Control in Atlanta, Georgia in April of 1989 and asked why the CDC consistently opposed premarital HIV testing. The response I got was really beyond comprehension and represented an intentional effort on the part of certain people within the CDC to distort reality with unsound arguments. But I am getting far ahead of my story.

✳✳✳

During one of the discussions at the convention when mandatory premarital blood testing was being discussed by public officials from Illinois, it was pointed out that premarital blood testing in Illinois revealed only .05% positive test results and, therefore, mandatory blood testing of marriage applicants was wasteful and unwarranted. In response to this statement, Colonel Donald Burke of Walter Reed Hospital (you will hear more of him later) rose to challenge the statistics.

"You insist on mandatory testing of blood specimens from blood donors when the incidence of infection is .05%. On the other hand, you say that premarital testing of marriage applicants is unwarranted because the incidence is only .05%. Isn't that inconsistent?"

The public health officials from Illinois had difficulty responding — because public health jobs are political jobs and public health officers want to keep them. That is why many public health officials publicly disavow testing, although privately they acknowledge that testing could save millions of lives.

✳✳✳

There was an art exhibit in the building immediately across the street from the Palais Des Congres. Here were a series of pictures aimed at desensitizing the viewer to the homosexual lifestyle. There was one picture of a man with his face in the crotch of another man — obviously engaging in oral sex. There were pictures of two young Oriental boys in bed, smiling at one another. There was another picture of two young Caucasian boys in bed — smiling and beaming. There were pictures of young men with their bodies intertwined in a strange, sensuous, passionate embrace.

Picture after picture demonstrating the loving relationships between men. This exhibit of "so-called" art was being presented as a "scientific exhibit" in an effort to desensitize the minds of the viewers and convince the public of the normality and acceptability of the homosexual lifestyle.

✳✳✳

From time to time the black-shirted young men would come into the major auditorium and take seats in the front. Their presence was sufficient to intimidate the organizers of the convention into acquiescence to any or all their demands.

On the second or third morning of the convention, a young man (who was not scheduled to be on the program) was suddenly the lead-off speaker. There was a band of black-shirted demonstrators in the front of the audience ready to disrupt the entire meeting if their spokesman was not allowed to speak. His subject was "discrimination" and how the speaker had encountered discrimination because he was HIV positive.

✳✳✳

As the days passed, it became increasingly obvious that the meeting was totally under homosexual domination. Time and again, if a speaker said something that the homosexuals disagreed with, the black-shirted young men from ACT UP would shout and scream and the speaker would generally apologize and concede that the real problem was not the virus but discrimination and that we needed antidiscrimination laws so we could begin to fight the epidemic.

It was late on Thursday afternoon, the final day of the conference, when I attended one of the seminars which was a discussion on "the danger to health care workers" and the general theme of the seminar was that **doctors should not test patients going into the hospital because doctors did not need to know who was infected.**

During the concluding remarks of the session, I rose to one of the microphones and asked a simple question.

"When are we going to stop treating this epidemic as if it were a civil rights issue and begin treating it as if it were a medical issue? When are we going to try to stop this epidemic?"

The audience broke into applause.

I went on to discuss the importance of knowing whether or not a surgical patient had an altered immune system before being subjected to surgery. After all, if a patient is HIV positive and has an altered immune system, his wound could break down and he could die unnecessarily of infection. Yet all the doctors on the panel objected to the testing of surgical patients. The representative from the CDC feigned surprise at the suggestion that those with an altered immune system might be endangered by surgery.

It is fascinating to look back at what happened during the next few minutes. As soon as the meeting broke up, a number of people came to speak to me. First there was a missionary doctor from Tanzania. He told me of operating on dozens of HIV-infected patients with altered immune responses and watching them die of uncontrollable infections.

The second person to approach me was a young man from Chicago. He remarked:

"You will be able to start treating HIV disease as a disease once we get our antidiscrimination law."

"An antidiscrimination law?" I responded. "You could have had an antidiscrimination law a year ago. The bill was on the governor's desk in California and Governor Deukmejian would have signed the bill if the California Medical Association and the AIDS Lobby had just allowed us to begin treating HIV as a medical condition, but they wouldn't make that concession. Discrimination isn't the issue. They just don't want physicians to address HIV as a disease."

The young man was quick and authoritative in his response.

"What we need is a national antidiscrimination law. It doesn't matter what happens in California. We need a federal antidiscrimination law and once we get a federal law, then you can begin treating the epidemic."

I looked at him incredulously as I contemplated the countless numbers of tragic people who have already been infected unnecessarily because AIDS and gay activists had effectively blocked doctors from doing what was medically sound. How many children have contracted the disease unnecessarily? How many marital partners have contracted the disease? How many people have been spreading the disease because they don't know they are infected? How many men have gotten the disease from prostitutes because houses of prostitution are still open? How many gay men have contracted the disease because gay bathhouses are open across our nation? How many more Americans are going to die unnecessarily because physicians have been blocked from addressing HIV disease as a medical issue?

My response was perhaps angry and ill-conceived, but faced with the nightmare of this epidemic and the unnecessary suffering and death that has occurred, I replied,

"And after we give you the antidiscrimination law — what next? The Manifesto of Montreal demanded that we subsidize AIDS care throughout the rest of the world. Do you really think that an antidiscrimination law is going to satisfy the people who have allowed the epidemic to spread this far?"

The young man looked at me, shrugged and walked off.

Next, a young lady came up to me and introduced herself. She was a medical student from McGill University.

"We had a speaker just last week at our medical school," she said. "He was an ethicist and he said that **doctors did not have the right to know whether or not their patients were infected.** Every student in our class thought that doctors should have the right to know who was infected, but the ethicist insisted that we were all wrong."

I smiled and told her reassuringly,

"You are right and he is wrong. You need to know for your own protection, for your marital partner's protection and for your staff's protection, but most of all, you need to know for the patient's protection and the protection of those people that he or she may infect unknowingly. You need to know, despite what the ethicist and all the people here at this convention and the CDC are telling you. Simply trust your own good judgment and intelligence."

I moved away from the conference hall, down the elevator and into the main lobby of the Palais Des Congres. Suddenly there was another young lady standing beside me.

"I followed you down here because I wanted to talk to you," she said quietly. "I'm a surgical nurse. I am worried to death, scrubbing in on cases when we don't know whether or not the patients are infected. We are not using any special precautions in surgery. We can't. There is no way we can protect ourselves unless we know who is infected. Why won't they let us find out?"

We talked for several minutes and as we did, I noticed a young man standing beside me, jotting down my name which he was reading from my name tag. I finished talking to the nurse, encouraging her to try to convince the doctors in her hospital to go against the recommendations from medical leaders and the so-called experts at the CDC. I told her that physicians must do what is logical and sensible. Doctors must begin trying to find out who is infected.

As the nurse turned to leave, the young man stepped forward. He was of medium height, handsome and neatly dressed with short cropped hair. He certainly looked like the college student who might have lived next door. He spoke clearly and concisely and I shall never forget his words.

"I followed you down from upstairs because I wanted to talk to you. I'm deeply concerned about what is happening and I thought I might somehow be able to help. I am quite articulate and people would probably listen to me...because I have the virus — I'm HIV-infected."

I looked at him and was suddenly overcome with a feeling of sadness. He was such a fine looking young man, clean cut, well spoken and as he said — articulate. My first impulse was to ask him how in heaven's name he had become infected, but my better judgment told me to refrain.

I began talking to him about our battle and how a small group of men and women across America were working to try to bring some logic into the handling of the epidemic. I told him that I would be glad to put him in touch with Shepherd Smith who headed an organization known as "ASAP" — Americans for a Sound AIDS Policy — which was one of only two organizations in our entire nation which were doing anything in an organized manner to try to approach the epidemic from a logical, medical point of view. I told him where to get the books to read about the epidemic and who the major players were. I pointed out Dr. Mervyn Silverman, the former public health officer from San Francisco, now President of Americans For AIDS Research. I pointed out Dr. Don Francis and Dr. James Curran of the CDC, who were there in the lobby. I mentioned the names of the various people who were at that meeting who played key roles in charting the course of the epidemic — most of them being on the other side and working to effectively block a logical approach to the epidemic.

As we talked on, the young man told me more about himself. He was a captain in the United States Army and had contracted the virus some years before, probably in college through heterosexual contact.

"You have no idea how irresponsible a lot of the homosexuals are," he said. "I had dinner just last night with the leader of the gay delegation from Vancouver. He told me he was going off to the gay bathhouse here in Montreal to find a partner for the evening and he wasn't going to bother to tell his partners that he had AIDS.

"I told him he didn't have a right to do that as we all have a social and ethical responsibility to one another. He got so mad at me that he started yelling and walked out of the room. But I feel strongly that we have to start doing something to address this epidemic and bring it under control.

"These activists who are demonstrating, yelling and screaming are accomplishing nothing other than discrediting themselves and blocking anything effective from being done. How can I help?"

I looked intently at this young man, a young man who was infected with a disease that sooner or later would reduce him to a pain-racked, demented, wasted remnant of humanity yet he wanted to help; he wanted to become involved in the battle.

Here was an ally who perhaps could be recruited into that small group of courageous men and women with whom I had had the privilege of working. A group of men and women so different in their backgrounds that it seemed almost incomprehensible that there could be a common bond between them.

For within that group was a left-wing Democratic Councilman from New York City who probably would not agree with any of the rest of us on most issues — except that he was overcome with a sense of grief and despair for his city which would soon be destroyed. There were several military officers, an insurance salesman, several women politicians, several doctors who specialized in sex and sex therapy and a handful of other physicians from across our nation, all working to try to begin addressing HIV disease as a disease and not a civil rights issue.

How many were there? Perhaps 15 or 20 people at the most. Twenty people with the courage to take a stand and upon whose shoulders lay the destiny of our nation. If they were to fail, then America as a nation would cease to exist, for the epidemic would destroy the stability of our society. We were all diverse, but in that diversity lay our strength. For we all knew, in our own way, that if we failed to bring some sanity to the handling of this epidemic, then the dreams that America represented would be lost, freedom would fail and America, as we have known it, would cease to exist.

As I looked at that handsome young Army officer who wanted so desperately to help, I reflected on the words of Randy Shilts, in his classic book, *And The Band Played On:*

> The bitter truth was that AIDS did not have to happen to America — It was allowed to happen by an array of institutions, all of which failed to perform their appropriate tasks to safeguard the public health...There was no excuse in this country and in this time for the spread of a deadly new epidemic.

---

1. The AIDS Lobby is made up of radical liberals, socialists and various revolutionary groups in America.
2. AIDS — *Sexual Behavior and Intravenous Drug Use* National Academy Press; Washington, D. C., 1989. pp 167-168

CHAPTER TWO

At what point should we expect the approach of danger? By what means should we fortify ourselves against it? Should we expect some transatlantic military giant to step the ocean and crush us with a blow? Never! All of the armies of Europe and Asia and Africa combined, could never, by force, take a drink from the Ohio or make a mark on the Blue Ridge, not in a thousand years.

Then at what point should danger be expected? I answer: if it ever reach us, it must spring up among us. It can never come from abroad. If destruction be our lot, then we ourselves must be its author and its finisher. As a nation of free men, we must live on through all time, or die by suicide.

— Abraham Lincoln in his address to the Lyceum in Springfield, Illinois, June, 1838

History records that during the plague epidemic of the 14th century, some 25 million people died in Europe. Indeed three-quarters of the population of some European countries died as a result of the "Black Death." At other times, in subsequent centuries, when the plague struck, it was always dealt with by using the force of government to isolate those who were infected to try to stop the spread of disease.

Sometimes whole sections of cities were burned to the ground, but always society moved to protect itself. Those who were infected were sometimes isolated until they recovered or died. In each instance, the spread of disease was stopped and life eventually went on as before.

There were outbreaks of syphilis in the 15th and 16th centuries and governments acted to close the brothels where sexually transmitted diseases were disseminated. Governments always reacted in an effort to protect the public health and preserve the structure of society.

The "great plague" that followed the First World War was the influenza epidemic of 1918-1919. Far more people died as a result of that epidemic than died during the hostilities of the "Great War." It is estimated that 20 million people succumbed to the complications of influenza worldwide. Here again, governments took steps to stop the epidemic.

People wore face masks in public to impede respiratory spread of the disease. Schools were closed, theaters and public meetings were cancelled to limit interpersonal spread of the virus.

In the 1930's, the spread of syphilis threatened our land and Surgeon General Thomas Parran launched an all-out attack on the disease. He encouraged doctors to do routine Wasserman (syphilis) testing on all patients in their offices and routine testing whenever a patient was admitted to the hospital. Premarital and prenatal testing were introduced. Identification of infected patients was followed up with contact tracing to determine who had transmitted the disease and who might have become secondarily infected. Syphilis was thus brought under control even before antibiotics were available — by using standard public health techniques and contact tracing to identify and educate those infected with the luetic spirochete.

By the mid 1940's, with the advent of antibiotics, doctors could treat almost all the common causes of infection.

By the beginning of the decade of the 1980's, it seemed that man had found the solution to all problems surrounding disease. Smallpox had been eradicated. Polio, measles and whooping cough could now be controlled with immunization. Mankind was entering an era of health and prosperity...or so it seemed. Now, pills or shots were readily available for syphilis and gonorrhea. We no longer had to fear the ravages of sexual promiscuity.

Indeed, in the Western World, abortion on demand was available and we no longer had to fear the complications of pregnancy. And so the "Sexual Revolution" began, encouraged by Planned Parenthood, by Siecus (Sex Information and Education Council of the United States) and by the Secular Humanists who told us there were no longer any barriers — we had entered the "Brave New World" of tomorrow and all the outmoded moral standards of the past had gone by the wayside.

By the beginning of the 1980's, no one had to be responsible for their actions. There was always a ready cure for any problem that arose...or so we thought.

Homosexuality came to be taught in our schools as an acceptable alternative lifestyle and we readily forgot the lessons of what had happened to Sodom and Gomorrah, Greece and Rome, when those great civilizations turned their backs on God's moral standards and repudiated the lessons of history and the Bible.

Tragically, Americans in the 1960's and 1970's did not have an inkling of what lay ahead. If someone had told you in the 1960's and 1970's that America would be visited with a horrible, deadly plague for which medical science would know no cure, most Americans would have ridiculed the idea. After all, Americans had gone to the moon. Americans had found the solutions to the problems of hunger and poverty. Americans had created a Utopian society ...or so we believed.

A plague that would destroy America? Ridiculous! It couldn't happen here. Everyone knew it couldn't happen here. Everyone knew that our government wouldn't allow it to happen. We would simply pass a law, spend enough money or do enough research. No infection could ever destroy America...or could it?

June 5, 1981 is the most significant date in contemporary American history. This was the date that marked the watershed for our society. Before this date America had evolved into a nation where there were no longer moral or sexual standards and where any form of hedonism or sexual excess was accepted as simply a deviation from the normal. Permissiveness, pornography, perversion and promiscuity had become the hallmarks of the American way of life.

June 5, 1981 was the date when the first published report appeared in American medical literature describing a new horrible, debilitating and ultimately fatal disease that was affecting homosexual men. Of course, no one was sure at the very beginning that it really was a disease. The first mention of the new condition was printed on the back pages of the weekly publication of the Centers for Disease Control's "Morbidity and Mortality Weekly Report," more commonly known as the "MMWR." That report was not felt to be of much significance. The really important articles on June 5, were:

1. The report of two cases of Dengue type 4 infection (breakbone fever) in U. S. travelers to the Caribbean and;

2. An update on the current trends in measles.

The third and final article in the MMWR was entitled, "Pneumocystis Pneumonia In Los Angeles" and simply stated:

> In the period, October 1980 — May 1981 — five young men, all active homosexuals, were treated for biopsy-confirmed Pneumocystis carinii pneumonia at three different hospitals in Los Angeles, California. Two of the patients died. All five patients had laboratory confirmed previous occurrence of cytomegalovirus (CMV) infection and Candidia (yeast) mucosal *infection.*

That was all that the article said. One short paragraph in the CDC's MMWR on June 5, 1981, introduced the "plague of the 20th century."

Less than one month later, on July 3, 1981, the MMWR weekly report announces;
26 cases of Kaposi's sarcoma were reported in homosexual men along with an additional ten cases of Pneumocystis pneumonia.
In the months that followed, young homosexual men all across America began dying from either Pneumocystis pneumonia (PCP) or Kaposi's Sarcoma (KS). Pneumocystis pneumonia was an extremely rare, parasitic infection seen only in patients with suppressed immune systems.

Kaposi's Sarcoma was ordinarily seen in men of Jewish or Mediterranean origin and then generally only in men over 60 years of age. Suddenly there were increasing numbers of cases of KS in gay men and even more startling was the fact that some patients were developing both KS and PCP. It soon became obvious that the common denominator between PCP and KS was a suppressed immunological system. It was found that the patient's T4 helper lymphocytes were suppressed and there was an alteration in the T4 (helper) to T8 (suppressor) lymphocytes so that the normal immunological response of the victim's body was paralyzed and could not protect him against disease.

Soon thereafter, a myriad of rare diseases began infecting homosexuals. There were infections with the cytomegalovirus producing blindness, infection with the Herpes virus producing horribly painful shingles, infections with yeasts and fungus, infections of the brain, bowel, heart and of almost every other organ system. There were strange and exotic diseases that had rarely attacked humans before. Tuberculosis began to appear with increasing frequency in the helpless young men. Peripheral neuritis and dementia destroyed their nervous systems.

The Centers for Disease Control is the department of the U. S. Public Health Service charged with investigating and monitoring disease in America. Almost immediately the CDC mobilized its resources to address the epidemic. Despite the protestation today by homosexual spokesmen that the disease initially was ignored by our government because it involved what the Reagan Administration looked upon as an undesirable element of society, nothing could be further from the truth. In fact, all the protestations that you hear to that effect today are simply aimed at covering up the involvement of the AIDS Lobby and the Gay Lobby in effectively blocking the use of standard public health techniques to monitor and control the disease during the decade of the 80's.

In October 1981, the Centers for Disease Control swung rapidly and efficiently into action. Trained epidemiologists and interviewers journeyed from one end of our country to the other to interview people with AIDS trying to find out if there were common denominators between the victims' lifestyles or their personal contacts.

Exhaustive interviews were carried out with written, informed consent and patients were asked to name their sexual partners during the five year period before they became ill. For those already dead, friends or close companions were interviewed and the information was compiled as quickly as possible.

What soon became obvious was that patients who had AIDS usually: (1) had met their partners in gay bathhouses; (2) had participated in the sexual practices of fisting (manual-rectal intercourse) or oral-genital sex.[1]

By April 1982, just seven months after the implementation of the interviews, Doctor William Darrow of the CDC in Atlanta had compiled all the information and realized that there was a common denominator among many of the patients. That common denominator was a French Canadian airline steward named Gaetan Dugas. The CDC referred to him as "Patient Zero" of their study.

In the classic article published by the CDC two years later in the American Journal of Medicine (March of 1984), Dr. Darrow outlined what was known in April of 1982.

(1) This new disease was sexually transmitted.

(2) It was spread in homosexual bathhouses.

(3) One man could be directly or indirectly traced to at least 40 cases of AIDS from New York City to Los Angeles to Orange County in California. Indeed, Gaetan Dugas was sometimes referred to as "The Orange County Connection."

According to the CDC:

> In Patient Zero, (Gaetan) Kaposi's Sarcoma had been diagnosed in May of 1980. He (Gaetan Dugas) estimated that he had approximately 250 different sexual partners every year from 1979 through 1981 and was able to name 72 of his partners for this three year period. 8 of those 72 partners were AIDS patients, 4 from Southern California and 4 from New York.

Subsequently, the CDC epidemiologists tracked down and identified 32 more people infected by the 8 initial contacts. Of these 40 AIDS patients, 24 had Kaposi's Sarcoma, 6 had PCP, 8 had both Kaposi's

Sarcoma and PCP, 1 had disseminated Cytomegalovirus and 1 had central nervous system toxoplasmosis. All of them would subsequently die because of the infection they acquired, directly or indirectly, from Gaetan Dugas.

In 1982, it was believed that the latency period for AIDS (i.e., the time interval between the initial infection and progression to the terminal stage, AIDS) was about 10.5 months with a range of 7 to 14 months. Unfortunately, the CDC's initial estimate was tragically flawed. The latency period for AIDS was not 10.5 months as thought in 1982 nor 5.5 years, as was believed in 1986. The latency period is now known to be as long as 10 years or more.

This means that the average individual who contracts the virus can live over 10 years before he comes down with that terminal stage of HIV disease which we refer to as AIDS. This also means that the average patient that Gaetan Dugas infected between April of 1982 (when he was identified as a primary vector) and March of 1984, when he died, has not yet come down with clinical AIDS.

Of course, many of his victims have already died — but the average victim he infected between April of 1982 and March of 1984, will not come down with the disease until 1992 or 1994 — and many of his victims will not develop clinical AIDS until the mid-1990's or even later.

That is what makes the rest of the story of the early part of this epidemic even more unbelievable. Because, you see, the Centers for Disease Control was so excited about its discovery of the link between Gaetan Dugas and the epidemic that in mid-1982, they invited Gaetan to come to Atlanta, Georgia to the CDC headquarters for examination and for interviews.[2]

Like so many homosexuals who are kind, considerate and thoughtful, Gaetan journeyed to Atlanta. He was informed that he must stop having sexual relations because he might be spreading the disease. Gaetan adamantly refused to control his promiscuity and CDC officials knew of his refusal.

After leaving Atlanta, Gaetan moved to San Francisco where he continued spreading the infection. He became somewhat of a legend in the bathhouses. The homosexual population came to recognize that he was actively and intentionally spreading the disease. He journeyed back and forth from San Francisco to Vancouver and, according to Randy Shilts in his classic book, *And The Band Played On,* Gaetan would openly admit to his homosexual partners, after he had finished with them, that he might have infected them with the gay cancer.

In November 1982, Gaetan Dugas was interviewed by a public health officer in San Francisco and was told that he must stop having unprotected sexual relations.

"I've got it — they can get it too," was his response.

And yet the public health officer did nothing to curtail Gaetan from continuing to spread the deadly disease. Public health officers (PHO's) have tremendous power at their disposal, but it is the saying among public health officials that if you have to use that power, you have failed.

Thus, the PHO in San Francisco made no attempt to use the power which was available to her. Gaetan Dugas continued to frequent the bathhouses of San Francisco and continued to spread the disease. Many of the people he infected during those months and up until the time of his death in March of 1984 will not come down with the disease until well into the 1990's.

Amazingly, it was not the public health officials who drove Gaetan out of San Francisco. It was a few concerned homosexuals who threatened him and let him know in no uncertain terms that if he did not leave San Francisco, there would be trouble.

Gaetan then moved back to Vancouver and from there he made journeys across Canada into other communities for sexual encounters. This man, who was known to be far more dangerous than Typhoid Mary could ever have been, was allowed to continue spreading HIV disease across the United States and Canada **for almost two years after the Centers for Disease Control determined that he had been responsible, directly or indirectly, for at least 40 known cases of the disease.**

Indeed, Gaetan was probably responsible for thousands of cases — either directly or indirectly. The problem was not the people he infected before the infectious nature of the disease was recognized in April of 1982. Those infections were tragic but unavoidable. The unbelievable part of the story is that there were CDC officials and public health officials who recognized the communicable nature of the disease in April of 1982 and knew that Gaetan was spreading it, yet they did nothing to stop him.

By June of 1982, the disease had been reported in IV drug users and in hemophiliacs, confirming the fact that there was a transmissible agent in the blood which could spread the infection from one person to another.

It was in 1982 that drastic steps should have been recommended to control the disease. Gay bathhouses, sex clubs and pornographic stores should have been closed. Houses of prostitution should have been closed and prostitutes taken off the streets. A massive drive against IV drug use should have been undertaken to close down shooting galleries, head shops and expand drug treatment programs.

That was the golden opportunity when the epidemic could have been readily stopped. However, it was not until March 14, 1986, almost five years into the epidemic, that the CDC issued weak recommendations suggesting that gay bathhouses and brothels be closed. Not until March 27, 1987, a year later, did the CDC make recommendations on the handling of infected prostitutes.

What did they recommend? The CDC, that department of the federal government which is responsible for protecting the health of our nation, recommended that if infected prostitutes would not stop soliciting customers, "They should insist on the use of condoms to prevent transmission of the virus to others."

Dealing with a rapidly spreading, almost universally fatal sexually transmitted disease, the CDC delayed 6 years in making their recommendations to the nation, then finally stated that…"Infected prostitutes should insist on the use of condoms."

It was during the period between 1982 and 1984 when the disease spread rapidly in the homosexual population of our nation. From statistics later obtained from the Cohort Study in San Francisco (a survey of 6700 homosexuals that began in 1978 as a hepatitis study), it is known today that by 1980, 25% of the homosexuals in the study groups in San Francisco were already infected. By 1984, 64% of them were infected.

It was during that period between 1982 and 1984 when closure of the bathhouses could have saved thousands of homosexual lives, but the bathhouses were not closed in San Francisco until late 1984. Bathhouses still remain open in many of the major cities of our nation today.

It is little wonder that many homosexuals are bitter over the way that the epidemic was initially handled by the CDC and the U. S. Public Health Service. Many young homosexual men are going to die in an epidemic that certainly could have been slowed in 1982, once the infectious nature of the disease was recognized. The tragedy is that the homosexuals never question why nothing was done. They think it was the apathy and indifference of the heterosexual population and the

Reagan Administration that rejected their lifestyle.

But is there another factor? Is there some other force that denies rational explanation which was intent upon preventing America from addressing this epidemic in 1982?

In June of 1982, the CDC published a report in the MMWR alluding to Gaetan Dugas and the fact that clinical AIDS might be related to a transmissible agent. Their article, however, concluded by suggesting that the disease might really be caused by the use of nitrates or other sexual stimulants or the use of drugs.

I have talked to present and past highly-placed officials at the Centers for Disease Control who have assured me that by June of 1982 they definitely knew that AIDS was an infectious disease. Then why did the CDC publish an article in June of 1982 intentionally deceiving public health officials and physicians across our nation, suggesting that the disease might be the result of the use of drugs? Why were no standard public health techniques used in 1982 to try to slow the spread of this sexually transmitted disease?

In our nation where couples are required by law to have a premarital blood test for syphilis before marriage; in our nation where children are required by law to have immunization and vaccinations before entering school to protect their health and the health of others; in our nation where most states require the wearing of automotive seat belts to protect the public health and where newborn children are usually required by law to have blood tests to diagnose a number of rare and exotic diseases; in our nation where hundreds of millions of dollars are spent yearly to monitor the spread and incidence of diseases and to protect the public health, why was nothing done to stop Gaetan Dugas who was intentionally spreading a deadly new disease that would eventually kill hundreds or possibly thousands of unsuspecting victims?

Tragically, the same story continues today. Nothing is being done to identify those irresponsible people who have the virus and are intentionally spreading it to others. In addition, most of the people within the heterosexual community who carry the virus do not know that they are infected because doctors are actively discouraged from trying to identify them. These people are unknowingly spreading the disease; yet, no effective efforts are being made to identify them or to stop them from spreading the epidemic.

Infected prostitutes are still allowed to continue plying their trade in most states across our nation. Gay bathhouses, sex clubs, crack houses and IV drug houses remain open and the disease continues to spread. Thus, the chain of transmission continues, the chain of death is unbroken and millions of Americans will die unnecessarily in an epidemic that never had to happen.

Gaetan Dugas was not an American citizen. He could have been deported as an undesirable alien if he refused to stop spreading the disease. There are laws to protect the public health. In California, an individual can be placed in jail for knowingly spreading an infectious disease, yet, for almost six months after Gaetan Dugas left Atlanta (after his interviews at the CDC), he lived in San Francisco, going to the bathhouses nightly and intentionally spreading a disease which he knew would kill many of his sexual partners. Existing laws in the State of California were ignored by local public health officials who knew that Gaetan was spreading the "plague of the 20th century."

In April 1989, I journeyed to Atlanta, Georgia to interview key personnel at the CDC to ask the question — Why? Why wasn't Gaetan stopped? Why weren't steps taken early in the epidemic to use standard public health techniques to monitor and control the epidemic? The answers I received defy the imagination. But, once again, I am getting ahead of my story.

✳✳✳

On **May 21, 1982** the MMWR reported the first cases of what came to be known as ARC or AIDS Related Complex. Of course, in 1982, no one realized the normal progression of this disease from:

(1) The initial infection with the HIV virus to,

(2) The stage where one develops swollen lymph nodes to,

(3) The gradual decline of T4 helper lymphocytes and the loss of the body's normal immune response to,

(4) ARC, the AIDS Related Complex with fever, malaise and weight loss to,

(5) The breakdown of the immunological system and the development of secondary infections, tumors and dementia (clinical AIDS) to,

(6) Death.

It was not until 1984-1985 that it came to be recognized that HIV disease was a chronic, progressive and eventually fatal infectious disease that was transmitted in a manner very similar to Hepatitis B, although HIV disease was considered nowhere near as infectious as

Hepatitis B.

※※※

By **September 24, 1982,** there were 593 cases of AIDS in America and 243 deaths from AIDS. 75% of the AIDS cases occurred among homosexual or bisexual men and 12% were among IV drug users. Haitians residing in the United States constituted 6.1% of cases and there were three hemophiliacs with AIDS.

※※※

By **January 7, 1983,** the CDC had discovered the disease among the female sexual partners of males with AIDS. At that point, it was possible to refer to the 5 H's of AIDS — **Homosexuals, Heroin users, Haitians, Hemophiliacs** and **Heterosexuals.** Years later, the Haitian category was dropped, because it came to be recognized that Haitians ordinarily acquired the disease by heterosexual contact.

※※※

On **March 4, 1983,** it was reported that there were over **1200 cases** of AIDS from 34 states, the District of Columbia and 15 countries; over 450 people had already died and the mortality rate exceeded 60% for cases first diagnosed over a year previously.

By March 1983, French researchers at the Pasteur Institute had isolated a retrovirus from the lymph nodes of an AIDS victim. It appeared that the disease was the result of a lentiviral infection...that type of retroviral infection which heretofore had only been found in animals. How had the lentivirus jumped the species barrier from animal to man? Where had the infection come from? The question of where and how this had occurred would challenge writers and investigators for years to come and distract doctors from the most important questions concerning this epidemic. Those questions were:

"Why weren't we trying to identify those who carry the infection?" and;

"Why weren't we trying to effectively stop the spread of the epidemic?"

※※※

By early 1984, Dr. Robert Gallo and his group of researchers at the National Cancer Institute had confirmed the French research and by May of 1984, they had developed a series of incredibly accurate blood tests which would allow physicians to identify those who were infected. After almost one year of clinical trials and delays, that blood test was ready to be released by the Federal Drug Administration in March, 1985.

But long before the release of the blood test, gay activists and leaders of the AIDS Lobby began to demand that **the tests only be used to test blood specimens in blood banks** and should **not** be used to screen the general population.

Suddenly there was talk of the possibility of violation of civil liberties and infringement upon civil rights. It was stated that if the blood test was used in the general population it could identify homosexuals and bisexuals and that lists of homosexuals could be compiled and utilized at some future date to discriminate against those within the gay lifestyle.

Homosexual spokesmen were quick to condemn the federal government, federal agencies and the President of the United States for their failure to act decisively during the early stages of the epidemic, but those same leaders never mentioned that it was often the same homosexual spokesmen who, in 1982, 1983 and 1984, had violently objected to any suggestion that gay bathhouses and sex clubs be closed in an effort to protect the lives of homosexuals.

By 1985 Dr. Mervyn Silverman, the former public health officer from San Francisco was the President of the U. S. Conference of Local Public Health Officers. Shortly before the scheduled release of the HIV blood test for general use, Doctor Silverman contacted the Centers for Disease Control and requested that the federal government issue guidelines to insure the confidentiality of HIV blood test results. Furthermore, he wanted funds for alternative testing sites where homosexuals and IV drug users and others could go to be tested.

The LAMBDA Legal Defense and Education Fund, a gay activist group from New York, threatened to bring legal action against the Federal Drug Administration to block release of the HIV blood test unless its use was restricted to testing blood for blood banks. Then, within a few days before the scheduled release of the blood test, the National Gay Task Force and the LAMBDA Legal Defense and Education Fund actually filed a lawsuit to block release of the blood test, a test that might have saved millions of American lives.

In return for withdrawing their suit, the gay organizations received assurance from officials at the FDA that the test was not to be used for testing the general population — it was only to be used to protect the nation's blood supply.

From that time on, there has been an organized, orchestrated, coordinated effort all across America to block the use of HIV blood testing in the general population and to block any efforts to identify those who are infected in order to stop the chain of transmission and death.

Just one month later, between April 15 and 17, representatives from the World Health Organization met in Atlanta. Representatives from Communist, Socialist and Western countries met to develop guidelines that were to be used to control the world-wide epidemic. Their concluding statement is recorded in the MMWR of May 17, 1985. It stressed the importance of the **confidentiality** of test results and the use of **informed consent** for testing.

Now these recommendations are indeed strange, because the confidentiality of test results and informed consent are never stressed in Cuba or behind the Iron Curtain. Testing in Eastern Bloc countries was simply carried out as for every other disease in an effort to stop the epidemic. In Russia, high risk individuals were forcibly tested and large segments of the population were screened; however, in America and in western European countries, the confidentiality of test results and informed consent were stressed and these barriers to testing have been used very effectively by the AIDS Lobbies to prevent physicians from addressing the epidemic.

Members of the AIDS and Gay Lobbies began to work to convince state legislators that HIV blood testing should not be used to identify those who were infected.

Starting in 1985, laws were passed in states all across America which served to effectively block doctors from using the blood test. As a result of this carefully orchestrated program, various state legislatures passed laws to:

1) Protect the confidentiality of blood test results.
2) Require written or informed consent before testing.
3) Require extensive pre- and post-test counseling.
4) Prevent the reporting of positive HIV test results to public health officers and block the use of standard public health techniques to break the chain of transmission of the disease.
5) Prevent discrimination in any form against those who were infected with HIV disease.

The Centers for Disease Control and the U. S. Public Health Service cooperated with this effort. Shortly after AIDS was recognized in our nation, the CDC requested that all state health departments declare AIDS to be a new disease and begin reporting AIDS cases to local public health officers. That information was then transmitted to Atlanta so that statistics could be compiled.

Every state complied with that request and, today, every state in the nation considers AIDS to be a communicable, reportable disease. Later, when it became apparent that AIDS **was not the disease but only the terminal stage of HIV disease** and a blood test became readily available to identify those who were infected, the Centers for Disease Control has steadfastly refused to ask state health departments to declare that **HIV disease** is a communicable, reportable disease so that the test results could be collected and forwarded to Atlanta.

As a direct result of this CDC policy, many states do not consider HIV disease as a disease; thus, it is not reportable. That is the reason there are no statistics available on the incidence of the disease in our nation today. Since the Centers for Disease Control has not requested that states declare HIV to be an infectious disease, many state health departments have no statistics on the incidence of the infection. As long as the states do not have any statistics on the incidence of the disease, the CDC can tell the citizens of this nation, year after year, that there are only a million to a million and a half cases of HIV disease. The truth is that the Centers for Disease Control has no idea what the incidence of HIV disease is in America and is specifically **not** trying to find out.

It was not until February 1989, eight years into this epidemic, when the CDC finally suggested that those states where there was some form of reporting should relay their statistics to Atlanta. However, officials from the CDC knew full well that in California and New York State and in the majority of the states with the major concentrations of disease, there was no mandatory reporting. Thus, CDC officials could be assured that any statistics they collected would show a low incidence of infection and the public would not be alarmed — they would not be alarmed until it was far too late to bring this epidemic under control.

What is so incredible about the whole story is that the Centers for Disease Control spends millions of dollars a year determining the incidence of every imaginable disease in America and throughout the world. They monitor every conceivable type of medical problem — from teenage pregnancies to the incidence of murders in blacks and Hispanics. The Centers for Disease Control monitored the incidence of tularemia in Tulare County, California two years ago. They monitor every imaginable type of disease and condition in this country...except HIV disease.

In California, in 1985, AB403 (Assembly Bill 403) passed the state legislature under the guidance of Assemblyman Art Agnos. In 1985, Mr. Agnos was the State Assemblyman from San Francisco, where his support came from the city's large gay constituency. The leaders of that constituency were intent upon preventing doctors from monitoring or controlling HIV disease as they do other communicable, infectious, sexually transmitted diseases.

AB403 was the cornerstone of the Gay and AIDS Lobby program in California. It was the barrier that would keep doctors from trying to stop the epidemic. There was no question that AB403 was designed to discourage doctors from addressing this epidemic. In summary, AB403 required that:

1. HIV disease was not to be dealt with like other diseases. No doctor could order a blood test for the disease without first obtaining a **written** consent from the patient. No other blood test requires a written consent — except the HIV blood test.

2. The test results were to be held in total **confidentiality** so that no one besides the doctor and the patient could know either that the patient had an HIV test done or what the results of that test were. If the doctor violated confidentiality, he faced a $10,000.00 fine and a year in prison.

3. Although the law did not specifically require pre- and post-test counseling, doctors were told by the CMA that counseling was required and that physicians must counsel their patients extensively both before and after the blood test had been done.

These requirements for HIV blood testing were introduced so that doctors in California would not carry out HIV testing on the general public. Why?

First of all, as far as the matter of consent is concerned, ordinarily, when you go to your doctor, there is an **implied consent** when you place yourself under your physician's care. If a doctor says to a patient that he wants to get a blood test, the patient will ordinarily ask what the test is for or what the doctor is checking. Ordinarily, the doctor will explain the test and if the patient doesn't want the test, he simply declines.

Usually the patient will agree and the test is performed, but in the case of the blood test for HIV disease, there would have to be a **written consent** and the doctor would have to stipulate a number of specific items on that written consent. Some years later, the AIDS Lobby was able to substitute "Informed Consent" for "Written Consent."

An informed consent is far more difficult for a doctor to administer than a written consent since it is much more time consuming and requires a physician to discuss with the patient all the possible harmful effects of having the test. By changing the requirement from a **written** to an **informed consent,** the objective was to make it even more difficult for doctors to do testing.

Secondly, doctors were told that they must counsel their patients both **before** and **after** the blood test was ordered. The counseling would be rather extensive and would require the doctor to tell his patient:

(1) HIV was a sexually transmitted disease;

(2) That the blood test was not totally accurate and that there might be false-positive and false-negative test results;

(3) That taking the blood test might well impact upon the individual's ability to get health or life insurance in the future;

(4) The implications of what it would mean if the blood tests were positive (i.e., the fact that the person might lose his housing, his job, his insurance and his personal relationships) if the result of the test was accidently released, etc., etc., etc.

Indeed, much of the initial counseling took 20 or 30 minutes if carried out as prescribed. One of the routine questions that physicians were told to ask was, "Are you emotionally able to cope with a positive test result and its implications for your life?"

Do you know a better way to frighten a patient out of being tested than to ask such a question? The format of the counseling that was recommended was not primarily educational. The counseling dealt with the social consequences of the test and the disease and not with the medical aspects of the disease.

In a busy doctor's office, such extensive counseling **before** a physician knew whether or not somebody had HIV infection was impractical. In fact, the concept of pre-test counseling was designed specifically to discourage doctors from testing.

The advocates of counseling said that it was much more important to counsel patients than to do testing. By requiring extensive counseling in the office of a busy doctor, the AIDS Lobby knew full well that the vast majority of physicians would not do blood testing on a routine basis and as a result, the objectives of the AIDS and Gay Lobbies would be carried out. The HIV test would not be used to identify those who were infected. The idea that a physician would be required to offer extensive counseling **before** he did a blood test is ridiculous. Could you imagine what would happen if a doctor were required by law to counsel a patient before he ran a large blood panel in his office? The large panel ordinarily covers screening for parathyroid disease, abnormalities of calcium and phosphorus metabolism, liver disease, diabetes, renal disease, etc.

If a doctor were required, by law, to counsel a patient as to the implications of parathyroid disease and what it would mean to the patient if he had parathyroid disease and what the treatment was for parathyroid disease; if the doctor then had to counsel his patient as to the implications of liver disease, the cause of liver disease, the treatment for liver disease, and the prognosis for liver disease; if the doctor then had to counsel a patient as to the meaning of an altered kidney function test, the causes of kidney disease, the treatment for kidney disease and the prognosis for kidney disease, etc., etc., no doctor would do a large panel in his busy clinical practice.

Could you imagine requiring a doctor to counsel a patient before checking their blood pressure? The doctor would have to say:

"Let me tell you all the causes of high blood pressure before I check your pressure... Now if I find your blood pressure is elevated it may be that you will die of a heart attack or a stroke. If your blood pressure is elevated, it could mean you would become uninsurable for life insurance and ineligible for health insurance in the future. Are you prepared to know that your blood pressure is elevated and that this could be a fatal affliction? Do you really want me to check your blood pressure?"

The purpose of counseling was to discourage doctors from using HIV testing to identify those infected with the virus. The plan worked very effectively.

In 1985, most doctors would have readily accepted the fact that it was only logical to try to identify those patients who were infected in order to try to stop the spread of disease. It would take several years of carefully programmed propaganda in medical journals such as the AMA News, from the leaders of organized medicine and from the U. S. Public Health Service and the CDC to convince many doctors that all the logical public health techniques that they had used in years past were no longer relevant and that physicians **should not** try to identify those who were infected because if physicians tried to identify infected patients, they would "drive the disease underground."

As far as the confidentiality component of AB403 was concerned, no one was to be allowed to know that someone had had the blood test. If a patient was to go to a clinical laboratory to have the blood test drawn, they would have to go with a **code number**. They could not use their own name. They could not pay for the test **by check** because someone would know their name. They **could not** have the test billed to their private insurance, since the insurance company would know they had had the blood test. The cost of the test **could not** be billed to a patient's home address, because the patient would have to give his name. All HIV testing had to be done in complete secrecy. Patients would have to pay for their blood test in cash. Then, when the report was sent to the doctor's office, no one working in the doctor's office could know who the patient was who had the blood test taken or the blood test results. If anyone in the doctor's office knew who the patient was or the test results, the physician was liable for a $10,000.00 fine and a year in prison. Only the patient and the doctor could know. The doctor was then supposed to counsel the patient again after the blood test came back.

Then, if the patient was going to be admitted to the hospital for surgery, no one at the hospital could know that the patient had a positive blood test. That meant that the nurses on the ward could not know, the laboratory technicians drawing blood could not know and the operating room personnel could not know that the patient was infected.

Since no one could know of the infection, no special precautions could be used to protect HCW's from infection. The idea of using routine precaution on **all** surgery patients is not only excessively expensive, but totally impractical.

For 50 years, doctors have used caps, masks and gowns in the operating room. What was desperately needed in 1985 was new technology and new equipment to protect the surgical staff from contamination by exposure to blood: to protect them from splashing, needle sticks or puncturing their gloves with sharp objects. The surgical staff needed protection from vaporization of blood associated with the use of power tools or the use of an electric knife (the Bovie).

However, if a surgeon were to suggest that the operating room staff use any special precautions on a case, everyone in the operating suite would know that that patient was infected and the doctor would face the threat of a $10,000.00 fine and a year imprisonment. Therefore, under no circumstances could the doctor, in any way, utilize the precautions necessary to protect both himself and his staff.

The situation was even more ridiculous in that if one of the operating room nurses were to stick her finger with a blood-covered needle, the doctor could not tell her that she might be infected with the HIV virus. (The chance of infection is now known to be 1 in 200 HIV contaminated needle sticks). It would be important to the nurse to know so she could monitor herself to determine if she had the disease.

It was even more important for her to know so that she could stop having sexual relations with her husband or boyfriend so that he could not become infected as well. But the doctor could not tell the nurse, the hospital personnel or anyone else that the patient had the disease without facing a **$10,000.00 fine and one year imprisonment.**

A doctor could not keep any record in his office chart that the patient had the disease. The record had to be secured in some hidden place.

Ordinarily, insurance companies and attorneys may subpoena medical records with the patient's permission. All information on that patient is available by subpoena — except for the fact that the patient had a positive HIV test.

If by one means or another, someone were to accidently find out from a doctor's records that a patient had a positive HIV test, the doctor would be subject to a $1500.00 fine, but if the doctor intentionally released that information, he would be subject to the $10,000.00 fine and one year imprisonment.

It was little wonder that doctors had no incentive to start doing blood tests to identify those who were infected.

Laws similar (although not identical) to AB403 were systematically enacted all across America in an effort to effectively block doctors from beginning to deal with this epidemic. These laws would ultimately result in the unnecessary loss of millions of American lives, but in 1985, few Americans were allowed to know what was really transpiring.

At what point should we expect the approach of danger? By what means should we fortify ourselves against it? Should we expect some transatlantic military giant to step the ocean and crush us with a blow? Never! All of the armies of Europe and Asia and Africa combined, could never, by force, take a drink from the Ohio or make a mark on the Blue Ridge, not in a thousand years.

Then at what point should danger be expected? I answer: If it ever reach us, it must spring up among us. It can never come from abroad. If destruction be our lot, then we ourselves must be its author and its finisher. As a nation of free men, we must live on through all time, or die by suicide.

— Abraham Lincoln in his address to the Lyceum in Springfield, Illinois, June, 1838

---

1. American Journal of Medicine, vol. 76; p. 487.Auerbach, Darrow, Jaffe & Curran
2. And The Band Played On, Randy Shilts, St. Martin's Press, 1977; p. 158
3. IBID, p. 200

CHAPTER THREE

"Those whom God wishes to destroy, He first makes mad."
— Euripides, Fragment

There are many reasons given by the AIDS Lobby, gay leaders, their surrogate public health officials and physicians as to why we cannot begin addressing this epidemic as we have other epidemics in the past. Of course, there are many health officials who do not agree with current policy, but most of them are afraid to speak out publicly.

On one occasion which I alluded to earlier, a public health officer from California came to me and told how he and other officers had been threatened and warned not to come forward and support my position within organized medicine. I have been told by another highly placed public health official from Colorado that he has had personal contact with physicians from the CDC who would love to tell the truth about what is going on — but they fear for their employment and their future.

Doctor James Curran, who heads the AIDS Division of the CDC in Atlanta, personally told me in April of 1989 that he supported more extensive testing and the use of public health techniques to control the epidemic. He went on to say, "Every time I talk about using testing to control the epidemic, I keep getting beaten up by politicians."

Thus, even the head of the CDC's Division on AIDS is unable to effectively influence the handling of this epidemic.

There are a number of reasons given by the media, gay activists and the AIDS Lobby as to why we have not addressed this species-threatening epidemic. The main justifications are listed below.

I. Physicians should not be ordering routine tests for the disease because of the inaccuracy of the blood test and the possibility of false negative and false positive test results.

II. If physicians did identify patients with the disease, what would they do with the information? After all, the disease is not curable.

III. If physicians try to stop the spread of the disease, they will simply drive it underground.

IV. The cost of trying to do widespread HIV testing is too expensive. In addition, if physicians did identify people with the disease, the cost of contact tracing to prevent further spread of the disease would be too expensive.

V. The reason that physicians should not perform testing is because they cannot insure the confidentiality of test results.

VI. If physicians identify those people who carry the virus, it would lead to discrimination.

VII. All that is really needed to stop the epidemic is education and behavioral modification.

VIII. It is not important to identify those who are infected because no one gets HIV disease unless they do something (i.e., have sexual relations). There is no such thing as casual spread of the disease.

You have probably read one or several of these arguments.

Let me address each argument in turn.

I. The first issue that has been raised by the Gay and AIDS Lobbies is to challenge the **accuracy of the blood test.** Blood testing for the HIV virus is not simply one test. It is a series of tests consisting of two antibody tests (the ELISA test) followed by a Western Blot test if the initial two Elisa tests are positive. Then there is a fourth confirmatory test which should be ordered if the previous three tests have all been positive.

How accurate is testing in the general population? Blood banks across America anticipate that they will miss infected individuals — about 1 in 100,000 transfusions that are drawn (a false-negative test). Admittedly, blood banks are dealing with a low incidence population and they try to screen out people who are IV drug users and homosexuals to decrease the chance that the blood donor could be in that window of infectiousness between the time when a patient has contracted the disease and the time when they develop antibodies to the retrovirus. However, if we are talking about general testing of the public, we would be dealing with a fairly low general incidence of disease. So the chance that we would miss a significant number of infected people by doing routine testing of the population is quite low. We could expect to pick up over 99.5% of those who are infected and might miss 1 in 100,000 but in that 100,000 people we could expect to pick up one hundred to several hundred people who carry the virus (depending upon the area tested) who are unaware of their infectious status and are spreading the illness unknowingly.

As far as false-positive blood tests are concerned, the AIDS Lobby has made a great issue of the fact that widespread testing might mistakenly identify people who were not infected and thus destroy their lives. The New York Times editorial, November 30, 1987, stated that doctors might very well come up with nine false-positive tests for every

true-positive test, thus unnecessarily shattering the lives of nine innocent people for every person who was accurately identified with the infection. The inference of the Times editorial was: "Why bother trying
to identify those who are infected?"

Although agreeing that testing was advantageous for homosexuals
and drug users, the Times steadfastly opposed general testing of our
population. The essence of their argument, published several months
before the release of the Presidential AIDS Commission's report, was
that the Presidential AIDS Commission must not advise general testing
to try to stop the spread of the epidemic. The Times editorial stated:

"If a low risk group in Peoria...were screened for AIDS...89 people
out of 100,000 would be labeled as carrying the virus. But the real
incidence of AIDS...is 10 per 100,000. The test would miss 1 of the 10,
catch the other 9 and falsely describe 80 other people as carriers."

That statement is totally erroneous; however, since it was printed in
the prestigious New York Times, most unsuspecting readers were
misled. In the mid-West, physicians could expect to find 300 infected
people per 100,000 and, chances are, they would pick up 298 or 299 of
them with testing. Secondly, there would be only 1 chance in 10 of
getting even one false-positive in 100,000 blood tests performed if the
proper sequence of 3 routine tests and one confirmatory test was
followed (1 chance in 1 million).

If testing were done in New York City (where the Times also opposed
routine testing) physicians could expect to find between 2,500 and 5,000
people testing positive per 100,000 tested—the majority of whom have
no idea they carry the virus. If physicians tested patients in many areas
of the Bronx, they could expect to find 25,000 cases per 100,000, but the
New York Times opposed testing in the Bronx as well.

The November 1987 editorial in the Times alluded to the work of
Colonel Donald Burke of Walter Reed Hospital and referred to him as
the Army's "Chief Tester," yet discounted his position favoring routine
testing. However, to date, the only large scale testing of the general
population done anywhere in the world (outside of the Soviet Union,
various Communist countries and the Red Cross) has been done by the
U. S. Army under Colonel Burke's personal supervision.

Colonel Burke is a research virologist at Walter Reed Hospital and
has personally supervised several million HIV blood tests. His statistics
initially showed that the Army, using a civilian laboratory had an
incidence of 1 false-positive in 135,000 blood specimens.[1]

Subsequent review of Army test results has revealed that the incidence of false-positives is actually much lower. By mid-1989, Colonel Burke estimated that Army HIV testing resulted in less than 1 false-positive in 1 million blood tests.[2] Thus, the issue of false-positives has been "laid to rest" scientifically. Still the New York Times, the AIDS Lobby and gay activists continued to echo the lie of "the danger of false-positive blood tests that are destroying lives."

II. The next question that is raised is — "Why bother to find out who has the virus? After all, you can't do anything about it. The disease is not curable."

Even before the proven success of Pentamidine and AZT in preventing Pneumocystis pneumonia in immuno-deficient patients and the success of AZT in slowing the progression of HIV disease, there were many reasons why physicians needed to find out who carried the virus.

First of all, if one person has the virus and gives it to just one other person in one year, at the end of one year you would have two people who were infected. If each one of these people gave the virus to just one other person the next year, at the end of two years you would have four people infected. At the end of the three years, if each one of those four people gave the virus to just one other person, you would have eight people infected. How many people would be infected at the end of ten years? You would have over 1000 people infected and spreading the disease. How many people would be infected at the end of fifteen years? Over 32,000 — all infected because physicians did not try to find that first infected case.

Of course, this example is somewhat exaggerated because many of the initially infected people would have long since died or become deathly ill by the end of that fifteen year period.

On the other hand, we have one instance in Belgium where one man from Africa — within the period of just a little over one year — gave the virus to nine separate women, one of the women gave it to her husband and her husband gave it to his mistress. That was eleven people, directly or indirectly, infected by one person within the period of a little over a year.[3]

Another case from Czechoslovakia was related to me by a Czechoslovakian physician who I met in Montreal. One infected young man he studied had given the disease to 16 girls. We know that Gaetan Dugas, the French Canadian airline steward gave the disease, directly or indirectly, to over forty people who gave it to other people who gave it to other people.

It is estimated that as many as 90% of the people who carry the virus (and perhaps even more) do not know they are infected. As a result, many people are spreading the disease out of ignorance. If someone is identified as having the virus, he or she can be educated as to their obligation to avoid spreading the disease. If information about their infection is recorded with public health officers and the infected individual intentionally continues spreading the disease, there must be legal resources to stop him (or her).

The first step in controlling any epidemic is to identify those who are infected. The members of the AIDS Lobby, however, insist that it is not important to identify carriers because **"physicians can't cure the illness."** They repeat: "Why bother to test? HIV disease is different from other sexually transmitted diseases. It can't be cured."

You have probably heard similar arguments used by those who oppose testing. For the average person, unacquainted with the true facts, it is very difficult to know how to respond. Allow me to outline just why it is so important to identify those with the virus — over and above the obvious benefits of preventing further spread of the disease.

First of all, diabetes is not a curable disease, but would anyone suggest that physicians should not try to identify those who have diabetes simply because diabetes isn't curable? Many times, cancer is not curable, but would anybody suggest that physicians should not try to identify those who have cancer because it may not be curable? Of course not. Both diabetes and cancer are treatable, and HIV disease is a treatable disease. Physicians may not be able to cure it as yet, but treatment can prolong patients' lives, maintain the quality of life and prevent unnecessary death from the development of Pneumocystis carinii pneumonia in patients who don't even suspect they have HIV disease.

Human lives can be preserved until better treatment becomes available. As noted in the last chapter, Pneumocystis carinii pneumonia was the first manifestation of the epidemic reported in June of 1981. It is a lung infection with a Protozoan organism which ordinarily is present in the environment, but which our bodies can fight off with a normal immune system; however, an immunosuppressed individual becomes susceptible to this illness.

Pneumocystis pneumonia carries a 20% mortality rate, even today. Yet this disease is preventable if physicians know that the patient has HIV disease and prescribes prophylactic medication (i.e., Pentamidine and AZT).

Because physicians have been actively discouraged from trying to monitor the disease and identify those who are infected, people who are apparently healthy, suddenly develop Pneumocystis pneumonia and 20% of them die — they die in America today of a disease which is largely preventable. Is this possible? Yes. In the 1990's, physicians are allowing people to die unnecessarily, suddenly and quickly — of a horrible, suffocating illness, because they have been persuaded not to try to identify those who are infected.

Up until 1989, most gay leaders opposed HIV testing to identify those who were infected. In April of 1989, when it became obvious that prophylactic treatment could prevent Pneumocystis pneumonia, some homosexual leaders began advocating routine testing (early diagnosis) for the gay population. Unfortunately those same homosexual leaders still actively oppose efforts to stop the epidemic in the heterosexual population. Why is "early diagnosis" important for the gay population, but not for the straight population?

A corollary to the arguments used by the AIDS Lobby is "because HIV disease is not curable (like syphilis and gonorrhea), physicians should not bother to do contact tracing to identify those who are infected." Public health officers routinely carry out contact tracing with most serious venereal diseases other than HIV disease. Physicians, however, have been told that there is no need to carry out contact tracing in cases of HIV disease because it is not curable.

In other words, public health officials should try to stop the spread of curable diseases but should not try to stop the spread of incurable diseases.[4]

In August 1989, the CDC released the report of their controlled studies showing conclusively that AZT could prevent progression of HIV disease from its latent stages to ARC and AIDS. Had physicians known the identity of the hundreds of thousands of infected HIV carriers in America, they could have placed them under treatment to prolong their lives.

However, in August 1989, doctors had little idea as to who carried the virus in the heterosexual and IV drug user communities and no treatment could be offered. Why? Because in August 1989, there was still an active coordinated program all across America to block doctors from carrying out routine HIV testing.

Why is it important to an individual to know that he or she is infected?

(1) No caring or moral individual would want to be responsible for giving a deadly disease to another person.

(2) If the patient is a woman, she should not become pregnant for two very important reasons. First, up to 35% of the children born to infected mothers will develop HIV infection and will die a slow, lingering and painful death. For their sake, pregnancy should be avoided. Secondly, it has been suggested that pregnancy alters the immune status of women and can convert latent HIV infection to full-blown AIDS, thus shorten ing the woman's life. Furthermore, if a woman has HIV infection and becomes pregnant, she should not nurse her child because many children are infected by breast feeding.

(3) If one has HIV disease, he or she should not take live vaccines because these vaccines produce an infectious state which challenge the immune system and can precipitate clinical AIDS.

(4) An infected person should avoid traveling to areas where para sitic infections are endemic since intestinal parasites can produce prolonged diarrhea and in immunologically impaired patients can precipitate clinical AIDS.

(5) If an infected patient contracts any infection, this infection should be treated much more aggressively than would be the case with a normal person. It is known that HIV-infected patients with other infections progress to AIDS much more rapidly.

(6) If a patient is to have elective surgery, the T4 helper lymphocytes should be checked preoperatively. If the T4 lymphocyte level is low, treatment with AZT should be instituted and surgery delayed to avoid infection and wound breakdown.

(7) People with HIV disease should actively work to maintain their physical health and nutritional status which may delay the progression of the disease.

(8) Smoking, alcohol and street drugs should be avoided since use of these products can influence the immune status.

(9) Patients with HIV disease should be under treatment to prevent Pneumocystis carinii pneumonia. Patients should be on AZT to prevent progression of their disease.

Since physicians are **not** doing routine testing to identify those in the general population who are infected, none of these logical steps are being carried out.

III. We are told that physicians should not try to do routine testing and contact tracing because by advocating testing and contact tracing, they would tend to "drive the disease underground."

That concept is simply a cliche. The disease is already underground. Over 90% of the people who have the virus don't know they are infected. Will testing with partner notification (contact tracing) be successful in identifying those who carry the virus? Certainly!

In Colorado, where public health officers began routine testing and mandatory reporting to the public health department in 1987, the number of people coming forward to be tested increased rather than decreased. In Colorado, HIV disease is considered an infectious disease by state law. In Colorado, the results of testing are routinely reported to public health officers. In March, April, May and June of 1987, Colorado performed almost twice as many HIV tests per 100,000 members of the population as were done in California during that same period.

In California, **public health officers refuse to consider HIV as an infectious, contagious, sexually transmitted disease** and there is no routine public health follow-up carried out. In Colorado, prior to the passage of legislation to allow reporting and partner notification, every effort was made by the gay community and the AIDS Lobby to frighten homosexuals into not being tested.

Homosexuals were told that if they were tested, they should **not** give their proper names because their identity could be discovered by homophobes and used to persecute them at some future date. As a result, many homosexuals **did** use false names, but it is interesting to note that virtually **all homosexuals** who came forward to be tested gave either their correct telephone numbers or addresses so that they could be contacted if their blood test was positive.

Furthermore, the vast majority of the homosexuals cooperated with public health follow-up and contact tracing. The original 282 patients with HIV disease who were interviewed named 508 sex partners. 81% had not been previously tested. Four-fifths of them were then tested.

Almost all those who were contacted accepted counseling and educational efforts to help protect themselves and their future sex partners. As a result of testing, 45 new cases of HIV disease were initially identified and counseling begun to stop the chain of transmission of HIV disease.[5]

Between 1987 and 1989, 13% of those interviewed and tested during contact tracing were found to have unsuspected HIV disease.

The idea that testing and contact tracing will drive the disease underground is a fallacy, but as Doctor Goebbels, the propaganda minister in Hitler's Germany, proved so well, "If you tell a big lie often enough, people will come to believe it."

You will find that those forces intent upon blocking testing will use the same cliche all across the free world. It was reported in the San Francisco Chronicle on January 19, 1989, that the Japanese government was attempting to enact legislation that would require physicians to report all AIDS cases and would empower authorities to stop people who tested positive for the AIDS virus from entering Japan. The article went on to say that:

> "The opposition Socialists, Communists and KOMEI parties opposed the legislation...the opposition charged that such a law would **drive AIDS carriers underground** as well as invade their privacy." (emphasis added.)

The same rhetoric is used by leftist groups throughout the world in an effort to prevent the use of standard public health techniques to stop the spread of this horrible disease.

The best evidence that reporting HIV disease will not drive the disease underground is the fact that in America today, all AIDS cases are mandatorily reported to public health officers and then to the CDC. AIDS is simply the terminal stage of HIV disease. Many patients go to the doctor and are tested and those test results are reported if the patient meets the CDC's strict criteria for the diagnosis of AIDS. What's the difference between HIV disease and AIDS? There is none. HIV and AIDS are the same disease. The early stage of the disease is not to be reported, while the late stage of the disease is to be reported.

> "Those whom God wishes to destroy,
> He first makes mad."

IV. Americans are told that it would be too costly to carry out widespread testing. We are told that the blood test ordinarily costs $20.00 to $25.00 in commercial labs, but **sometimes** it can cost $100.00 to $300.00. Furthermore, we are told that **health care dollars** are too scarce to use for general testing. Thus, physicians should **not** try to identify those who carry the virus and are spreading it...because of the tremendous cost that would be involved.

Rather, the federal government, in 1989, spent one and one-half billion dollars for education and treatment of those who have become infected unnecessarily. In 1990, 2 billion dollars was appropriated. In addition, individual states spend hundreds of millions of dollars yearly on treatment as the epidemic continues spreading across our land.

In 1990 an additional 2.5 billion dollars was appropriated for emergency relief to cities that faced financial catastrophe. The State of Florida estimates that it will be spending 2 billion dollars yearly by the year 2000 to care for victims of the epidemic.

The cost of testing is really not a factor. If public health authorities really intended to stop the epidemic, they could have undertaken testing of our population just as the Army does for less than $4.00 per person.

If the U. S. Public Health Service wanted to identify those who are infected, they could test every citizen in our nation for $4.00 each. For 3/4 of a billion dollars (a fraction of what we are spending yearly) we could test every American at risk. Tragically, physicians have not been encouraged to carry out routine testing.

Public health authorities have not recommended what is logical. Rather, our nation is spending exorbitant amounts of money on counseling, sex education, anonymous testing centers, gay and AIDS organizations and providing treatment for the tragic victims of this unnecessary epidemic.

The American public perceives that a great deal is being done, but they do not realize that doctors are being actively discouraged and prevented from doing what is really necessary.

Physicians are also told that if they do testing and report infected cases to public health officers, it would be far too expensive to carry out contact tracing.

In February of 1989 Dr. Donald Francis, the West Coast representative of the Centers for Disease Control, was asked on a San Francisco radio program why doctors were not doing testing in California and trying to identify carriers.[6] His reply:

"If we did widespread testing and reporting in California, we would have to put 200,000 to 300,000 names in computers and public health authorities would have time for nothing other than putting names into computers."

He went on to say, "If we tried to do contact tracing on all those infected, there is simply not enough money." Of course, what Dr. Francis neglected to state was that the reason no money was available was because public health authorities had repeatedly stated that our nation does not need general testing and contact tracing. Because CDC and public health officers have not requested money for contact tracing, it is not available. Because money is not available, public health officers cannot recommend contact tracing. Thus, you see the philosophy of those intent upon blocking routine testing and reporting of the disease.

The AIDS and gay Lobbies keep telling us, **It's too expensive to try to stop this disease. Prevention is far too expensive. Our nation should simply wait and watch as more and more of our young people come down with this fatal illness...and then try to take care of them.**

What logic is there in this policy? When has any logical person ever suggested that prevention is too expensive and our nation should simply allow an epidemic to take place? Yet this is the philosophy that is being espoused today by the U. S. Public Health Service and many state health departments. Our nation faces a major epidemic. For the first time in all history, public health authorities are **not trying** to stop its spread, because it would be **too costly.**

Physicians are told that the real expense involved in doing testing involves counseling and that physicians should never do blood testing without counseling. Counseling may cost as much as $50.00 and will raise the price of testing (if done in mass numbers) from $4.00 to $54.00. It is this cost (which includes counseling) which is often used to dramatize the exorbitant costs of universal testing.

Why is counseling important? Do we counsel everyone before we test for cancer or diabetes? Of course not. As I noted earlier, the whole concept of pretest counseling was specifically designed to discourage doctors from performing blood tests on patients in their offices.

The President's AIDS Commission recognized the absurdity of pretest counseling and recommended using a simple brochure in low risk patients in a doctor's office.[7] But if you were to look back in your magazines and newspapers to the reports on the President's AIDS Commission, you will never find that fact mentioned.

The AIDS Lobby didn't want physicians or the public to challenge the absurdity of their pretest counseling requirements which were utilized to effectively block testing. Isn't it strange that physicians have never been required to do counseling before drawing a blood test for syphilis or doing a smear for gonorrhea? Isn't it strange that it wasn't until HIV disease appeared in America that it was suddenly necessary to counsel people **before** blood testing?

There is no question that physicians should counsel those with a positive HIV blood test, but why must physicians counsel before performing an HIV blood test? Pretest counseling was recommended simply to discourage physicians from testing.

In Colorado, Dr. Tom Vernon, the state public health officer, estimates that for every dollar spent on contact tracing, the state saves $5.00 in treatment costs. Yet physicians across America are assured that it is too costly to carry out contact tracing.

The last fallacy in the arguments of the AIDS Lobby against testing "because of cost" is the simple fact that **government doesn't usually pay for the tests.** The cost of testing is ordinarily taken care of by patients. The inference of the AIDS Lobby is that government will finance testing and there will be expenditures of the government's limited resources which are needed elsewhere for other, more important activities. Of course, that isn't true.

All of the arguments of the AIDS Lobby are based upon illusion and delusion, deceit and deception — and intentional lies — because the AIDS and Gay Lobbies have perpetuated this unnecessary epidemic. The cost of the care of the tragic victims of this epidemic will eventually bankrupt our society...an epidemic which we are told we cannot fight because it would be "too costly."

V. We are told we must not do testing because physicians cannot insure the confidentiality of test results. We are told that physicians must be extremely concerned about patient confidentiality.

No one ever mentions that there is a tradition in medicine and that tradition requires that anything a patient tells a doctor must be kept in strict confidence. If a doctor were to release information on a patient to an employer, a relative or even to a patient's wife without the patient's specific permission, that doctor would be performing an unethical act and would be liable for civil action.

Never, until the HIV epidemic, was it suggested that doctors did not keep patients' records confidential. We have done blood tests for syphilis for years, but no one ever suggested that information on syphilis testing was released outside the confines of the medical profession.

For years, physicians have done smears for gonorrhea, but no one ever suggested that special confidentiality laws were needed to protect that information. Suddenly, **faced with this epidemic,** an epidemic that threatens to destroy our nation, confidentiality has become a prime factor in dealing with disease.

The passing of confidentiality laws has made it so difficult for physicians that, at least in the State of California, most doctors have avoided testing because by ordering the blood test (or even finding that the patient has had the blood test elsewhere), a physician could expose himself to a $10,000.00 fine and a year in prison.

At the California Medical Association conference in 1987, Dr. Seymour Alban from Southern California reported that he was asked to examine a patient as an impartial examiner by both sides in a litigation. As part of his examination, he drew a blood specimen for a series of blood tests, including an HIV test. The test was run in his office laboratory by his technician. Because Dr. Alban's technician **knew the patient's name,** the doctor was sued for $150,000.00 and a $25,000.00 settlement was paid. The reason for the settlement? The laboratory technician knew the patient's name.

An orthopedic surgeon in Santa Cruz, California, Dr. Paul Clayman, simply mentioned in a report to an insurance company that a patient had told him of his HIV status. A suit was filed and a $15,000.00 settlement was paid. Why? Because Dr. Clayman truthfully mentioned in his report exactly what the patient had told him.

In my own practice, I had a patient with HIV disease. I did not record anything in my office chart about his disease, but a local hospital sent a copy of the patient's records to my office which included mention of the patient's HIV status. I did not know that this report was even in my chart when it was subpoenaed because the patient was involved in litigation. Records were subpoenaed from three other doctors' offices as well.

As a result, the patient demanded $1500.00 from each doctor. One doctor paid. I refused to pay the $1500.00 and as a result, I and one other physician spent three days in court before the case was ultimately heard and found in our favor. All across the State of California and the nation, doctors have been harassed and intimidated with confidentiality laws.

All information in a medical chart must be released when subpoenaed...that is, all information **except** information on the status of HIV disease. On one hand, doctors are told on a subpoena that they must release every bit of information they possess on a patient or face prosecution. On the other hand, the law in California (Agnos' AB403) prevented physicians from releasing any information on a patient's HIV status. Which law were physicians to obey?

Do you think, for one minute, that all this confidentiality legislation would have been passed if this disease had not initially involved homosexuals? Certainly, the homosexual is fearful and paranoid. Homosexuals are concerned that people will use information on their disease to discriminate against them. But is there another factor? Do you know of a better way to destroy our nation than to allow this epidemic to continue its unchecked spread within the heterosexual population?

VI. The concepts of confidentiality and discrimination go hand in hand. Physicians have been told that they must keep information on who is infected absolutely confidential so that no one will know who has the virus. Information was not to be transmitted to public health officers. There must be no public health lists of those who carry the virus because the homosexuals believe that lists may be used at some future date to publicly identify them.

Indeed, according to Randy Shilts, the homosexuals fantasize that it will be "out of the bathhouses and into the concentration camps; out of the bathhouses, into the ovens." And so homosexuals are fearful and their fears are constantly inflamed by those who would use this epidemic for their own political purposes. Many of the homosexual leaders and gay publications constantly reinforce those fears, telling homosexuals that anyone who wants general testing of our population is their enemy, that those of us who want to stop the spread of this plague are really motivated by a desire to see homosexuals herded into prisons and quarantine camps.

This is the first epidemic in all history where the population is being told that the major problem is not the virus, the major problem is "discrimination."

I should point out that there are already extensive public health lists of those with the infection. AIDS is a reportable disease. We have mandatory reporting of the terminal stage of HIV disease in every state in the Union and lists of patients with AIDS are in the files of public health officers in all 50 states. Yet, the presence of these lists has never led to discrimination. There is not one reported instance that I know of in America where release of the names of AIDS patients reported to public health officers has ever led to discrimination.

The blood banks keep computerized lists of those who have been found to have HIV disease so that infected patients cannot donate blood in the future. No one has ever suggested that this information has been used to discriminate against those who are infected.

Rectal gonorrhea in males is a homosexual disease. There are extensive public health lists kept on patients with rectal gonorrhea, but no one has ever suggested that those lists have been used as a basis for discrimination.

Discrimination is something we must all be concerned about. Certainly, the tragic victims of this disease must be cared for and **should not be discriminated against.** On the other hand, people must be concerned about the potential for the spread of the disease. This does not mean that infected people cannot, in most instances, continue working on their jobs or that they cannot live in their homes or that they need to be put into concentration or quarantine camps. The disease is not that infectious. What we do need to do is report those infected with the disease to public health officers so that they can do contact tracing and identify those who are spreading the disease knowingly and unknowingly.

In 1987, when Colorado was trying to enact public health laws which would allow an intelligent approach to the epidemic, the Colorado Chapter of the ACLU denounced the bill as a gross invasion of privacy and threatened litigation should the bill become law.

Opponents of the bill argued, "...that the bill should not be passed since the confidentiality of testing and reporting could never be guaranteed." According to a May 1, 1987 article in the "Rocky Mountain News," some homosexual activists went so far as to attempt to gain access to confidential hospital records of AIDS patients — "...just to show there is no such thing as confidentiality."

Apparently radical opponents of the Colorado law (HB1177) contacted a record clerk at Denver General Hospital (who acknowledged he was a homosexual) at least six times. At first they had said: "Hey, why don't you just pull a few records for us?" the clerk related. "Then they started to get heavy with me." The activists accused the clerk of being disloyal to the gay cause because he refused to turn over records. They also threatened to undermine his reputation in the gay community. Despite this effort to subvert the confidentiality of AIDS records and the ACLU and Gay opposition to HB1177 in Colorado, the bill passed in both legislative chambers.[8]

❋❋❋

Very often, in debates with members of the AIDS Lobby, they will point out that it is easy to steal hospital records. They point out that on one occasion, records were stolen from an office of a public health department in Northern California. They, of course, at no point questioned who stole the records and at no point were they able to show that any discrimination occurred because records had been stolen.

Many times, homosexual groups will actually go in and steal records in order to illustrate that records can be stolen...to justify the charges that discrimination could occur because medical records are vulnerable. The tragic part of the story is that because the gay groups have effectively blocked public health officers from addressing the epidemic, tens of thousands—probably hundreds of thousands—of homosexuals have contracted the disease and will ultimately die. Had public health officials begun using standard public health techniques early in the course of this epidemic, the epidemic could have been stopped and the lives of hundreds of thousands of homosexuals spared.

Instead, the homosexual community has been manipulated by its leaders. As a result, the epidemic continues unabated, spreading through the homosexuals, into the drug abusers, and now, into the heterosexual community.

Despite homosexual and AIDS Lobby charges about the dangers of discrimination — and discrimination is not entirely imaginary — the dangers of discrimination should never have kept physicians from using public health techniques to stop this epidemic.

Discrimination usually has occurred only when people have announced publicly that they have the virus or when one of their friends (who **they** have told of their HIV status) tells others. Discrimination occurs because most people are frightened by this disease, but they are frightened for the wrong reasons. This disease is hard to get. The danger from this disease is not from casual contact. The danger is from the intentional efforts to block the use of time-proven techniques to stop its spread — efforts that will ultimately result in the unnecessary deaths of millions of Americans.

※※※

Probably one of the most widely known and tragic incidents in America was the burning of the home of the Ray family in Arcadia, Florida in August of 1987.

"Discrimination, house burning, prejudice against innocent children, throwing innocent children into the street," are images created in the minds of the American public as the media hammered away at that unfortunate event. Strangely, the media has never told you the whole story of what really happened in Arcadia, Florida in 1987. The media would have you believe that the act of arson was the work of bigots — and perhaps it was. But, still, we do not know who set the fire and one might ask, "Who would benefit from burning down the home of a family with three HIV-infected hemophiliac children?"

The tragedy began in August 1986 when Louise Ray, the mother of Randy, 8, Robert, 9, and Richard, 10, discovered that all three of her sons had been infected with the virus from taking Factor 8 — a blood product used to prevent bleeding in hemophiliacs. At that point, Mr. and Mrs. Ray went to the school board and acknowledged that their children carried the virus. The school board asked if they would keep their children out of school in the fall of 1986 while a committee was set up consisting of the family pediatrician, members of the school board and other medical experts in the field, to determine whether or not it would be safe for the children to enter school.

It was decided by the committee that young children, many times, do not act responsibly. Furthermore, these children were hemophiliacs with recorded instances of recurrent bleeding. Since the infected children's blood on the skin of others could lead to infection, it was felt that it would be best to educate the children at home. Arrangements were made for a full-time tutor. From the fall of 1986 until the spring of 1987, the children remained at home with a teacher provided by the local school district.

After five months, the family became dissatisfied and decided to move to Bay Minette, Alabama, to start over. They went to the local school board in Bay Minette and asked if their children could be admitted to school. Once again they informed the school board that their children carried the virus. In this instance, the school board formed a committee, but included Mr. and Mrs. Ray on that special investigative committee.

The committee decided that **the children could be admitted to school** and they were simply awaiting the next regular meeting of the school board before the children could start attending regular classes. At that point, the Rays decided they would move back to Arcadia, Florida. The following reason was given by Mrs. Ray in her deposition which was part of their law-suit against the school district in Arcadia:

> After the Mobile meeting, I called our doctor (a physician in St. Petersburg, Florida, who had treated the children and was opposed to the home-bound instruction that was offered in Arcadia) to ask him if he would send a letter to the Alabama School Board. He said he would, but also said that he had found a lawyer to represent us free if we wanted to come home...Because it was going to take so long for the Bay Minette School system to decide, we had thought about moving to another county in Alabama and starting again. We realized

it wouldn't work, because the school records would follow us. We decided that if we had to fight we might as well fight at home in De Soto County.

The children were about to be admitted to school in Alabama and would have been in school, presumably, within a few weeks; however, there were forces that were not necessarily interested in solving the problem, but were interested in creating a media event. Thus, free legal counsel was provided to encourage the family to return to Arcadia to promote a suit against the local school district.

Did the AIDS Lobby want to create an issue, a law-suit, a confrontation? Certainly! Confrontation is the standard technique used by those intent upon creating publicity. And who were to be the losers? The Ray children could have been admitted to public schools in Alabama. Instead, they returned to Arcadia, where they were kept out of school for another semester and put into direct confrontation with the local school district. When it appeared that the problem was about to be solved by court order, a fire strangely occurred in their home and a national media event resulted.

This event allowed Senator Edward Kennedy (the hero of Chappaquiddick) to say on September 11, 1987: "This family tragedy confirms everything we know about the need to fight hysteria and fear with education...It demonstrates the destructive forces that can be readily unleashed when people react to fear with hatred and discrimination."

As a result of the lawsuit that was brought against the school district in Arcadia, a temporary injunction was delivered by the court requiring that the three children be admitted to school. On August 5, 1987, the court's decision included the following statement:

> Whatever their chronological years, these three boys must take on adult responsibility for protecting themselves from substantial risk at school, the school population from risk of exposure to the HIV virus and the possible consequences which might occur from such an exposure.

Now how can boys 8, 9 and 10 years of age take on adult responsibility? What was the danger to young children in school, playing side by side with hemophiliac children who had the virus? In 1986, there was still a very real concern about casual spread of the disease. School districts were being told that there was no reason to be concerned about having infected children in school but in New York City, teachers were each being issued pairs of rubber gloves in case an infected child had a nose bleed or got a cut.

In 1986, a book was widely circulated in America entitled The AIDS Cover-up, which gave the impression that the disease was much more contagious than the public had been led to believe. In 1986 most people really didn't believe what our government told them about the epidemic.

I will cover the matter of casual spread of the disease later in our story, but I can assure you that casual spread of the disease is very rare and that most **mature** children **can** attend school safely without danger to their classmates if they are carefully monitored, do not have a bleeding tendency, do not get into fights or participate in contact sports and have no other communicable diseases.

In 1986 and 1987, however, there was still a serious and justifiable concern about the danger to school children from casual spread of this fatal disease.

In any event, the Ray children were to be admitted to school on August 24, 1987.

A boycott of the school was organized by concerned parents to coincide with the court-mandated admission of the Ray children. On Monday, August 24, the first day of school, "only 337 of an expected 632 students attended classes."[9] Dozens of reporters came to Arcadia to report on the school boycott and decry the bigotry of parents who kept their children out of classes. Every day that followed, more and more children attended school, until by Friday, things were almost back to normal and many of the reporters had left.

That is, things were almost back to normal until shortly after 10 p.m. Friday evening...when a fire broke out at the home of the Ray family. Neither the parents nor the three boys were at home when the fire started. The family charged that their house had been firebombed, yet looking at the pictures of the house it is quite obvious that the fire started inside.

There was an extensive investigation by the County Sheriff's Department and the State Fire Marshall. Three weeks later, when the investigative report was released, information came out that the fire had originated inside the house and that there was no evidence that the fire had started outside. The question of arson was raised.

There was a question raised as to how an arsonist gained access to the home. The major question, however, is "Who benefited from the fire?" Was it citizens of Arcadia, a city which has been vilified and attacked by the media all across America? Was it the citizens who organized the

student boycott? Was it the Ray family—a tragic family who obviously
had been manipulated into coming back to Arcadia from Alabama?
Was it agents of the AIDS Lobby, an organization which has been
coordinating efforts all across the nation to dramatize the dangers of
discrimination and to use the specter of discrimination to justify the fact
that we should not address the epidemic? Who benefited from the fire?

I do not know the answer to that question. Certainly, if law enforcement agencies in Arcadia cannot determine who started the fire, I
cannot. But I would ask you to keep that question in mind as our story
continues to unfold and I take you behind the scenes onto the battle-
fields where few have stood, to meet the enemy who has perpetuated this
epidemic.

✳✳✳

One very important fact should be kept in mind. That fact is that
homosexuals are constantly reminded by gay publications and gay
leaders that there is a very real danger of quarantine for anyone infected
with or suspected of being infected with the virus (i.e., all homosexuals).
The specter of quarantine is used to reinforce homosexual fears that they
will soon be rounded up and incarcerated. This may seem a foolish and
unfounded fear to the straight community, but it is of grave concern to
the gay community which is made up of young men and women who
already feel alienated from society because of their lifestyle.

Homosexual fears are reinforced by the actual confinement of HIV
infected individuals in Cuba.

Homosexual fears were further reinforced by Lyndon LaRouche's
ballot initiatives in California in 1986 and 1988 (Propositions 64 and 69)
which simply stated that HIV should be treated like any other disease
and those who were infected should be reported to public health officers.
But Lyndon LaRouche and his followers kept talking about the necessity of "quarantine." Their mention of quarantine served to reinforce the
homosexuals' convictions that anyone who wanted public health reporting and monitoring of this disease — also wanted quarantine.

All responsible medical authorities have agreed that quarantine is not
necessary to stop this epidemic — except for those people who are
intentionally spreading the disease.

Yet the Cuban action and the words of Lyndon LaRouche have
convinced the homosexuals of America that anyone who favors routine
testing and public health follow-up really wants to "quarantine" them.

Have you ever wondered why the Cuban government quarantines those with HIV infection when all medical authorities have said it is unnecessary? Have you ever wondered why Lyndon LaRouche advocated quarantine when there was no possible medical justification for that position? As our story unfolds, you will, hopefully, come to understand their motives.

❋❋❋

Is discrimination the real issue? Will antidiscrimination laws solve the problem and allow physicians to begin addressing this epidemic?

If the people within the AIDS Lobby were really concerned about discrimination, why is it that they would not withdraw their opposition to routine testing, contact tracing and the use of standard public health techniques in exchange for an opportunity to have an antidiscrimination law signed by Governor Deukmejian of California in the fall of 1988?

California State Senator John Vasconcellos authored an antidiscrimination bill which cleared both houses of the California legislature in 1988. Conservative Republican, Senator John Doolittle offered to make a political deal. The antidiscrimination bill would be signed by Governor Deukmejian if the California Medical Association and the AIDS Lobby would give up their opposition to Proposition 102, a State Initiative to allow routine testing and contact tracing. The CMA (which works closely with the AIDS Lobby) refused. Discrimination was not the real issue. In 1990, the "Americans With Handicaps Bill" became law. This was a gay-AIDS antidiscrimination law. Despite the passage of this law, the AIDS Lobby continues to oppose testing and contact tracing.

The real issue was that physicians were not to be allowed to use time proven standard public health techniques to stop this epidemic. Nothing effective would be done. Billions of dollars would be spent, volumes would be written, demonstrations would occur and the media would lament the ever continuing expansion of AIDS, while never mentioning that AIDS was not the epidemic — just the end stage of HIV disease.

VII. Education is the answer to the epidemic. Education and behavioral modification will stop the spread of the disease. That is the current party line of the representatives of the U. S. Public Health Service, the Gay and the AIDS Lobby.

"Knowing the facts about AIDS can prevent spread of the disease," stated Surgeon General C. Everett Koop in the Surgeon General's

Report. "It is the responsibility of every citizen to be informed." (See Appendix I).

Now, one might ask why we never tried to control tuberculosis with education or why we never tried to control syphilis, leprosy or gonorrhea simply with education? Certainly, as a physician, I am required by law to report cases of syphilis, gonorrhea, tuberculosis, tularemia, typhus, typhoid and Toxic Shock Syndrome, measles, meningitis and whooping cough to the public health officer.

Why is it that, by law, we have always had mandatory reporting of these diseases, but with HIV disease (an almost 100% fatal disease) we are **not** required to report cases? Indeed, until January of 1989 in California, a physician was liable for a $10,000.00 fine and a year imprisonment if he reported a case of HIV disease without the written permission of the patient.

At the present time, in California, a physician may "voluntarily report" the disease to the public health officer if he chooses — but very few physicians do report because of the doctor's fear of fines, imprisonment and confusion about the new laws. Why must physicians report so many nonlethal diseases, but are discouraged from reporting lethal HIV disease? The reason is quite simple. It has been determined that America will not use standard testing and follow-up to stop **this** epidemic.

So how effective is education and behavioral modification in stopping the epidemic? The members of the AIDS Lobby will point, with great pride, to the drastic drop in rectal gonorrhea in the homosexual population in San Francisco. "Education works," they repeat over and over again — and always they allude to the drastic drop in rectal gonorrhea and the new cases of HIV disease in the homosexual population of San Francisco.

Their statistics are really quite accurate. The incidence of rectal gonorrhea **has** dropped in the homosexual community in San Francisco. In addition, the incidence of new cases of HIV infection **has** drastically dropped in the homosexual population in San Francisco, but to understand what has happened in San Francisco, you must understand the "cohort study" and its results.

In 1978, over 6700 homosexual men in San Francisco volunteered to enter into a **hepatitis** study. The purpose of that study was to determine whether or not homosexual men who were immunized with a vaccine against hepatitis would come down with the illness. Hepatitis is much more prevalent within the homosexual community because of their promiscuous lifestyle.

Investigators wanted a large number of gay men in their study so blood specimens were drawn and stored. Of the 6700 men evaluated, only 350 were not already infected with Hepatitis B. These were the least promiscuous of the 6700 men studied.

The members of the group of 350 who were not Hepatitis B antigen positive received either the hepatitis vaccine or a placebo to determine the effectiveness of the vaccine. When the HIV epidemic became apparent, the original frozen serum specimens were tested for HIV antibodies and many of the participants have allowed investigators to draw regular blood specimens from them to monitor the course of the epidemic within the original 6700 members of the cohort. Thus it has been possible to follow the clinical course of the epidemic in this large group of homosexual men. As of 1987, 75% of the 6700 members of the cohort were infected with the HIV virus.[10] That means that three-quarters of those 6700 homosexuals are infected and are going to die.

By March 1988, they had tracked these patients even further. During the preceding year, an additional 1% of the cohort group had contracted HIV disease.[11] Now 1% doesn't sound like a very large number of new cases, but if you realize that there are only 25% of the original 100% who were uninfected, to infect 1% means that 4% of the **uninfected** homosexuals within the cohort population in San Francisco contracted the disease during that year. Certainly, there is no better educated, better informed group of citizens anywhere in the country than the homosexuals of San Francisco. In addition, homosexuals are usually very intelligent people. If intelligence and education are sufficient to stop the epidemic, why did 4% of the uninfected homosexuals in the cohort study group of 6700 homosexuals in San Francisco acquire the disease between 1987 and 1988? The answer is quite simple. Education and information alone will not stop the spread of this disease.

Why has the number of new cases of HIV disease decreased in the homosexual community in San Francisco? Because over three-quarters of the promiscuous homosexuals are already infected. Why has the incidence of rectal gonorrhea dropped? First, the venereal disease rate was astronomically high during the early 80's. It has been estimated that the rate of venereal disease among homosexuals in San Francisco was twenty-two times higher than in the general population. Thus, a significant drop in the rectal gonorrhea rate has little meaning. There is still a significant incidence of rectal gonorrhea in San Francisco in 1991. Also, in recent years, many homosexuals have given up sodomy and now practice fisting, oral sex or mutual masturbation to fulfill their sexual craving. Also, with over three-quarters of the homosexual population of San Francisco infected, many of the tragic young men do not participate in sexual orgies as they have in the past.

※※※

A survey of 1,481 men carried out by the National Opinion Research Center was reported in September of 1988 by the CDC. They found that 14.0% of single men, ages 18 to 29 who had never married, reported having sex with 5 to 10 or more women during the previous year. That was during the years 1987-1988, when maximum AIDS education was being carried out.

Calculating these figures on a nationwide base, that meant that there were almost one million of our young people at major risk for contracting the virus and spreading it to 5 or 10 women a year. Despite these figures, the Centers for Disease Control and the AIDS Lobby tell us that **all that is necessary to stop the epidemic is education.**

Even U. S. Surgeon General C. Everett Koop who keeps reiterating that "our only weapon with which to fight this epidemic is education," noted in January of 1989 on a television interview, **"We do know that teenagers are not listening."** He noted that 3 out of every 1,000 college students in one study were seropositve and that it is probable that most of these young people contracted their HIV infection while still in high school. "Teenagers are risk takers," he said. "They feel they are immortal. They don't like any admonition that begins with the word 'Don't.'"

In a letter to the American Medical Association, Dr. Steven Keller of the New Jersey Medical School in Newark, New Jersey, noted that a survey of teenagers showed that they had excellent knowledge of the fact that sexual activity could lead to HIV disease, but that programs "focusing on increased AIDS awareness are unlikely to substantially reduce sex risk behavior in sexually active adolescents."

In study after study after study...in survey after survey after survey which have been carried out by responsible authorities, it has been shown that education alone has failed to influence the sexual activity and promiscuity of our young people.

Tragically, even in the homosexual communities where education has been the most intense, it has not been effective. In 1989, in Seattle, gonorrhea in homosexuals was up 400%. In 1989, in the 350 members of the cohort still being closely followed, an additional 3% became infected. But that is the story that the AIDS Lobby does not want you to hear as they continue to reiterate that "all we need to control this epidemic is education and behavioral modification."

✻✻✻

We have no idea how rapidly the epidemic is spreading in our nation, but we can look at the incidence of sexually transmitted diseases to see how effective education has been in changing the sexual habits of our population. If one studies what has happened to the spread of syphilis in our nation, we find that syphilis was declining in the early part of the 1980's, but that trend reversed itself in 1986 when the massive AIDS educational program began.

Concurrent with all the TV ads and education on the sexual spread of HIV disease, the incidence of syphilis began to climb. The more you talk about sex and AIDS without stressing morality and abstinence, the higher the incidence of promiscuity and the higher the incidence of syphilis.

Syphilis rates were up between 1986 and 1987, up again between 1987 and 1988 and up between 1988 and 1989. These rates continue rising higher in the 1990's reflecting an increase in promiscuity on the part of certain segments of our population. However, the media doesn't tell you that. They lead you to believe that all we need is education and behavioral modification to stop the epidemic.

A massive new educational program has been mandated for our schools. Our Surgeon General has advocated that we start teaching children about sex in the lower grades and teach them about sex and AIDS, every year, up until the time they graduate. We are going to talk about sex, and talk about sex, and talk about sex, and talk about sex.

We are going to place young boys and girls in the same classroom and strip away their modesty and embarrassment. We are going to discuss every intimate and personal aspect of sex — oral sex, vaginal sex, masturbation and rectal sex. We are going to concentrate their attention on sex — without mention of God or morality. The public is assured that by talking about sex and spending a great deal of money on sex education and by desensitizing our children to the subject of sex, we are going to cut down on the promiscuity of our young people. Tragically, that will not occur.

What is the relationship between sex education and promiscuity? The more sex education you get, the more promiscuity you will have. To document this, one has only to refer to the work of Doctor Jacqueline R. Kasun published in "The Family Resource Center News" in the summer of 1987.

Using the statistics from the Guttamacher Institute, a creation of Planned Parenthood, she was able to show that sex education and contraceptive education increased the odds of starting intercourse at age 14 by a factor of 50%.

In addition, in a paper available from the "American Life League," Doctor Kasun used Planned Parenthood's own statistics to show the direct relationship between per capita expenditures on birth control information and the rate of abortion plus unmarried births in white girls between the ages of 15 and 19. Progressively, the more money that a state government spent on sex education, the more abortions and births occurred in girls 15 to 19 years of age.

When one analyzed Maine, which was spending 106% of the per capita rate of the nation, they had a figure of 46 pregnancies per 1,000. In South Carolina, where they spent 114% of national per capita expenditure, the rate was 47 per thousand. In Vermont, where they spent 116% of the national per capita expenditure on sex education, they had a figure of 60 per 1,000. In 1980, Utah spent only 31% of the average national per capita expenditures on birth control education and had a rate of abortion and birth rate of 30 per 1,000.

It is very easy to see in this study that the more money that was spent on sex education, the higher the rate of promiscuity as reflected in the rates of abortions and unmarried pregnancies.[12]

What needs to be done to stop the epidemic? The people who can best be educated are those who have the virus or who know somebody else who has the virus. Those easiest to educate are those who know someone who has died of this horrible disease. Thus, we must try to find out who carries the virus and then educate them as to their responsibility to stop spreading the disease. Furthermore, there must be legal recourse to take against those infected people who knowingly have sexual relationships with unsuspecting partners and endanger their lives.

What should the message of education be? Having sex outside marriage is playing Russian Roulette in the Lottery of Death, a lottery in which there are no winners, only losers. And if you lose, your reward is a slow, lingering, painful death. This is a horrible and frightening message. But allowing our young people to believe that sex with condoms is "safe sex" is criminal negligence. Yet this is the message being presented to the youth of America today, orchestrated by the AIDS and Gay Lobbies and the U. S. Public Health Service.

What is "safe sex"? Safe sex is sex with someone wearing the wedding ring that you gave them when you were married. The message that should be presented in schools today is that there is a God, that every individual is important to God and there are moral standards that have existed down through all ages. Violation of God's codes for sex leads to syphilis, gonorrhea, chancroid, lymphopathy venereum, lymphogranuloma venereum, venereal warts, herpes, hepatitis, cervical cancer, Chlamydia, Trichomonas vaginitis, monilia vaginitis, pregnancy, emotional disorders and guilt.

Pelvic infection from promiscuity can lead to sterility and the inability to have children. In addition, if you get HIV disease, you should never marry, you should never have children and you can look forward to a slow, lingering, painful, demented death.

A return to the teaching of moral standards and morality is the first step in "sex education." We need to talk about chastity education and sexual responsibility, about a sense of personal worth, personal values and personal morality. We need sex education programs that emphasize sex in the context of marriage — not the values neutral humanistic programs being presented in schools all across America today.

※※※

There is one more factor as far as education is concerned. The homosexual agenda today is designed to teach young people about homosexuality at a very young age. The homosexual agenda intends to implant in young people's minds the possibility that they might be homosexual. The homosexual lifestyle is presented as a happy, successful one. Indeed, a program called Project 10 (also referred to as Gay and Lesbian Education — GALE) has been introduced into the Los Angeles City School System with similar educational programs being introduced all across our nation.

The basic precept of Project 10 (GALE) is that 10% of our children are homosexual and that these latent homosexual children must be identified and must realize that they are homosexuals so they can be released from their fears and frustrations. They must learn their true sexual identity early so they can begin to express themselves freely. In this program, young people are asked such questions as: "Have you ever wondered if you are homosexual?" "Have you ever wondered if any of your friends are homosexual?" "Have you ever had any strange sexual feelings?" "Would you like to meet some successful homosexuals?"

The children, without parental permission, are required to attend classes where successful homosexuals — doctors, lawyers and teachers — tell about their happy lives. Homosexual role models are being presented to your children without your knowledge or consent. Children are told that they should not tell their parents about the classes.

You see, the homosexual population is being decimated by HIV disease. If the homosexual lifestyle is to continue, they must have new recruits. The homosexual has been told over and over again, that homosexuality is a trait that he is born with and thus he can justify his lifestyle. Your children are being taught that as well.

That concept is being used to implant the idea in many children's minds that they may be homosexual...in an effort to bring those children into the homosexual lifestyle. Yet, statistics have shown that if your first sexual experience is a homosexual one, chances are that you will remain homosexual throughout the rest of your life, whereas, if your first sexual experience is heterosexual, you have relatively little chance of becoming a homosexual.

Tragically, they never teach our children in schools that male homosexuality involves fisting (inserting one's fist and forearm into another man's rectum), rimming (licking about a man's anus with ingestion of feces), golden showers (lying naked while others urinate on you and may involve the drinking of urine) and sodomy (penile-rectal intercourse).

Education on homosexuality never tells our children **what homosexuals really do,** it only serves to convince them how nice and pleasant homosexuals are. The fact that 25% of homosexuals practice sado-masochism or that the North American Man-Boy Love Association (NAMBLA) of homosexual pedophiles is actively seducing your children is never mentioned.

Children are never told that homosexual practices lead directly to Hepatitis B infection, a massive incidence of venereal disease and a compulsive, addictive sexual lifestyle with severe emotional problems.

Children are never told of the high suicide rates among homosexuals or the sadness and isolation felt by these tragic people. They are educating our children only about the positive aspects of the homosexual lifestyle in order to encourage the curiosity of youth and lead our young people into the homosexual way of death.

"Those whom God wishes to destroy, He first makes mad."

VIII. We are told that it is not important to identify those who are infected because no one gets this disease unless they do something (i.e., have sexual relations). There is no such thing as casual spread of HIV disease.

Is there casual spread of HIV disease? When Doctors Masters, Johnson and Kolodny suggested in their book, *Crisis,* in March of 1988 that there was some question as to the mode of transmission of this disease, they were attacked by the Surgeon General, the Centers for Disease Control, the media, the AIDS and the Gay Lobbies. For no one is to raise the question of casual spread of HIV disease. You will recall that in Chapter One, we listed the demands presented in the Manifesto of Montreal. The second item in that manifesto proclaimed:

"Governments must recognize that HIV disease is not highly infectious. Casual contact presents no threat of infection and irrational fears of transmission must be fought."

Despite the gay proclamation laid out in that Manifesto, one must look at the medical facts that are known. First of all, we know that HIV disease is primarily transmitted by sexual relations, but it can also be transferred by blood or blood products and from a mother to her child. HIV disease is spread in exactly the same manner as infectious Hepatitis B, although fortunately, HIV disease is felt to be less contagious than Hepatitis B.

How is Hepatitis B known to be spread? In addition to spread by sexual and blood products, Hepatitis B can be spread by close and intimate contact in families, in hospitals for the mentally defective and in institutional settings. Does this method of spread hold for HIV disease?

The Centers for Disease Control always reports that 3% of their cases do not fit into any one of their risk groups. Careful analysis of that 3% reveals that a significant number of the patients have acquired the disease from prostitutes and many of them have had other sexually transmitted diseases suggesting that patients acquired the disease because of promiscuity. However, there are always a few cases that the CDC cannot explain, although that number, fortunately, is small. In addition, you will recall that AIDS statistics only tell us what happened in the epidemic ten years ago. They do not tell us what is happening today. Ten years ago there were relatively few people infected with the virus and little chance for casual spread. Today there are probably 20 or 30 times as many people infected who have the potential for infecting others.

When we talk about **casual spread** of the disease, we have one major problem. Is **casual spread** of disease the type of infection that we would expect to see among health care workers? Is casual spread of disease possible from deep and passionate kissing? Is casual spread of disease something that occurs when you shake hands or when you sit down next to someone who is infected? Nobody has ever defined what is meant by **casual spread.**

I agree with Surgeon General Koop when he says that you aren't going to get the disease by shaking hands or by going into a restaurant. In all probability, this type of spread of the disease is extremely rare — and would probably be as likely as getting struck by a meteor or by a bolt of lightning. Although casual spread occurs, it occurs very infrequently. But certainly there is the potential for the spread of this disease when you are in constant close and intimate contact with someone who harbors the virus. When spread occurs it is usually within families.

Many times, I have sat next to those who were infected, I have shaken hands with those who carry the virus and I have eaten with them. I have taken care of infected patients in my practice and I have operated on them. I believe that the risk of spread of the disease is infinitesimal under most circumstances. But the public is being lied to about a number of major issues and these issues must be addressed.

First of all, there are two major hazards to the average person who comes in contact with people with HIV disease. The first problem is the possibility of developing one of the associated infections carried by those with an altered immune system. The second possibility is the remote possibility of getting HIV infection by nonsexual contact.

As far as the danger of secondary infection is concerned, you must understand that people with an altered immune system are unable to resist infections. As a result, virtually all those with full-blown AIDS are infected with the cytomegalovirus. Although cytomegalovirus is of little danger to the average person with a normal immune system, if a pregnant woman contacts cytomegalovirus infection there is a good chance that her child will be born with horrible congenital deformities. There is an instance in San Francisco, where Mrs. James Watson, a pregnant nurse working on the AIDS Ward at San Francisco General Hospital, was denied permission by her gay supervisor to wear a mask and gown when caring for AIDS patients. Despite Mrs. Watson's protestations, her supervisor threatened disciplinary action if she dared to wear protective clothing. As a result, when her child was born, the child had cytomegalovirus infection, microcephaly and the typical deformities which are well described in the pediatric literature.

Yet despite this recorded instance of secondary infections of a pregnant woman, HCWs are told that there is absolutely nothing to worry about from being in contact with those who have AIDS. As late as 1988, an article appeared in the New England Journal of Medicine stating that female doctors who were pregnant had **no right to refuse** to take care of AIDS patients. Such statements are criminal negligence — or worse.

A significant number of AIDS patients carry the acid-fast bacteria of tuberculosis. In fact, most identified AIDS patients are routinely placed on anti-tuberculous therapy. As long as that therapy is effective and their sputum is not infectious, there is little to worry about from caring for AIDS patients. However, there is one instance reported in Pennsylvania where eleven nurses became infected with tuberculosis while caring for a tuberculous AIDS patient.

Much more dangerous than the identified AIDS patients are those patients who have an altered immune system where HIV disease is not recognized and patients are not under anti-tuberculous therapy. These patients will continue to spread tuberculosis in the general population until they are identified. Today, all across America, there is a resurgence of tuberculosis, a disease which had almost been eradicated a decade ago. The incidence of tuberculosis is rising significantly and is threatening the health of our nation. Yet doctors are constantly being discouraged from identifying those who are infected with the HIV virus who often carry infectious tuberculosis.

There is a very real danger of the spread of Pneumocystis carinii pneumonia to anyone with an altered immune system. There was one instance reported from England where AIDS patients had been placed into a hospital with cancer patients being treated with immuno-suppressant therapy. An epidemic of Pneumocystis carinii pneumonia broke out among the immuno-suppressed cancer patients with devastating results.

Most AIDS patients are infected with the hepatitis virus and because of their altered immune system, they cannot deal with the virus efficiently. About 10% of AIDS patients become chronic carriers of the hepatitis virus and are potentially infectious to those who are in close and intimate contact with them.

A report from France by the Pasteur Institute documented the high incidence of the hepatitis antigen among non-HIV-infected children living in a boarding school with a number of hemophiliac children who acquired HIV virus from taking blood concentrates. Today there is a very real danger of infectious hepatitis in our nation.

Patients with an altered immune system often carry the pneumococcus bacteria in their nasopharynx. If transmitted to older people, it can result in pneumococcal pneumonia.

Most AIDS patients are infected with the Epstein-Barr virus which can be transmitted to those they come in contact with. Patients with altered immune systems often carry salmonella, giardiasis, amebiasis and other intestinal parasites which can be passed on to others with improper hygiene. Fortunately, the majority of the other infections that attack the immuno-suppressed bodies of AIDS victims are not transmissible to those in the general population and thus, are of no major concern.

❋❋❋

Then the matter of transmission of the HIV virus by nonsexual means must be addressed.

First of all, an article appeared in the Lancet magazine from the Pasteur Institute in September 1985. This report showed the "unusual stability" of LAV, HTLV-III virus at room temperature. It was shown that the virus could survive in dry form for seven days and in liquid form for ten days. Although the number of viral particles decreased dramatically, HIV disease can be produced by only one viral particle entering the human body.

Thus, what you have probably read or heard stating that this virus will not survive outside the human body is not true. Indeed, IV drug users across America are being told that all they have to do is wash out their needles with bleach and they will have nothing to worry about. But late in 1989, articles were published in medical journals pointing out that some IV drug users who regularly use bleach to cleanse their needles were still coming down with HIV infection.

The second important fact to realize is that the Langerhans cells which lie in the subcutaneous level of the human skin and beneath the surface of the mucous membranes of our mouth, bronchia and lungs is the primary cell that is infected by the HIV virus. Recent studies at the University of Oslo have shown that the Langerhans cell sends dendrites out to the skin level and if the HIV virus is on the human skin, it can be channeled into the Langerhans cell and then into the lymphocytes of the body.

It is by this means that blood contamination of the skin can lead to infection of health care workers as was documented in the three "splash cases" which were reported by the CDC and which I will cover later. A case was published in Lancet in 1990 from Varese, Italy reporting an Italian man who became infected during a soccer game from colliding with an HIV-infected drug user when both players incurred cuts and bleeding.[13]

There was a separate report of an American traveling on a train in Africa. His train collided with another train. Many people were injured and bleeding. The American became infected from contact with the blood of his fellow passengers. Thus, infected bodily fluids on the skin or mucous membranes can lead to infection.

✳✳✳

The American public has been told by the Surgeon General and public health authorities that it is impossible to contract HIV disease from kissing. To justify their conclusions, they report several medical studies where children have lived in homes with infected parents. The children ordinarily were kissed on the cheek and occasionally kissed on the lips. Over a period of one to two years, none of the children converted to a positive HIV test. However, there has never been a study of people who engaged in deep and passionate kissing (without sexual intimacy) as is carried out so commonly by our youth today.

Yet, the Centers for Disease Control, the U. S. Public Health Service and the Surgeon General have assured the youth of our nation that they have absolutely nothing to fear from kissing. The problem is that one kisses their grandmother on the cheek far differently than young people kiss one another in the back seat of a car on Saturday night.

All the evidence points to the fact that exchange of saliva and blood, which are present in the oral cavity, can lead to infection. Tragically, irresponsible public health officers continue assuring the public that kissing is completely safe. Why? To avoid irritating the AIDS and homosexual contingent who insist that the public must be convinced that there is no possibility of casual spread of the disease.

In an article in Science magazine in February of 1988, Doctor James Curran, Director of the Centers for Disease Control commented: "HIV disease has been recovered from saliva but the isolation rate is much lower than that from blood."

In the San Francisco Chronicle on June 24, 1989 it was reported that 27 babies had been infected in the southern city of Elista in the Soviet Union. All the infants were under two years of age and had been infected because of the use of a common syringe that had been contaminated with HIV infected blood. The article then stated that:

"Four mothers apparently picked up the virus through cracks in their nipples while breast feeding their babies, **although Western experts discounted this.**" (emphasis added)

Now you might ask why Western experts insisted that those infected children could not transmit HIV disease to their mothers via saliva? Why? Because if Western AIDS experts were to admit that salivary transfer of HIV disease was possible from infants to their mothers, they would have to admit that saliva in the mouth of anyone infected with the virus could transmit the disease to others. You must understand that Western AIDS experts **must convince the public** that there is no way that saliva transmits this disease.

There have been a number of instances where mothers have received HIV-infected transfusions immediately after they delivered their children. The previously uninfected mothers then contracted HIV disease. They nursed their children and the children got the disease from either their mothers' milk and/or bleeding from the mothers' nipples. Certainly this is an example of transmission of the disease across the mucous membranes of the mouth or the gastrointestinal tract.

Tragically, many homosexuals have believed the lie that oral sex was safe. In the Lancet magazine, December 7, 1988, a case was reported of a 29-year-old homosexual who had had no sexual contact other than oral-genital sex and had never had anal intercourse. After oral receptive sex one evening, his partner told him that he was HIV seropositive. Later testing of the 29-year-old homosexual revealed that he had been infected.

In January, 1989, an article was published in the Journal of the

American Medical Association by Italian investigators. They reported that in studying couples who had engaged in deep, passionate kissing, they found evidence of red blood cells and bleeding of the gums in 91% of the cases. Certainly we know that blood can transmit this disease and the virus does not differentiate between vaginal, rectal or oral mucosa. Blood-tinged saliva from an infected individual would certainly pose the danger of transmission of disease to an uninfected partner.

In May of 1988, the majority of American households received a message from Surgeon General Koop. On page three of that document, the statement was made: "You won't get AIDS from insects — or a kiss." The report goes on to say, "No matter what you have heard, the AIDS virus is very hard to get and is easily avoided. You won't catch AIDS like a cold or flu because the virus is a different type...You won't get the AIDS virus through everyday contact with people around you, in school or the work place, at parties or at child care centers or stores...You won't get AIDS from a mosquito bite, you won't get AIDS from saliva, sweat, tears, urine or a bowel movement...You won't get AIDS from a kiss."

Now much of what was said is probably true. To date, we have no evidence of spread of the disease from passing someone in a store or from a mosquito bite. But there is absolutely no evidence that you won't get this disease from deep and passionate kissing. Yet, the U. S. Public Health Service, with absolutely no documentation or controlled studies of the spread of HIV disease by deep and passionate kissing, made a totally unfounded statement to the youth of our nation. This is not only bad medicine, it is criminal negligence.

In the Lancet magazine, September 20, 1986, (page 694) a case of horizontal transmission of HIV disease between two siblings was reported. Apparently, the younger child developed the disease after a blood transfusion during cardiac surgery. After the boy's death, the other members of the family were tested and the older brother was found to be infected. The mother suggested that the younger brother had bitten his older brother and that she had seen the bite marks.

In Lancet, June 18, 1988, (page 1395) there is a report of HIV transmission between five homosexuals who had engaged in no type of sexual activity other than oral sex over a period of three years. Two of those infected had only engaged in insertive oral sex and, therefore, would have gotten the disease from contact between their skin or mucous membranes and the saliva of their infected partners.

According to Dr. Lorraine Day, Dr. James Curran of the CDC had assured her that saliva can transmit the virus from one person to another. Yet, faced with the overwhelming evidence of the salivary transmission of the disease, young people all across the nation are repeatedly assured that there is no danger from deep, passionate kissing — and the dying continues, the death continues as the disease spreads among our youth.

Is there a danger from living in close contact with or caring for someone who carries the HIV virus? For many years, the experts have assured health care workers and family members there was no cause for worry. More recently, AIDS experts have begun telling health care workers that they should have known there was a risk when they went into their profession and HCWs have to be prepared for possible infection and death. They are told that it is part of their professional obligation, part of their professional duty and they certainly should not complain.

For years, health care workers were told that there was absolutely no danger of getting the disease from a single needle stick. When it was ascertained that the chance of getting the disease from a contaminated needle stick was 1 in 200, health care workers were assured that this was really only a "low risk" situation.

How many health care workers are infected with the HIV disease today? No one knows because hospitals are consistently told that health care workers **should not be tested** for HIV disease unless they have some specific exposure. Then, if they do have an exposure and are found to be infected, it can be suggested that they may have had the infection all along and probably became infected from some illicit behavior. By not routinely testing HCWs and determining the incidence of disease among those in the medical profession, experts can assure medical personnel that there is absolutely nothing to worry about.

First of all, you must understand that for some strange reason the Centers for Disease Control separates AIDS cases from those infected with HIV disease. The Centers for Disease Control will admit that there are over 6,000 health care workers dead and dying of AIDS — but insist that the vast majority of these are homosexuals or IV drug users or promiscuous people. They will admit, however, that there are a significant number of HCWs with AIDS whose disease cannot be explained. While there are only 3% of the overall AIDS cases that are unexplainable, there are approximately 5% of AIDS cases among health care workers that cannot be explained. Then the CDC admits there are another 25 cases of unexplained HIV disease in HCWs.

On the other hand, OSHA suggests, in the Federal Register, that there may be 150 or more HCWs infected. No one really knows the incidence of infection in HCWs because the CDC objects to routine testing of HCWs.

Is transmission of HIV disease in the hospital setting truly casual transmission? I don't believe so. I believe that when one works in the hospital with blood and body fluids and in close and intimate contact with patients, one is in much more danger than the average citizen would be—especially since HCWs are not allowed to know which patients are infected so that they can protect themselves.

I have tried long and hard to document incidences of casual transmission of the disease in America. I have been assured by several responsible investigators (who I trust) that they have tried to find evidence of horizontal transfer of the disease and have been unable to document such an occurrence. Indeed, the only case that I have been able to document was the case of Craig Stenger.

I will tell you this tragic story for several reasons. First of all, I think it is important that you understand that the Centers for Disease Control knows of this case and of a few similar cases but has specifically suppressed such information so they would not offend the Gay and AIDS Lobbies.

Secondly, the Gay and AIDS Lobby representatives within the media across America carefully censor information. Although the story of the Stenger family was well publicized in Pennsylvania, it was intentionally deleted from the wire services so that the information could not be disseminated across the nation. The Gay Media Task Force has done an excellent job of controlling what the American people are allowed to read, see and hear.

Third, I wish to let you realize that with all the extensive contacts that I have been able to develop over four years, I can only find this one (and perhaps two other cases) where it would appear that there has been casual transmission of the disease within families. That means that casual transmission, although it does occur, is very uncommon.

The story of the Stenger family started when Mrs. Donna Stenger, who lived in Brodheadsville, Pennsylvania received a transfusion at the LeHigh Valley Hospital Center in Pennsylvania in 1984. The transfusion apparently carried the HIV virus and shortly thereafter, Mrs.

Stenger became increasingly ill.

Her husband contracted the disease from Mrs. Stenger through marital relations. The problem for AIDS investigators was their son, Craig. Craig also contacted HIV disease, but he was four years old when his mother became infected. The question is raised as to how Craig contracted the virus.

I should point out that Craig's case is currently under litigation in Pennsylvania. I have been in contact with the family lawyer and have been assured that Craig, now 10 years old, is in excellent health which would tend to rule out the possibility that he had contracted the disease earlier in life.

Newspaper articles on this case were repeatedly published across Pennsylvania. A number of public meetings were held by concerned parents in Brodheadsville where Craig was to be registered for school. Many of the parents questioned whether or not this disease could be spread by casual transmission and they objected to their children going to class with a child who carried the virus.

At one of the meetings, there were members of the state public health department who assured the parents that there was absolutely nothing to worry about because neither New Jersey, New York nor Pennsylvania considered those who carried the virus as contagious.

The parents who attended the meeting were not convinced. They asked over and over how Craig had gotten the virus when his mother had not become infected until Craig was four years old. School officials insisted that they could not discuss this one case because of confidentiality restrictions, but they could assure the parents that there was absolutely nothing to worry about because AIDS experts insisted that you could not get the disease by casual transmission.

Despite the assurances from school and public health officials, the parents simply wanted to know how Craig had gotten infected. They were told that there was absolutely nothing to worry about and that if any parents withdrew their children from school, they would be subject to prosecution.

As a result, many of the parents took their children out of that school and put them into private schools, because no public health official could ever answer the question, "How did Craig Stenger get the virus?"

By late 1989, Julie Stenger was dead, Mr. Stenger was seriously ill, but Craig was still healthy and active. Hopefully, the new treatments which became available in the fall of 1989 will prolong his life until such time as better treatment is available.

Does the CDC know that there is such a thing as casual transmission? Certainly they do. But all material released by the CDC must be cleared by committees which are influenced by the policies of gay and AIDS activists. When I talked with Dr. James Curran in April of 1989, he made this statement:

"What are we going to do when the first infected surgeon infects one of his patients? Because it is going to happen sooner or later. This disease is spread in the same manner as infectious Hepatitis B, and we certainly don't let a surgeon who has hepatitis continue practicing surgery."

A year-and-a-half later, the CDC reported that Kimberly Bergalis of Florida had contracted AIDS from her infected dentist during a routine dental extraction despite the fact that the dentist used a mask and gloves.

Not until we have done general testing of our population and have adequate information in the hands of responsible researchers who have no political connections can we have any hope of assuring the nation as to the true risk of casual transmission. Not until this disease has been depoliticized and treated as a medical illness rather than as a civil rights issue can we really be certain that we are obtaining accurate facts about its spread. Why hasn't the American public risen up and demanded that we address this epidemic?

"Those whom God wishes to destroy, He first makes mad."

1. Colonel Donald Burke's presentation at ASAP meeting, November, 1987.
2. Colonel Donald Burke presented his material at the 5th International Conference on AIDS, Montreal, June, 1989.
3. CDC AIDS Weekly, December 25, 1989; p. 7. (The man actually infected 11 of 18 women he had sexual relations with.)
4. Most venereal diseases which are monitored by public health departments are curable, except for infectious hepatitis which is a reportable disease and is spread in a manner identical to HIV disease. Several venereal diseases such as herpes simplex and Chlamydia are not traced, but these diseases do not threaten a patient's life.
5. Vernon & Juston, "American Journal of Public Health," April, 1988.
6. Don Francis, M.D. radio broadcast, January, 1989.
7. Presidential AIDS Commission Report, June 4, 1988. p. 115.
8. Rocky Mountain News, May 1, 1987.
9. Article in "The New American," October 26, 1987.
10. MMWR, September 27, 1985; vol. 34 and 38, pp. 573-564.
11. Talk by Dr. Rutherford, CMA Convention, Reno, Nevada, March, 1988.
12. Copies of this paper are available at $1.00 each from the American Life League, P. O. Box 1350, Stafford, Virginia 22554.
13. CDC AIDS Weekly, May 21, 1990; p. 11

BOOK TWO

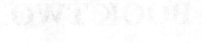

CHAPTER ONE

Keep your honor like your saber bright.
Shun coward's fear and then,
If we must perish in the fight,
Oh let us die like men.

— George Washington Patton, (1808-1882)
"Oh let us die like men," Stanza 4

The history of the AIDS epidemic, to date, is the saga of malice and mistakes, illusion and delusion, deceit and deception, of dying and death. It is the story of young, homosexual men filled with fear, resentment, anger, hostility, isolation and pain.

This is the story of just a few men and women of courage. It is also the story of efficient organizations all across our country intent upon blocking a logical public health response to the epidemic, and the story of a great number of equivocal men who were unwilling to take a stand in a time of crisis.

The history of this epidemic records a total failure on the part of the leadership of much of organized medicine. There have been consistent efforts on the part of the leadership of organized medicine in California to block the wishes of the duly-elected representatives of the physicians of California, physicians who hoped to begin dealing with the HIV epidemic as a medical issue in 1986 and 1987. But I will tell you more of that story later.

The history of this epidemic is the history of the failure on the part of many public health officers and of the leadership of the Centers for Disease Control, but most of all, it is the record of the failure of leadership on the part of the former Surgeon General of the United States, C. Everett Koop. Surgeon General Koop was the one man who had the respect of our nation and could have mobilized the forces of the U. S. Public Health Service during the early years of the epidemic to slow the spread of this horrible disease.

It was his opportunity; it was his responsibility; it was his obligation to offer moral and spiritual leadership during the early years of challenge and controversy. But unlike Surgeon General Thomas Parran, the man who led America's battle against the syphilis epidemic in the

1930's and demanded the use of strong public health measures to control the spread of disease, Surgeon General C. Everett Koop has won the undying gratitude of the AIDS and Gay Lobbies by embracing their programs requiring **consent, confidentiality and counseling** before testing for the virus.

Instead of emphasizing the moral and religious implications of this sexually transmitted epidemic, Dr. Koop, in his Surgeon General's Report (see Appendix I) recommended that we contact various gay and lesbian organizations across America to learn of more efficient and safer techniques for sexual relations.

Instead of stressing marriage and morality, he laid his stress on condoms and safer means of coitus. Instead of recommending moral education in our schools, he recommended sex education starting with younger children, sex education which presents homosexuality as a normal, healthy, alternative lifestyle.

It is little wonder that gay leaders and the media elite across America have lauded and praised the Surgeon General for his enlightened position.

✳✳✳

The story of the epidemic can be divided into four parts.

1. The period of **challenge.** (June 5, 1981—April, 1982)
2. The period of **controversy and concession.** (April, 1982—March, 1985)
3. The period of **confrontation, confidentiality, counseling, consent and condoms.** (March 1985 to the late 1990's)
4. The period of **conflict and crisis.** (Late 1990's and beyond)

The first time period was that period of **challenge** — between June 5, 1981 (when the first cases were reported in the MMWR) and April of 1982 — when the Centers for Disease Control determined that AIDS was a sexually transmitted disease. It was during this time period that the Centers for Disease Control functioned well and appropriately and carried out its assigned task to safeguard the public health.

The second time period was between April 1982 and March 1985 when the HIV blood test became available. This is the period that I have labeled **Controversy and Concession.** It was during this period that the U. S. Public Health Service and the Centers for Disease Control should have insisted that appropriate public health measures be used.

It was here that public health policy began to fail because gay leaders objected to the closure of gay bathhouses, sex clubs, gay bars and houses of prostitution where the disease was being spread. As a result of demands from gay leaders and members of the AIDS Lobby, no effort was made to stop those who were infected from transmitting the disease to others.

Although the Centers for Disease Control eventually suggested the closure of gay bathhouses and houses of prostitution in 1986, their recommendations were far too late and were never made authoritatively. In 1983, when it became obvious that the disease could be spread heterosexually, there should have been a massive educational program to reinstitute moral teaching and moral values into our society in an effort to try to stop sexual promiscuity and save human lives; however, almost no one in our government wanted to talk about morality. No one in a position of authority in government wanted to talk about God and, certainly, no one in government wanted to advocate marriage as the only form of "safe sex."[1]

The third stage of the epidemic began in March 1985, when the HIV blood test was released for general use. This was the period of **confrontation.** In 1985, widespread routine testing should have been encouraged across our nation to identify those who were infected, educate them and stop further spread of the disease. This was not done because of the fear of **confrontation.** This was the time period when liberal and homosexual organizations mobilized to influence state governments to pass legislation discouraging physicians from using HIV testing to stop the epidemic.

It was during this period that our Surgeon General and the U. S. Public Health Service failed so tragically in their responsibility to protect the public health. It was during this period that Surgeon General Koop issued his report (1986), a report which is still available from the U. S. Public Health Service. (See Appendix I).

In this document, the Surgeon General told Americans that if they wanted to learn more about the epidemic, they should contact various gay groups for information. The Surgeon General then gave addresses and telephone numbers so that concerned Americans could contact such organizations as the National Coalition of Gay, Sexually Transmitted Disease Service, The National Association of People with AIDS, The Gay Men's Health Crisis, The American Association of Physicians for Human Rights, The Los Angeles AIDS Project, the National AIDS

Network, etc. (See page 35 of the Surgeon General's Report, Appendix I).

It was during that same period that the Surgeon General assured the American public that "There is no danger from kissing," (see page 3 of the Surgeon General's Report) that there is "No danger from casual contact," (see page 13 of the Surgeon General's Report); and the reason that dentists started wearing masks and gloves was because they wanted to protect "you...from hepatitis, common colds or flu," (see page 23 of the Surgeon General's Report).[2]

The Surgeon General's picture appeared on the front of the circular from the U. S. Public Health Service which was sent to every home in America in early 1988. This circular told Americans that, "You can't get AIDS from a toilet seat, from eating in a restaurant, from shaking hands or from kissing." Furthermore, the public health service suggested that "Before having sex, couples should openly discuss their past sexual activities."[3]

It was during this period of **confrontation** when death threats and threats of reprisal were made against anyone who dared to suggest that our nation should begin addressing HIV disease as an epidemic. This was the time when demonstrations were used to intimidate politicians and citizens. It was during this period that demonstrators jeered at the President of the United States and the Prime Minister of Canada and other leaders who wanted to use accepted public health techniques to control the epidemic.

This was the time when the average American was so busy being busy and leading the good life that he/she could not find the time to be concerned about those who were contracting the disease unnecessarily...as long as it was somebody else's son or daughter. If the disease did affect a loved one — then they couldn't understand how it ever happened.

The fourth stage of the epidemic will occur in the late 1990's. That will be the period of **conflict** and **crisis.** If the Centers for Disease Control's estimation is correct and by the end of 1993 there are 435,000 people dead and dying of AIDS, then by the mid-1990's we can anticipate 500,000 to 600,000 Americans ill and close to a million dead or dying in the late 1990's.

Of course, those will only be the people in the terminal stages of HIV disease. By then there will be countless millions who will be infected.

At that point, our whole system of health care delivery will begin to crumble because there will be inadequate funding to care for all the tragic victims of this epidemic.

As I write this book, in many of the major hospitals in New York City, it takes three days to get from the Emergency Room onto the wards, because there are no hospital beds available. People are dying in emergency rooms in America today because they can't get to the wards for medical treatment. Imagine where we will be by the late 1990's.

By that time, our nation may well be spending hundreds of billions of dollars yearly, caring for the tragic victims of an epidemic that never had to happen. The spirit of our nation will be broken. Our people will be disillusioned and angry. Taxes will be increased to offset the ever increasing spiral of governmental costs which will be demanded by those who are infected — costs not only for caring for people medically, but for providing them with welfare and hospice care, and ministering to their social, psychological and physical needs.

Homosexual groups have already talked about the fact that they may have to arm themselves and take to the streets to get what they are entitled to. At their rallies, they often carry signs proclaiming "Civil Rights or Civil War."

As the tempo of violence and demonstrations increase, the heterosexual community will lash back in anger and blame the homosexuals for the crisis that we face — without realizing that the homosexuals have been manipulated and used by the AIDS Lobby — a group which is utilizing this epidemic for their own political goals and objectives.

Senior citizens will demonstrate to demand that their needs be met. The black and Hispanic communities will feel that their youth has been allowed to acquire the disease because of a lack of concern by the white community. Each group will lash out at other groups during the coming period of conflict and crisis.

✳✳✳

It was not until the third stage of this epidemic that I personally became involved. Little did I imagine when I first sat in my study in November of 1985 and wrote out a simple resolution to be presented to the House of Delegates of the California Medical Association in March of 1986 that my life would change and change dramatically.

Little did I understand that I would be entering back into a conflict that I had abandoned over a decade before. Little did I realize that I was being propelled back into the nightmare that I felt I had turned my back on in the early 1970's.

To understand the story I am about to tell, you will need to know of my past life. It will be important that you understand the philosophy that I embrace, to be able to understand the incredible events as they have occurred.

I attended the University of California as an undergraduate at the very end of the Second World War and in the immediate post-war years. I graduated from college when I was 20, incredibly immature and naive. Although I minored in history and had a Phi Beta Kappa key, I was totally committed to socialist concepts and fully embraced the liberal lie that government can solve the problems of mankind.

I had somewhat of a belief in God carried over from my youth, but no firm commitment to a religious structure of life, nor did I realize that the heritage of America was based upon the Judeo-Christian concepts of liberty under God, rather than freedom derived from government benevolence.

I graduated from medical school when I was 23 and went on to specialize in orthopedic surgery.

It wasn't until I had been in the private practice of medicine for several years that I began reading of America's history and I came to understand that centralization of power in government always leads to tyranny — no matter how well motivated the ruler may be. I joined a patriotic national organization, intent upon trying to restrict the power of government in order to preserve our freedom.

I worked very hard for many years, but totally unsuccessfully. I became the best known conservative voice on talk radio in the Western United States and for years I attempted to awaken my fellow citizens from their complacency. When one takes a stand against the forces of liberalism and socialism in America, one comes under tremendous personal pressure. The midnight telephone calls, the hearse that arrived because there was a report of a dead body; the bomb squads coming in the middle of the night because they have been informed that there were bombs planted in the basement; the ambulance arriving because there is a report of someone injured and the Sheriff arriving in the middle of the night because they have reports of a murder.

This form of harassment eventually takes its toll. The death threats, the threats against one's wife and children — all of this is part of the pattern of intimidation waged against anyone who takes a position in the battle for traditional values against those forces moving us towards a collectivist tyranny in our land.

Few people realize that this battle goes on or the terrible toll it can take on one's family. When my wife became depressed (as a result of this harassment) and died, I remarried and went to Africa where I taught in a medical school. I returned to America in 1977. At this point, I decided to withdraw from the political arena and spend my time studying and researching the forces which were destroying the fabric of our society.

I intended to leave the battle to others — or so I thought. However, in the late 1970's I was selected to be one of the representatives from my county medical society to the House of Delegates of the California Medical Association. Supposedly, the House of Delegates is the ruling body within organized medicine in California. It is widely believed to be an organization which works to preserve the private practice of medicine and strives to preserve the health of the public. Of course, many times perceptions are far different from reality.

As I attended meetings of the House year after year, I found that there were forces within that organization which were intent upon undermining and destroying not only the private practice of medicine, but also our American way of life.

On one occasion, when the subject of a bilateral, verifiable nuclear freeze was brought before the House, I questioned whether doctors were really knowledgeable enough to take positions on nuclear warfare and military strategy. When I suggested we should support a strong military defense for America rather than recommend a nuclear weapons freeze, I learned just how democratic organized medicine really was. Although there were six resolutions supporting a bilateral, verifiable nuclear freeze and all the proponents were allowed to speak, I, as the lone dissenter who wanted a strong military defense, was prohibited from speaking. Although proponents of a nuclear freeze were allowed to project slides, I was refused even the use of the microphone and told by the Speaker of the House, "Sit down, since what you are going to say is political."

The outcry of indignation from both liberal and conservative members of the House to the speaker's remark has prevented the leadership from ever again utilizing such flagrant abuse of power. However, there have been other, far more subtle techniques used to prevent me from expressing my views. After that meeting, the official position of the CMA came to be one of support for a bilateral, verifiable nuclear freeze. Every year after that I would ask for permission to present a resolution to the doctors supporting a strong defense for America. Every year I was refused.

On one occasion, I went to the conference hall before the meeting convened and left printed fliers on all the seats to give my side of the defense debate. Monitors were promptly sent by CMA leadership to pick up those fliers so that the delegates could not read them.

On other occasions I tried to rent a meeting room at the hotel where the CMA Convention was held in order to invite delegates to come so that I could express my views on certain issues. CMA officials told the hotel management not to rent me a conference room. On several occasions I have had to rent meeting rooms in adjacent hotels to have an opportunity to speak. You see, the leadership of organized medicine really did not allow any effective opposition to their policies.

When it came to preserving the free practice of medicine, it was incredible how our leadership betrayed the physicians. In the early 1980's when the California State Legislature passed laws that allowed corporations to move into medicine and begin controlling private practitioners, I campaigned actively to get the CMA leadership to oppose those disastrous new policies. To my amazement, when I intercepted the private communications among the hierarchy, I found that there was a tacit approval of the new direction towards corporate medicine and an absolute refusal on the part of CMA leadership to use the tremendous political and financial clout of organized medicine to counter this disastrous move.

With the support of the governing board of the Santa Cruz Medical Society, I attempted to call together the leaders of the various county medical societies throughout California in an effort to make them realize what was happening. Tragically, two members of my own medical society, working with CMA leadership, managed to delay the meeting and so weakened my position that I was unable to accomplish my goal.

And thus it was that the first steps towards the destruction of the private practice of medicine were carried out — with the approval of the leadership of organized medicine — leaders who informed physicians across our state that they were actively fighting corporate intrusion into private practice while secretly condoning it. (See Appendix 8)

As I attended meetings of the CMA year after year, I came to realize that certain leaders of our organization had fully embraced the programs of the far left. Organized medicine supported sex education without moral values, the homosexual lifestyle and abortion on demand. They advocated ever more governmental control and regulation over every aspect of our lives to preserve the public health. These were the programs of the radical left and these came to be the policies of the CMA.

Year after year, the doctors in California paid their dues to CALPAC — the political arm of the CMA. Year after year, CALPAC gave $25,000.00 to the left-wing speaker of the State Assembly, Willie Brown, a man committed to destroying the private practice of medicine.

In 1986, the CMA rated California Legislators as to how they voted on CMA supported legislation. Tom Hayden, Jane Fonda's husband, got a 100% rating for supporting the CMA's legislative positions. That should have told physicians what the CMA and organized medicine really supported. Tragically, most physicians were too busy making a living to be concerned.

❋❋❋

In November 1985, I regret to say, I was really unconcerned about the HIV epidemic. Like most Americans, I was primarily concerned with what affected my family and my patients and what affected those with whom I shared the responsibility for caring for my patients.

When word of the new AIDS legislation came to my attention, I was perplexed. With the passage of AB403, I found I would be subject to a $10,000.00 fine and a year imprisonment if I were to tell my surgical nurse that we were operating on an HIV-infected patient. What would happen if my nurse or assistant stuck themselves with a sharp object and were inoculated with the virus? Certainly they would go home and infect their husband or wife. If their wife became pregnant, their children could become infected. Yet, I faced draconian punishments and possibly even the loss of my medical license if I warned anyone that they might be infected.

In November 1985, physicians knew very little about the true danger from needle-stick injuries. Medical experts had repeatedly told physicians that there was **absolutely no possibility** of getting the infection from a needle stick, but by November 1985, there were five known cases of HCWs who had converted from a negative to a positive blood test after such injuries. One of these cases had been reported in the Lancet, a British medical journal. The other four cases had been reported in November 1985 in the Journal of the American Medical Association. Based upon this information, I wrote the following resolution:

> Be it RESOLVED:
> That the California Medical Association advocate that an admission HTLV-III (HIV) Antibody test be drawn on all patients entering the hospital for surgery and if that test is positive then the medical personnel involved be informed so they may be better able to protect themselves from contamination and infection.

It seemed only logical that if there was a needle stick injury involving an infected patient, the injured nurse or doctor had a right to know. It seemed like such a proper step to take — but in 1985, I was ill-informed as to the forces that were organizing to prevent physicians, health care personnel and concerned public health officers from addressing this epidemic.

By March 1986, I was the senior delegate from Santa Cruz County to the House of Delegates of the CMA. I closed my medical practice and journeyed to Los Angeles. It was there that I would have my first experience with the sarcasm and ridicule which would be used so frequently in the years that lay ahead. It was there that I would catch my first glimpse of what lay in store for anyone who dared to challenge the authority of those who controlled the management of this epidemic.

Most of the doctors arrived at the CMA Convention Friday evening. Early Saturday morning, the delegates met in a large auditorium. There were introductory remarks and then the doctors dispersed to the various Reference Committees. Ordinarily, there would be 11 Reference Committees, each committee with 5 physicians and 1 representative from the full-time paid staff of the CMA.

In my experience, the important Reference Committees were usually packed with several liberal physicians who were dependable and would predictably recommend positions compatible with those of the CMA hierarchy. There would always be a small number of impartial physicians on the committees (those without any truly preconceived notions) but ordinarily there were enough "dependable" physicians to convince the Reference Committees to accept policies which were acceptable to the hierarchy.

The format of the Reference Committee involves the 6 committee members sitting at a table in the front of a meeting room while those doctors who wish to speak sit in the audience. When a resolution is called, the author rises and addresses the Reference Committee; afterwards other physicians can comment on the resolution. I shall have to admit, looking back over many years, that I do not recall the details of what was said that Saturday morning; however, I do remember my amazement at the intensity of the attack on my simple, straightforward resolution.

I recall some of the people who spoke that Saturday morning in March of 1986. There was the leader of the California Chapter of Gay and Lesbian Physicians and a representative from the Gay and Lesbian House Officers Association. Other doctors in the audience rose to vilify me, to challenge my goals, impugn my motives and to ridicule the idea that physicians should try to remove the restrictions which had been placed on HIV testing. The hostility, anger and bitterness that were expressed that morning was my first inkling that there was an organized force that opposed a logical approach to dealing with this epidemic.

There were public health officers who spoke vehemently against me. There were members of the CMA Council[4] who attacked me. There were only one or two doctors who dared to openly support my position (i.e., Dr. Carl Treiling).

I shall have to admit that my first impulse was to recoil from the attack, the vilification, the charges of bigotry and homophobia. My better judgment told me, however, that somehow this must be an important issue and it was best to hold my position. This I did, simply pleading that we needed to address HIV disease like we have addressed other diseases.

Ordinarily, the members of the House of Delegates have Sunday off while Reference Committees meet to work out a statement on each resolution. Because the House of Delegates annual meeting corresponds with the general meeting of the CMA, there were medical meetings and medical exhibits to attend.

On Sunday morning, as I walked through the exhibits, I reflected back to a meeting several years previously in that same exhibit hall where I had encountered Larimore Cummins, a gastroenterologist from Santa Cruz, California. Larimore had been a CMA delegate in years past but had quit in disgust.

During a discussion at a Reference Committee meeting in 1984, he had backed a resolution supporting the right of patients to have self-directed blood transfusions, (i.e., to have friends or relatives donate type specific blood for their use). Although self-directed transfusions are generally accepted in the 1990's, in 1984, the AIDS Lobby actively opposed the thought that anyone had the right to have friends or relatives donate blood for their personal use.

Larimore had been attacked at the Reference Committee meeting as a racist and a bigot and accused of wanting to avoid having black or Jewish blood transfused into his body. He was accused of wanting to call blacks "niggers" simply because he wanted people to have the right to have their relatives donate blood for their personal use. The same attack was renewed at our District Delegation meeting.

When Larimore tried to defend himself against the vilification, he was denied an opportunity to speak. Following the confrontation, he asked the Chairman of our delegation why he couldn't respond and was told, "What you had to say would be better off not said."

That was too much for Larimore. He promptly submitted his resignation.

Truly a man of many and varied talents, Larimore had put together four complicated medical computer programs which he demonstrated at that CMA Convention, hoping to interest investors in financing his initial venture into the world of programming. He recruited several investors and for two years he was involved in marketing computer programs. But just as my destiny changed in 1986, so Larimore's destiny would change shortly thereafter, and we were both drawn into the swirling vortex of the AIDS confrontation.

Soon thereafter, Larimore would be offering advice to a United States Senator, acting as a personal consultant to one of the leading conservative senators in California and providing suggestions to policy makers in the White House.

However, on that Sunday in March 1986, neither one of us realized that our lives were about to change dramatically from the humdrum existence of medical practitioners in the seaside town of Santa Cruz to become players in the dangerous game that would ultimately determine what course our nation would follow in the decades to come.

Larimore is short in stature with brown curly hair and graying sideburns. His face is characterized by high cheekbones and a broad, youthful grin. He speaks, sometimes hesitantly, yet I have learned to value what he says, for he has an uncanny ability to crystalize ideas and a unique talent of being able to put aside all side issues and zero in on major problems with a clarity I have always envied.

I am sure it was that ability that attracted his counsel to both Senator Doolittle and Congressman Dannemeyer — and even into the White House itself. In the years that lay ahead, highly placed Washington officials would check with him for information and for approaches that were used in Senate debates on the AIDS issue.

※※※

The Reference Committee reports were available early Monday morning. Members of our 7th District delegation[5] met to review the reports. I quickly turned to Reference Committee G to see their recommendations on my resolution — 708-86. I was pleased to see that they had accepted at least part of my suggestion and had recommended:

> Be it RESOLVED:
> That CMA support legislation to modify current restrictions on communication of HTLV-III test results among medical personnel for the purpose of diagnosis, treatment and infection control.

Looking back on that event, I now realize that the Reference Committee had specifically deleted that portion of my resolution calling for routine testing of surgical patients. In 1986, I did not realize that the intent of the AIDS and Gay Lobbies was to prevent routine testing of our population in any form. Also, the Reference Committee had failed to address the threat of a $10,000.00 fine and a year's imprisonment for a physician breaking confidentiality.

Early Monday afternoon, the House of Delegates convened. One of the first issues that was taken up was that of AIDS. There were several other resolutions. One dealt with AIDS education. Another advocated that the CMA "produce guidelines for making HTLV-III antibody data available to public health authorities for contact tracing." In 1986, this resolution passed without opposition, yet many years later, routine contact tracing is still not used to stop the epidemic in California.

Then the discussion turned to my resolution. Doctor Carl Treiling from South Hollywood moved to amend my resolution to read:

> Be it RESOLVED: The CMA support legislation to delete the requirement to require consent to perform HTLV-III testing and to

modify current restrictions on communication of HTLV-III test results among medical personnel for the purpose of diagnosis, treatment and infection control."

Several doctors spoke against his amendment. Then the Chairman of the CMA Council, Dr. Laurens White was recognized by the speaker. Doctor White is a large, burly man with bushy, graying hair. As Chairman of the Council he was the second most powerful man in organized medicine in the State of California and one of the six members of the CMA Executive Committee.[6]

"I am opposed to both this substitution, any likely substitution and the resolution as originally written and the recommendation of the Reference Committee. I think...the amendment is absurd and if that is defeated I assure you that the resolution itself is absurd."

This commentary on my resolution, delivered in a booming voice by the Chairman of the ruling Council of the CMA, tended to awe the audience.

Doctor Treiling countered this attack stating, "The test for HTLV-III antibody is the only blood test in the physician's armament that requires written consent to perform."

A representative from the Speciality Delegation rose to speak:

"This amendment, like everything else related to 708-86, is feeding on what is unscientific hysteria about AIDS. The evidence is preponderant that AIDS is not transmissible except by sharing needles and in high risk populations, primarily homosexual...I think that in any kind of situation...there has to be balanced public good, social good and the individual good. I think that the weight of scientific evidence is that social good is not met by this or any of these other kinds of requirements...we must come down for the protection of the individual...Therefore, I ask that this amendment be defeated...and the resolution be defeated."

Then it was my turn to reply. I argued that we had an obligation to protect our staff. I pointed out the fact that the epidemic had been politicized and physicians needed to practice logical medicine. The full text of my remarks are included in Appendix III. My remarks were met with applause.

A surgeon from San Francisco rose to challenge me and to insist that, "There is no evidence that you get AIDS by sticking your finger with a needle." He was adamant in his statements and urged the delegates to vote against the amendment and the original resolution.

An unnamed delegate rose to say, "I have serious doubts this is even legal. This is assault and battery...You can't do an invasive test on patients without their consent."

The acting Speaker of the House, Dr. Charles Plough, immediately called on the CMA lawyer. The lawyer (an employee of the CMA hierarchy) insisted that it was illegal to draw a blood test for HIV disease without (written) consent. It is obvious that the acting Speaker of the House was using a clever ploy to convince the delegates that somehow physicians would be assaulting their patients by performing an HIV test without written consent...despite the fact that **all other blood tests are** drawn without written consent.

There is no question that the delegates wanted to do away with the written consent requirement in 1986 and treat HIV disease (HTLV-III) as physicians dealt with all other diseases. There was no question that Doctor Treiling's amendment dealt with the written consent requirement of AB403.

The amended version of 708A-86 was presented to the House of Delegates for their decision.

Despite the attack by the Chairman of the Council, Doctor White, and the confirmation by the CMA lawyers who assured the delegates that physicians would be assaulting their patients if they ordered an HIV test in the same manner as they ordered any other blood tests, the support for my resolution was overwhelming and it was voted in by the House of Delegates.

✳✳✳

As I waited at the airport in Los Angeles two days later, I had a feeling of elation. For the first time in my many years of attendance at meetings of the California Medical Association, I had actually accomplished something which was important.

Through my effort and the efforts of Carl Treiling, the members of the House of Delegates had the courage to take a stand against the leadership of the CMA and support a logical, reasonable approach to the AIDS epidemic. The House of Delegates had spoken with a unified voice. There was no question as to what they wanted. They wanted to make HIV testing readily available without the requirement for **written** consent and confidentiality mandated by AB403; they wanted to stop the epidemic; they wanted to stop the dying, the suffering and death.

As I climbed the stairs to my waiting airplane I felt as though I was walking on air. Soon doctors in our state (and perhaps all across the nation) would be able to identify those who were infected. Then public health officers could do contact tracing and identify other people who had the disease. Before long, physicians could begin to break the chain of transmission of the epidemic.

In my own small way, I believed that I had actually accomplished something that would have an effect on the course of the epidemic, an epidemic which I little understood, but which I sensed, even at that time, might have a profound impact on the very survival of our nation. But in March 1986, I was incredibly short-sighted. At that point in time I could not possibly have understood the magnitude of the forces which I had inadvertently engaged and what would happen in the months and years that lay ahead.

I could not have imagined in my wildest nightmares in 1986 the events that would follow and just how futile my effort had been. For everything that had been said and done at that CMA meeting in reference to the epidemic would be for naught, and the epidemic would continue running its course and the suffering, dying and death would continue. Eventually, millions of Americans would die...they would die in an epidemic that never had to happen.

✳✳✳

Physicians who are members of the House of Delegates get monthly reports on the activity of CMA lobbyists in Sacramento and the legislation that the CMA promotes. Almost immediately after our meeting in March, I learned that the CMA was supporting legislation to carry out the programs which had been adopted by the House. Month after month, I kept waiting for the bill to pass through the state legislature. I assumed that legislation would change consent and confidentiality requirements for HIV testing so that this disease could be treated like other diseases.

In March 1986, there were slightly over 17,000 reported AIDS cases in America. It had been just one year since the ELISA blood test had been released for general use.

At that time, it was feared that many homosexuals would donate blood at blood banks to find out their HIV status. To avoid further contamination of the blood supply, **alternative testing sites** were established across America where concerned homosexuals (and heterosexuals) could go for testing.

Despite numerous articles in homosexual magazines and newspapers designed to frighten homosexuals and discourage them from being tested, most homosexuals wanted to know if they had contracted the disease. Some who were tested and were negative could breathe a sigh of relief. Those who were not tested or those who tested positive lived in perpetual fear. That fear, combined with the threat of discrimination and quarantine, was subtly used to mobilize homosexuals into an active political force to control the subsequent course of the epidemic.

Most states set up alternative testing sites. Most of the clients were homosexuals or bisexuals. Pretest counseling was administered and much of the counseling was designed to frighten patients. They were told that a break of confidentiality could result in the loss of their jobs, their insurance and their homes.

Then they were asked how they would feel if they were to find that they had a positive blood test and if they were emotionally prepared to know that they had a disease which might well kill them.

As a result of the counseling, many of the frightened young men refused to be tested. Pretest counseling was initially provided for 93,900 people. After counseling, 79,100 people agreed to be tested. The percentages of positive blood tests was overwhelming. By December 1985, 17.3% of those tested in alternative test sites across our nation were found to carry the virus. 41.5% of those tested in Colorado were HIV positive while 30.7% of the people tested in New York City carried the virus and 39% of those tested in Utah were infected.[7]

✳✳✳

There was a growing fear across our nation in those days. In March 1986, a group in Kokomo, Indiana was raising funds to try to keep thirteen-year-old Ryan White, an AIDS victim, out of school. In April 1986, there was increasing concern over a California ballot initiative that was gathering signatures in an effort to declare HIV disease an infectious, contagious, communicable disease that should be reported to public health officers. The sponsor of the bill was a left-wing revolutionary named Lyndon LaRouche, an old line Stalinist turned Democratic politician. His ballot initiative was referred to as Proposition 64.

✳✳✳

On May 28, 1986, the Washington Post reported that the City Council of Washington, D. C. had given final approval to a bill prohibiting health and life insurance companies from turning away those who tested positive for exposure to the AIDS virus. The so-called AIDS Insurance Bill (AIB) was passed unanimously by the city council and provided fines of up to $300.00 a day for insurance agents who denied coverage to anyone who tested positive for the HIV virus.

Indeed, the city council was in effect requiring that "anyone who already had the disease could automatically go out and buy health and life insurance because that was their right." That is similar to saying that anybody whose home is burning has a legal right to buy fire insurance and the insurance agent would be fined $300.00 a day if he didn't provide a policy.

In May 1986, AIDS was the leading cause of death in men between ages 21 and 44 in New York City, yet insurance companies in Washington, D. C. were forced to provide health and death benefits for anyone infected.

❋❋❋

In the latter part of May 1986, there was a meeting in Philadelphia of public health officials from across America. These men were intent upon blocking the use of HIV testing for routine screening and opposed the use of standard public health techniques to stop the epidemic. What was their rationale? One public health officer was quoted as saying:

"The appeals for screening are seductive, but the results can only prove catastrophic."

Another health officer said:

"Quarantine or isolation of AIDS patients in the community is doomed to failure as the method to control the spread of this disease."

Why were they discussing quarantine? By 1986, physicians knew that quarantine was unnecessary to control this epidemic and that mature, responsible children could attend school. By 1986, physicians recognized that HIV disease was a difficult disease to acquire. Then why were public health officers raising the specter of quarantine?

By raising the question of quarantine, they could effectively discourage any efforts to try to use standard public health techniques. The experts at that conference in Philadelphia recognized that by early 1986, there might already be a million and a half people infected with the virus. In San Francisco, New York and Los Angeles, surveys suggested that as many as 70% of promiscuous homosexual men were already infected. AIDS experts stated that there were just too many people to test, and because of the large numbers of infected homosexuals, physicians should not try to carry out testing of the general population.

Then there were the ethical aspects of blood testing. Representatives from New York's Hastings Institute, an organization usually affiliated with the far left, raised the question as to whether testing the general public was justifiable. Members of the institute condemned HIV testing because of the danger of false-positive test results and insisted that contact tracing in the homosexual population was doomed to failure because homosexuals had so many sexual contacts, the latency period of the disease was so long, and homosexuals couldn't possibly remember all their previous sexual contacts.

In view of these facts, why should physicians even try to stop the epidemic in the homosexual *or* heterosexual populations?

Their arguments were somewhat valid as far as the homosexual populations in New York City, San Francisco and Los Angeles were concerned. By May 1986, the majority of homosexuals in these three large population centers were already infected. But certainly their arguments were **not** valid as far as doing testing and contact tracing on homosexuals in most other cities in our nation.

In addition, testing and tracing should have been used in the heterosexual population to try to stop the epidemic, but by pointing out the absurdity of testing in the three cities where the majority of promiscuous homosexuals had already become infected, the AIDS Lobby could utilize a "leap in logic" and discount the necessity for testing our population as a whole. Why?

There were forces in 1986 intent upon blocking efforts to stop this epidemic. Those forces purposely confused the issue of contact tracing in the homosexual population in New York, San Francisco and Los Angeles with testing of the general population. Since many would agree that contact tracing in homosexuals in the three largest cities was not applicable, why suggest testing in the general population?

That was the line of reasoning that was used so effectively. The arguments were intentionally complex and confusing and the average American could not possibly understand the significance of what was happening. By May 1986, this misguided philosophy had been adopted by members of several public health organizations and it was decided that our nation would not use standard techniques to try to stop the epidemic.

*** ***

By 1986, it was obvious that there was not one but three major epidemics. The first was the homosexual epidemic which had infected the majority of promiscuous homosexuals in New York, San Francisco and Los Angeles. The second was in the IV drug users. The third was the spread of the disease into the heterosexual population as had occurred so disastrously in Africa.

By 1986, the first epidemic had already peaked out; the majority of homosexuals in our larger cities were already infected. The second epidemic was on the rise with the majority of the drug users in New York and along the Eastern Seaboard soon to be infected. But the third epidemic — that epidemic which would destroy our nation — was just beginning to permeate the youth.

It was in 1986 when measures should have been taken to stop the spread of disease into our youth. Tragically, all efforts to adopt a logical public health program were blocked by the AIDS and Gay Lobbies.

*** ***

By May 1986, there were 20,776 reported cases of AIDS. In May, the Centers for Disease Control recommended that gay bathhouses across our nation be shut down. Over 400 new cases of AIDS were being reported every week and more than 11,000 Americans had already died.

In May 1986, some CDC officials were considering the use of widespread testing of our population to stop the epidemic, but members of the AIDS and Gay Lobbies were intent upon blocking any such action.

Doctor James O. Mason, Director of the CDC, sent a letter to public health officers in which he suggested that there should be widespread testing of people in high risk groups in an effort to identify and counsel people who were infected. He recommended encouraging people to have voluntary antibody testing and counseling.[8]

However, the Association of Local Public Health Officers, strongly influenced at that time by the leadership of Dr. Mervyn Silverman, actively opposed the tracing of sexual partners to control the spread of AIDS. The Association said that a positive antibody test **should not** be classified as a reportable condition. The group further said that private physicians should *not* be required to report test results to public health officials.

Paul Boneberg was the coordinator of the "San Francisco Mobilization Against AIDS." He openly criticized the CDC for daring to suggest that public health officers should expand testing. He brought up the fact that children were being thrown out of schools, people were losing their jobs and soldiers were being discharged from the Army. Faced with attacks from all sides, CDC officers backed away from their position on testing.

In the years that followed, responsible, embattled physicians at the Centers for Disease Control retreated again and again under the onslaught of gay activists and their political supporters on Capitol Hill. CDC officials backed away from premarital, prenatal and routine testing to try to stop the epidemic. As a result, the disease has continued to spread and spread across our tragic land.

※※※

By mid-June 1986, there were over 21,000 cases of AIDS. At that time, it was announced that Proposition 64 sponsored by Lyndon LaRouche had qualified as a ballot initiative for the November election in California. To those readers who are unacquainted with the concept of ballot initiatives, California has a unique provision in the State Constitution that allows concerned citizens to submit various issues to the public for a vote.

If a group can get enough signatures, measures can be brought before the public. Once voted in by the populace, that measure becomes law and cannot be reversed by the legislature. The initiative process has allowed the citizens of California to circumvent a corrupt and oppressive liberally dominated legislature.

It was because of the Jarvis-Gann Initiative passed by the voters in the late 1970's (Proposition 13) that the citizens of California were able to restrict exorbitant property tax increases. It was through similar efforts that the citizens were able to do away with the State Inheritance Tax.

In June 1986, a new state initiative (Proposition 64) qualified to be placed on the ballot in November. The initiative stated that::

> Acquired Immune Deficiency Syndrome (AIDS) is an infectious, contagious and communicable disease and the condition of being a carrier of the HTLV-III virus is an infectious, contagious, communicable condition and both should be placed and maintained by the Director of the Department of Health Services on the list of reportable

diseases and conditions mandated by Health and Safety Code Section 3123... and all personnel of the Department of Health Services and all health officers shall fulfill all the duties and obligations specified in each and all the sections of said Statutory Division and Administrative Code..."

The initiative really said very little. The purpose of the initiative was to declare HIV disease an infectious, contagious, communicable disease and have it reported to public health officers as was done with AIDS and 57 other reportable diseases.

There was **no mention of quarantine in the initiative;** there was no mention of restricting the rights of infected people. According to the text of the AIDS initiative, management of the disease was to be left completely at the discretion of locally appointed public health officials.

Had the initiative passed, physicians would have:

1. Started reporting of the disease to determine the incidence of the infection as is done with all other serious diseases.
2. Started contact tracing to break the chain of transmission.
3. Public health officials would have been able to identify infected individuals who were intentionally spreading the disease.
4. The ability to get infected patients under medical treatment.

The unfortunate thing about Proposition 64 was that it was introduced by a political extremist. The initiative had been written by one of Lyndon LaRouche's followers, Khushro Ghandi, Chairman of the "Prevent AIDS Now Initiative Committee," referred to by the acronym, PANIC.

Lyndon LaRouche was running for the Democratic nomination for the Presidency of the United States and the California AIDS Initiative was one of his basic platforms. Although the position outlined in Proposition 64 was logical and medically sound, Lyndon LaRouche and his supporters persisted in calling for "quarantine" and stated over and over that once Proposition 64 was enacted, California could begin to isolate those who were infected.

Lyndon LaRouche was well known for his extremist positions, such as his statement that the Queen of England was involved in a vast conspiracy to rule the world. Some of his rhetoric was similar to that of conservative groups in that he called attention to the influence of the Council on Foreign Relations and the Trilateral Commission within our government; however, Lyndon LaRouche was so radical in most of his views that even the Democratic Party wanted nothing to do with him. According to a booklet distributed by the CMA, Lyndon LaRouche had published his AIDS plan in the Executive Intelligence Report (EIR) magazine. The plan outlined "a program to stop the AIDS pandemic." LaRouche referred specifically to Proposition 64, tying it into the larger issues of international monetary policy, neo-Nazi groups, twentieth-century fascism, bolshevism, the "neo-Malthusian" movement centered around the Club of Rome and its interface with the Soviet KGB.[9] As soon as Proposition 64 qualified for the November ballot, gay groups began organizing. Leaders from across the state assembled in Los Angeles to plan their strategy to defeat the initiative. According to the San Francisco Chronicle (June 21st) representatives of the California Department of Health Services stated that:

"Because the HIV test measures antibodies and not the virus itself, test results could not legally be used to implement the initiative's mandate of screening out AIDS virus carriers."

Of course that statement by California State Health Department officials was simply a smoke screen, another example of the sophistry that would be used so effectively in the months ahead to confuse the public. The antibody test was used by physicians to identify those with the virus and public health officers certainly knew that.

The Orange County Chapter of the American Civil Liberties Union issued a press release stating:

"A stringent interpretation of Proposition 64 could lead to travel limitations, job restrictions and even indefinite isolation of people carrying the AIDS virus."

Immediately, liberal public health officials and gay activists organized against the initiative and attacked the concept that HIV disease should be considered an infectious, contagious, communicable disease — even though it was an infectious, contagious, communicable disease.

Those who attacked the initiative pointed out that there was no reason why HIV infected people couldn't act as food handlers, yet there was absolutely nothing in the initiative suggesting that infected people couldn't work as food handlers.

The media labeled the initiative "The AIDS Quarantine Act" and the public was told that if the initiative passed, it would lead to the quarantining of all HIV carriers. It was interesting that whenever one listened to Lyndon LaRouche or his followers, they would always allude to the fact that the initiative would allow quarantine of those who were infected.

I kept wondering why LaRouche and his followers were talking about quarantine. Over and over again LaRouche's supporters called for quarantine. Their statements seemed to justify the fears of gay activists who were convinced that anyone who supported declaring HIV disease as an infectious, contagious, communicable illness was an extremist and supported quarantine.

San Francisco gay Supervisor, Harry Britt, branded Lyndon LaRouche as "a political fanatic who is trying to stir up fear of AIDS in order to advance his political agenda."

Gay leaders attacked the initiative saying it would lead to "witch hunts."

On June 29, gays and lesbians marched down Market Street in the nation's largest gay and lesbian celebration, demonstrating against the LaRouche Initiative. On that day, an estimated 250,000 people lined Market Street to watch the six hour parade, hear the speeches and enjoy the entertainment.

This was the 11th annual San Francisco Gay-Lesbian Freedom Parade and the major thrust of the demonstration was opposition to Lyndon LaRouche's initiative and his PANIC Committee. Literally thousands of signs attacking the initiative were passed out to parade marchers by the San Francisco Community AIDS Network and the California AIDS Network.

The signs carried such messages as, "WITH LAROUCHE, EVERYBODY IS SUSPECT" and "DEFEAT THE LAROUCHE BIGOTRY" and "EDUCATE DON'T SEGREGATE" and "DOUCHE LAROUCHE." Gay and lesbian organizers came from all across the nation to help in the celebration and encourage their supporters to defeat the AIDS initiative — to defeat anyone who wanted to declare HIV disease to be an infectious, contagious disease.

Mayor Dianne Feinstein sent a proclamation to the parade organizers, and Supervisors John Molinarie, Louis Rene and Richard Hongisto rode in their convertibles through the streets of San Francisco along with the gay activists. Assembly Speaker, Willie Brown, rode in a convertible with San Francisco's gay Supervisor, Harry Britt. State Senator Milton Marx walked with his gay friends down the street.

Three hundred motorcycles led the parade with a banner proclaiming: "DYKES ON BIKES." "Sister Boom Boom" rode in the parade. The Gay Men's Choir was there along with a group of lesbians carrying their placards, "LADIES AGAINST WOMEN." The sadomasochists were there, carrying their whips, studs and chains and signs proclaiming "SM IS SAFE SEX."

The gay and lesbian atheists were there. The underlying theme of the parade that day was to show the gay community unified in opposition to the LaRouche Initiative and any effort to deal with HIV disease as if it were really a disease.[10]

✳✳✳

In the latter part of 1986 there were many events that should have begun to give physicians some insight into the magnitude of the epidemic but the major issue before the public in California was the LaRouche AIDS Initiative — Proposition 64. That initiative came to be the focus of an intensive media attack. The initiative was opposed by gay activists, the American Civil Liberties Union (ACLU), the California Medical Association (CMA), The California Hospital Association (CHA), The Union of American Physicians and Dentists (UAPD), The California Dental Association (CDA), and the California Teachers Association (CTA), along with dozens of moderate and left-wing organizations including the Communist Party (CPUSA).

It was during these months that I began to catch my first glimpse of the forces that were aligned in an effort to stop sound medical measures from being used to stop this plague.

✳✳✳

In June 1986, initial reports were released by the U. S. Military on the results of testing military recruits across America. Among 237,000 whites tested, the rate of infection was .9 per thousand or about 1/10th of one per cent, (0.1%). Among 55,000 blacks tested, the rate was 3.9 per thousand, (0.39%). The army report revealed that across the nation, 25% of all HIV infection occurred in black males, and black women accounted for 52% of all female cases. Representatives of the National Coalition of Black Gays immediately organized a conference to dramatize the fact that the disease seemed to be affecting blacks more than whites and to demand that something be done to stop its spread.

In June 1986, the results of military AIDS testing were presented before the Second World Congress on Acquired Immune Deficiency Syndrome in Paris. It was reported that 2% of military applicants in Manhattan were infected, 1% of military applicants in Washington, D. C. and almost 1% in Puerto Rico were infected.

Colonel Donald S. Burke of the Walter Reed Army Research Institute, the physician who supervised the U. S. Army testing project, noted that the figures were "higher than the experts...had predicted." He reported the ratio of men to women infected with the virus was 2.5 to 1 and was much lower than the ratio of men to women noted in AIDS cases (13 to 1). This meant that the disease was rapidly spreading into the heterosexual population. It was not just a homosexual disease or an IV drug users disease.

Those infected were young, healthy military recruits who now carried the virus. Since HIV disease was not considered an infectious disease in most states in 1986, the cases identified by army recruiters were not reported to local public health officers. As a result, those infected young people who were irresponsible could continue spreading the disease to others without fear of punishment.

No one was allowed to know who the majority of those young people were and the Army could not notify public health authorities in most states because of **confidentiality restrictions**. And so, there were thousands of young heterosexuals who carried the virus. How many were irresponsible and continued to spread the disease? In 1986, nothing could be done to keep those irresponsible young people from intentionally infecting others to gratify their own sexual cravings.[11]

✳✳✳

It was also at the 2nd International AIDS Conference in Paris that Doctor Margaret Fischel, an AIDS researcher from Miami, Florida, announced that 35% of her AIDS cases were females — double the percentage that she had seen just one year earlier. She felt that 8% of the AIDS cases were actually instances of heterosexual transmission.

Tragically, in mid-1986 most Americans were still oblivious to the danger that they faced. After all, this was a disease of homosexuals, this was a disease of IV drug users and hemophiliacs, it was a disease of blacks and Hispanics and that really did not affect white America. People had not yet realized that this was also a disease of heterosexuals and it would soon involve their children and their grandchildren. However, in mid-1986 most Americans simply ignored the epidemic because it was somebody else's problem.

✳✳✳

In the fall of 1986, Lyndon LaRouche became the subject of an organized, coordinated attack and Lyndon LaRouche was a very easy person to attack. Some of the attacks were justified — some of them were not. Lyndon LaRouche was branded as a "kook" for suggesting that he believed that the Rothschilds helped assassinate Abraham Lincoln, started the Ku Klux Klan and that Henry Kissinger and Walter F. Mondale were agents of the KGB.

Regular meetings were held by the American Civil Liberties Union, various Democrat organizations and gay activists to stop Proposition 64. Lyndon LaRouche was characterized as a "monster" and a "dangerous animal" and was equated with Joe McCarthy and Adolf Hitler. It was open season on Lyndon LaRouche and his initiative.

❊❊❊

By September 1986, a number of states had passed laws related to AIDS discrimination. Americans were told that we were only going to be able to stop further spread of the disease by passing antidiscrimination laws which were being introduced by the National Gay Rights Advocates and similar gay organizations.

There were hundreds of gay organizations across the country which were using the AIDS epidemic as a vehicle for introducing gay antidiscrimination laws and other legislation to carry out the gay agenda for America. Gay activists were far more concerned with passing antidiscrimination legislation than with stopping the epidemic.

I certainly do not think that anyone should be discriminated against, whether they be homosexual or a victim of AIDS. If their working does not endanger someone else's health, AIDS patients should be allowed to stay on their jobs. But what happens if those who are infected do endanger somebody else's health? What happens if they have some other disease that is dangerous to others or their mental status has begun to deteriorate to the point where they cannot perform their regular job?

In mid-1986, the U. S. Justice Department released a directive which stated that if a public health officer felt that an infected individual was dangerous to others in the work place, then that worker could be discharged or reassigned; however, if the worker represented no danger to himself or others, he should be allowed to stay on his job. This was not the policy that gay groups wanted.

The gay groups' attitude was that it didn't matter how dangerous an individual might be to someone else; if he had AIDS (and was presumably gay), they **must** be allowed to work. Benjamin Schatt, Director of the AIDS Civil Rights project of the National Gay Rights Advocates commented on the Justice Department directive:

"The U. S. Justice Department and others have injected politics into the issue and distorted the law. I am pleased that many states haven't followed the poor example of letting prejudice and fear interfere with their obligation to enforce the law."

And so it was that across the nation, anti-handicap laws were introduced to forbid bias against anyone with HIV disease or AIDS and any form of discrimination became illegal. It didn't matter how sick somebody with AIDS might be, no employer had a right to take an AIDS patient off the job. Officials from states across the nation announced that discrimination was prohibited by law. Eight states expressed willingness to investigate complaints of AIDS related discrimination. Only two states — Kentucky and Utah — said that AIDS itself "cannot be considered a handicap."[12]

***

On September 29, 1986 Dr. John Seal, an English specialist in venereal disease, held a press conference in San Francisco under the auspices of PANIC, Lyndon LaRouche's committee supporting Proposition 64. Doctor Seal disavowed support for Lyndon LaRouche, but stated that he thoroughly supported Proposition 64 because, "The illness is a species threatening disease" and "Public health authorities must be given power to fight a scourge that politicians are not taking seriously enough."

The San Francisco Chronicle which reported the interview attempted to discredit Dr. Seal by pointing out that he had not done any laboratory research and his only knowledge of HIV disease was from reading medical literature and treating AIDS cases in London. The article went on to say:

"If passed, Proposition 64 would...require that all persons who carry the AIDS virus...be removed from public schools and banned from food handling jobs."[13]

There was absolutely no basis for these statements since AIDS patients were allowed to work in restaurants and attend school but the average person reading the article would have no way of knowing that. So the media began to build up mass hysteria about Proposition 64, claiming tremendous expense would be incurred if it became law and physicians began trying to identify those who carried the virus.

On radio, television, in newspapers and magazines — in pamphlets and at meetings during October one found article after article, speaker after speaker — all condemning Proposition 64 and claiming horrible discrimination and injustice would occur if it passed and physicians began treating HIV disease as an infectious, contagious, communicable disease.

※※※

By October 1, 1986 there were approximately 25,000 people in America diagnosed with AIDS. I was overcome with a sense of urgency, frustration and anger. I could see how the media was manipulating the public to believer that truth was falsehood and falsehood was truth. By repetition, the media, gay activists and their liberal allies were creating a specter of fear and hysteria as far as Proposition 64 was concerned.

It was because of my growing concern about the epidemic that I wrote a letter to the editors of a number of newspapers in California. Several of them published it. The basic text stated that California must declare HIV disease to be a legal disease so that we could begin to save lives. Although disavowing Lyndon LaRouche, I gave full support to the wording of Proposition 64. (See Appendix III for the text of the letter).

What was the result? I received death threats and hate mail. A doctor in Santa Cruz wrote a letter to the editor in the local newspaper to condemn me for daring to support Proposition 64, an initiative which was being openly opposed by the CMA.

One of the few public figures with the courage to take a stand in support of Proposition 64 was Congressman William Dannemeyer, the Republican representative from Orange County. Although also carefully disassociating himself from Lyndon LaRouche, the Congressman wrote a position paper supporting Proposition 64 for the California Voters Guide which was sent to all registered voters. In his argument in favor of Proposition 64, Congressman Dannemeyer stated:

> California law today makes it illegal for public health authorities to be informed of a large number of those (about 385,000) who can spread the deadly AIDS virus to others. How can they take the necessary steps to slow its spread as long as this is true? Under existing law, a physician who encounters any one of 58 reportable diseases is required to report them to...public health officials. Included are several venereal diseases such as syphilis and gonorrhea. Contact tracing is conducted, but for those with the AIDS virus not yet developed into AIDS, a special state law, passed at the request of the

male homosexual lobby, prohibits contact tracing. Proposition 64 will require that those infected with the AIDS virus will be reported as other communicable diseases. It does not require quarantine. The cost of the AIDS epidemic in California, it is estimated, will be at least 59,400 lives by 1991 and almost 6 billion dollars to be paid out by insurance and/or tax payers. Let's reduce this statistic by voting YES on Proposition 64.

Congressman Dannemeyer was subsequently vilified, attacked as a homophobe, a bigot and likened to Joseph McCarthy and Adolf Hitler. Nothing too horrible could be said about him — because he openly supported Proposition 64.

※※※

On October 23, 1986, the Surgeon General's Report on AIDS was released to the public. By then over 15,000 Americans were dead. The report was conveniently timed to be used in the defeat of Proposition 64 — just as 2 years later — Surgeon General Koop would come out with public statements aimed at defeating Proposition 102 (the Gann AIDS Initiative).

In his 1986 report the Surgeon General laid out his plan to fight the disease. How were we going to stop the epidemic? We were going to use education. We were to start sex education as early as possible in school and then educate and desensitize our children to sex year after year after year.

For those interested in documenting the homosexual control of public health policy during this era, I suggest the book, *Private Acts, Social Consequences — AIDS and the Policies of Public Health* by Ronald Bayer.
1. Secretary of Education, William Bennett was the only highly placed government official to publicly stress concepts of morals and values. This placed him in direct opposition to Surgeon General Koop who rarely mentioned abstinence and seldom used the words "marriage" or "morality" publicly. Although the Surgeon General is a professing Christian, he refrained from stressing moral and religious values presumably to avoid offending members of the AIDS and Gay Lobbies.

2. Certainly the Surgeon General did not really believe what he told the public. I tried to relay information to him on a case of HIV disease which appeared to be an instance of casual spread of the disease by kissing (the case reported by Doctor Illa to which I will refer later). Repeated letters to the Surgeon General were never answered so I relayed information on the case through one of his friends who worked in the White House and knew him personally. According to this woman, when she told him of the case, the Surgeon General commented: "Casual spread really is very uncommon." Yet in his Surgeon General's Report, Dr. Koop emphatically stated that "There is no risk from casual contact." (See Appendix I).

3. There is overwhelming evidence to suggest that deep, passionate kissing can spread the virus. The virus can cross any mucous membrane — vaginal, rectal, oral. There are no studies to confirm the Surgeon General's position — yet he allowed his name and position to be used in the U. S. Public Health Department pamphlet to mislead the public. (See Appendix II).

4. The council is made up of 33 councilors. In Southern California, councilors run for election and are elected by practicing physicians. In Northern California, councilors are appointed by the district delegations and physicians are unable to run for election in their districts.

5. San Mateo, Santa Clara, Santa Cruz and Monterey County delegates make up the 7th District delegation to the CMA.

6. The Executive Committee consists of 6 members. The Chairman and Vice-Chairman of the Council, the President and President-elect of the CMA, the Speaker and Vice-Chairman of the House.

7. MMWR, May 2, 1986; vol. 35/17, p. 285.

8. AMA News, February 14, 1986; p. 59.

9. CMA booklet on the "Background of Proposition 64" CMA; p. 10.

10. Santa Cruz Sentinel; June 30, 1986; article by Herbert Michelson and McClatchy News Service; p. B16. (Reprinted with permission).

11. San Francisco Chronicle; June 26, 1986; p. 9.

12. San Francisco Chronicle; September 4, 1986; p. 6.

13. San Francisco Chronicle; September 30, 1986.

CHAPTER TWO

It was in the fall of 1986 when newspapers reported that Governor Deukmejian of California was about to sign the legislation (AB3667) which had been supported by the California Medical Association. This was the bill that I had been waiting for. This was the bill that had resulted from the passage of my resolution in March of 1986. This was the bill that would do away with the requirement for a written consent for HIV blood testing. This was the bill that I assumed would change the confidentiality requirements so that doctors would no longer face the threat of a $10,000.00 fine and one year imprisonment if they told a surgical nurse who had a cut or a needle stick that she was potentially infectious. This was the bill that would promote contact tracing and allow physicians in California — perhaps all across America — to begin addressing HIV disease as an epidemic.

For this reason, I waited with anticipation for the Governor to sign "my" bill. There are very few times when an average citizen has the opportunity to influence legislation that may have a profound impact on society. The majority of legislation that is passed — at the state or national level — is relatively unimportant and usually deals with issues that benefit one group or one industry or one community. But "my bill" could possibly save the lives of hundreds of thousands of people. If a doctor, during his entire professional career saves a few hundred lives, it is a great accomplishment. In this instance, with the passage of AB3667, I might play a small part in saving tens of thousands of lives.

I shall have to admit that I looked forward with anticipation to the Governor signing "my bill." It was not that I looked for any personal accolade or notoriety, it was simply the personal satisfaction of knowing that my actions at the House of Delegates had really made a difference.

When I picked up the newspaper one morning in the fall of 1986, I could not believe what I read. It seemed beyond comprehension that it could have happened, yet there it was in the headlines. Governor Deukmejian had vetoed "my bill," (AB3667). George Deukmejian is one of those rare politicians who is generally a man of principle and integrity. Although I do not always agree with him, I have never questioned his honesty.

In fact, as our story unfolds you will find that Governor Deukmejian was willing to take a heroic stand on the HIV epidemic in the fall of

1988, knowing full well that almost all the newspapers in California would oppose and vilify him. But George Deukmejian, in stark contrast to many politicians, often does what he thinks is right rather than what is expedient.

What was so incredible in the fall of 1986 was that George Deukmejian vetoed the California Medical Association's bill (AB3667) which I assumed would have done away with written consent and some of the confidentiality requirement for HIV blood testing.

I hurried to my office and wrote the governor an angry letter demanding to know why he opposed a logical, public health approach to the epidemic.

It was several weeks later when a letter arrived from one of the governor's aides. It was a polite letter that explained that the governor agreed with certain parts of the CMA sponsored bill, but there were certain parts of the legislation with which he could not agree and it was because of the objectionable parts of the bill that he had vetoed it. A copy of the bill was included.

I read the legislation with disbelief. I suddenly felt disillusioned, for the legislation that the CMA had passed did not include the positions supported by the House of Delegates. The legislation was an AIDS Bill of Rights. It was aimed at expanding antidiscrimination laws for AIDS victims and those perceived as having AIDS (i.e., homosexuals). The bill did to some extent expand confidentiality so physicians could tell nurses in the operating room that the patient was infected, but the bill in no way addressed the requirement for a written consent for HIV blood testing and there was still a $10,000.00 fine and a year imprisonment for physicians who released information on HIV test results. Routine reporting and contact tracing were also ignored.

I did not understand how this could have happened. How could the hierarchy of the CMA totally disregard positions taken so clearly by the House of Delegates? Didn't the House set policy or was that simply a facade? I began to wonder if the meetings of the House were simply window dressing while a small, well-organized minority carried out their own programs. Were we simply play-acting at our meetings, pretending to be a democratic organization while all the time the major policy decisions were made by others?

Months later, I was able to obtain copies of the minutes of the CMA Council meeting of July, 1986. The following is the summary of those minutes:

CMA Council at its July, 1986 meeting did not implement...resolution (708-86) on advice of our legal counsel, (i.e., removing the written consent requirement), because the first part appears *to advocate what is essentially patient assault.* (emphasis added)

The CMA Council's action followed a recommendation of the CMA Committee on AIDS and Sexually Transmitted Disease.[1]

Up to this point, I had always felt that the reason I had not been able to sway CMA policy was that I had not been able to reach members of the House of Delegates and convince them of my positions. Ordinarily, I had been prevented from disseminating information. On one occasion, I was prevented from speaking and from passing out fliers. On other occasions, I was prevented from renting meeting halls at the conventions. As a result, I was never able to put forward my views effectively. Yet here was an instance where my position had been overwhelmingly supported by members of the House and, despite that fact, the Council had seen fit to override the policies adopted by the House.

What was their rationale? It was the fact that removing the requirement for written consent to perform an HIV blood test "appears to advocate what is essentially patient assault."

As the story began to unfold, it became increasingly obvious that there were those within leadership positions who had one primary goal and that goal was to prevent doctors from using the HIV blood test. They consistently placed barriers in the way of physicians. They did this in 1986, 1987, 1988 and again in 1990. For you see, physicians were not to use blood testing to try to identify those who were infected in order to stop this epidemic.

It was in November 1986 when the state election was held on Proposition 64, the LaRouche Initiative. As expected, the initiative went down to defeat. There were a number of factors that bothered me about the handling of that initiative in the final weeks. First of all, during the last three weeks of the campaign, Lyndon LaRouche spent almost no money on advertisements or TV commercials to try to get his initiative passed. After initially spending almost one-quarter of a million dollars to get the initiative onto the ballot, Lyndon LaRouche and his supporters made no effort to convince the public that passage of Proposition 64 was important or that physicians needed to start addressing HIV disease as an infectious, contagious, communicable disease. Rather, Lyndon LaRouche and his associates kept hammering away at the importance of quarantine.

What bothered me most was the simple question — "Why would anyone spend almost one-quarter of a million dollars to get an initiative on the ballot and then spend almost no money to support that initiative?" That really didn't make sense. Was it that Lyndon LaRouche didn't have funds? Not likely, since two years later, in 1988, Lyndon LaRouche was back, once again, with Proposition 69 which was almost identical to Proposition 64. He had the funds to run another initiative two years later — an initiative which would also lose when Lyndon LaRouche and his supporters raised the issue of quarantine.

Lyndon LaRouche ordinarily had large sums of money to spend. He published a number of expensive, slick magazines including "Fusion," Executive Intelligence Report," "The Campaigner," and "Young Scientist." In addition, he published the tabloid, "New Solidarity." Any one of those magazines or the tabloid would cost tens of thousands of dollars a month to print and distribute.

LaRouche had an international organization with extensive research facilities and a large, full-time, paid staff. In 1986, he lived in an expensive, heavily guarded, 171 acre estate in Leesburg, Virginia. People have questioned where LaRouche's money comes from. He may well have obtained some of it from the illicit use of credit cards, but long before his followers used that scam, Lyndon LaRouche had large sums of money coming from somewhere in the world. I have heard Senator John Doolittle suggest that there was evidence that some of his money may have come from East Germany or other communist countries.

In October 1969, the New York Times reported that some of the funding for LaRouche came from "3 cult members' corporations" in Manhattan that performed works for Mobil, Citibank, AT&T, the Ford Foundation and the Bristol Meyers Corporation (which today manufactures AZT).

Whatever the source of LaRouche's funding, he did not spend any of that money to get Proposition 64 passed. In fact, the result of his efforts can be summarized in an editorial which appeared in the San Francisco Chronicle shortly after Proposition 64 was defeated. That editorial said in effect:

"The people of the State of California have spoken. They do not wish physicians to treat HIV disease as they do other diseases. They do not want to use the same public health approaches to control this disease as are used with other diseases."

The average citizen of California did not understand the implications of the defeat of Proposition 64. The average citizen who opposed Proposition 64 was supporting the position of the CMA, the CNA, the CHA, the UAPD, the CDA, the ACLU and a myriad of other radical left wing organizations including the CPUSA. In defeating Proposition 64, the people of California had, in reality, voted that they did not want to use standard public health techniques, HIV blood testing or contact tracing to try to stop the spread of the disease.

In the months that followed the defeat of Proposition 64, I reflected back on what had occurred. The more I reflected, the more frightening were the implications. I had studied Lyndon LaRouche and his movement for many years. Contrary to what the liberal media tells you, **Lyndon LaRouche is not a right-wing extremist.** Lyndon LaRouche is an old-line Stalinist.

He started his political career in the Socialist Labor Party and then joined the Worker's League. The Free University of New York, where he taught in the mid-1960's, listed him as a "Professional economist and a Marxist." During the turmoil of the 1960's, he founded the U. S. Labor Party and the International Labor Party. In January of 1973, in his publication, "New Solidarity," he called on Gus Hall of the U. S. Communist Party to form a united front with his revolutionary group. Gus Hall and his followers rejected the offer.

Lyndon LaRouche gathered his followers from The Students For A Democratic Society — the left wing revolutionary movement of the Vietnam War era. These young people were disillusioned with America. They were intent upon overthrowing what they perceived as a corrupt, capitalist society and hoped to replace that society with a new social structure — a new Socialist Order which they would lead.

They circulated materials showing that there was a small group of wealthy capitalists who dominated both the Democrat and Republican parties and consistently were able to plant their members in key cabinet posts and advisory positions in successive administrations. The LaRouche publications attacked the Council on Foreign Relations and the Trilateral Commission and its members for having gained clandestine control of the reins of power of the American Government and using that power to further their own political agenda. LaRouche's followers wanted to overthrow those wicked capitalists and gain power for themselves.

According to their publication "The Campaigner," LaRouche's followers looked upon themselves as the true "epistemological brother-hood of Plato," a group of idealists who would bring to America the Philosopher King that Plato had written about in his classic, "The Republic." And their Philosopher King, the so-called "Just Ruler," the man who would lead America to Plato's Utopia, was none other than their leader...Lyndon LaRouche.

LaRouche's Revolutionary Movement is simply one of a number of revolutionary groups that exists today within our society. The leading revolutionary group in America is the Communist Party, U.S.A. (CPUSA), which is under Russian domination and works to bring about a socialist America.

In addition, there are the Maoists, the Trotskyites and certain other smaller socialist revolutionary groups. One of the most formidable and subtle of these smaller groups is the U.S. Labor Party under the leadership of Lyndon LaRouche.

All these various revolutionary groups are intent upon the overthrow of our government by democratic means, if at all possible, but if they cannot convert our nation to a socialist dictatorship by peaceful means, they will ultimately resort to violence.

As I contemplated the strange facts surrounding Proposition 64, I wondered how Lyndon LaRouche could ever hope to gain political power? Many of his extremist views were certainly well known, his followers were few and even with the vast amounts of money that he had spent through the years, he could not possibly hope to gain power via the democratic process.

By what means then could LaRouche ever hope to have any signifi-cant influence on our national policies? I reflected on what will happen ten years hence, as the HIV epidemic begins killing hundreds of thousands of our citizens. What will happen when it becomes apparent that the epidemic resulted because political leaders refused to try to stop the spread of this disease?

After all, Adolf Hitler came to power as a direct result of the chaos in Germany in the 1930's. Benito Mussolini came to power as a direct result of the chaos in Italy during the 1920's. Could it possibly be that LaRouche ran Proposition 64, intentionally, to lose with the hope that our nation could one day move into a period of chaos and conflict?

Could it be that he talked about quarantine simply to inflame the fears of gay activists in order to mobilize them as a political force to block the use of blood testing? Could it be that he was far more clever and diabolical than anyone ever imagined — and that he realized that his only hope for gaining power lay in that period of chaos and conflict which looms ten years hence?

Why else would anyone with great wealth and power spend almost one-quarter of a million dollars to get Proposition 64 on the ballot and in the last three weeks before the election spend virtually nothing to insure its passage? Why would LaRouche and his followers keep talking about quarantine when every medical researcher agrees that quarantine is unnecessary?...Why?...

After November of 1986 and the defeat of Proposition 64, few politicians had the courage to step forward and say that our nation should begin addressing HIV disease as an infectious, contagious, communicable disease. As a result, the epidemic, the dying and death continued.

❊❊❊

As of December 8, 1986 the U. S. Public Health Department reported 28,098 patients with AIDS. Of these, 15,757 were known to have died, including 79% of those patients diagnosed before January of 1985. During the preceding three months, an average of 58 AIDS cases had been reported to the CDC daily, compared with 35 cases reported during this same period in 1985 and 20 cases in 1984, and 10 cases in 1983.[2]

❊❊❊

It was in January of 1987 when **bleach** became a new weapon in the battle against AIDS. Groups in San Francisco, New York and other cities began passing out bleach to IV drug users so they could sterilize their needles and cut back on the transmission of the AIDS virus when sharing needles with fellow drug users. Two other events occurred during the month of January which began to change my perception of the epidemic. The first event involved the flagrant misuse of power within another medical organization. The second involved a physician being threatened by the west coast representative of the CDC for daring to speak publicly about what he perceived as a case of casual transmission of HIV disease from a wife to her husband.

It was in mid-January of 1987 that I went to a hotel at the San Francisco International Airport as a delegate to the convention of the Union of American Physicians and Dentists. The UAPD is an organization created by Dr. Sanford Marcus, a surgeon from South San Francisco. Doctor Marcus had managed to recruit thousands of physicians from across our land into the UAPD, which purported to truly represent the interests of the medical profession.

By 1987, many doctors had become disillusioned with traditional medical organizations, recognizing that the CMA, the AMA and many state medical societies were not effectively opposing America's move towards socialism and the control of health care. As a result of their disenchantment, a number of physicians dropped out of their county and state medical societies and joined the UAPD. Doctor Marcus had spoken across our nation, warning of the danger of the move towards Health Maintenance Organizations (HMO's) and Preferred Provider Organizations (PPO's). He warned of the danger of the corporate takeover of American medicine.

It was Doctor Marcus's words of concern and the eloquence of his presentation that convinced many conservative physicians from California and across the nation to put aside their feeling of repugnance towards the concept of a medical union and join the UAPD.

The basic theme which Doctor Marcus presented was that the UAPD was a medical organization dedicated to the preservation of the public and private practice of medicine so that physicians could continue serving as the advocates for their patients rather than becoming employees of government or corporations.

By January 1987, I was appointed to be a representative to the National Convention of the UAPD. One of my objectives was to present a resolution supporting the concept that HIV disease should be legally considered as an infectious, communicable, sexually transmitted disease. Since the UAPD had been one of the organizations which opposed Proposition 64, I hoped to get the Union to publicly support the concept of declaring HIV disease as a "disease," independent of the "quarantine" rhetoric of Lyndon LaRouche and his radical supporters.

Much to my amazement, when I attended the appropriate committee meeting and brought up the subject, I was informed by the committee chairman that the UAPD did not take positions on medical matters. When I pointed out that the UAPD had joined in condemning Proposition 64 and that Proposition 64 was a medical issue, I was again told that the union did not take positions on medical matters and that I would not be allowed to present my resolution or to bring up the subject at the general meeting. I was reminded of the time, many years earlier, at the House of Delegates of the California Medical Association, when I had tried to speak in favor of a resolution supporting a strong defense for

America and been told, "Sit down. You cannot speak because what you are going to say is political."

I had come to expect that type of undemocratic action in the House of Delegates but I was shocked to find that the UAPD Committee Chairman was just as intolerant of conflicting viewpoints and that the UAPD was really no more democratic or representative than the traditional houses of organized medicine.[3]

✳✳✳

The most significant event of January 1987 was my contact with Doctor Robert Illa, a physician from Burlingame, California. The story he told gave me my first glimpse of the frightening tactics which were being used all across the nation to silence opposition. It was one thing to circumvent the democratic process within organized medicine by refusing to carry out a directive of the House of Delegates. It was an entirely different matter to threaten physicians with reprisal in order to silence them. But that would be the recurrent story which I would hear over and over again with minor variations in the months and years that followed. What was happening was not accidental for there were forces at work, powerful forces, which were intent upon silencing anyone who spoke out on the epidemic and differed with "the official party line."

In 1985, an article appeared in the San Francisco Chronicle which I had read and filed. It was the story of a physician who had cared for an elderly woman with AIDS. The patient subsequently died. Then her husband came down with a disease which appeared to be AIDS and also died. The physician felt that the husband's illness might be a case of casual transmission of AIDS. That was all the article said.

By January 1987 I was increasingly convinced that there was a cover-up at the national level. I did not understand the cover-up nor the true nature of what was transpiring so I decided to try to track down that story. I found the article and noted the doctor's name. I was able to get his telephone number. I went through his "physicians exchange" and finally I could hear the phone ringing on the other end of the line.

"Doctor Illa?" I said, introducing myself. "I am calling you about an article in the San Francisco Chronicle two years ago concerning a patient where you thought there might be casual transmission of AIDS. I want to ask you about that case."

There are very few conversations from years past that I can recall word for word but I remember Dr. Illa's response as if it was yesterday.

"God bless you!" the voice at the other end of the line responded. "You are the first person in two years to ask me about that case. That case destroyed my life." Then he began to tell me his story, a story which I subsequently repeated before a Congressional Committee, discussed before legislators of the State of California and which I alluded to in my testimony before the U. S. Civil Rights Commission. Despite the fact that TV cameras recorded my testimony on two occasions in Washington, D. C., I am sure that you have never heard this story mentioned by the media.

Doctor Illa's story was essentially this: He was an internist practicing in Burlingame, California. He cared for a woman who contracted AIDS from a transfusion. She became increasingly ill and subsequently died. Her husband took care of her during her prolonged illness. He was impotent because of diabetes so there was no sexual contact. The only intimate contact between the man and wife was kissing.

After the wife's death the husband's condition began to deteriorate. It appeared that his immune system was malfunctioning and he became susceptible to a series of infections. His clinical course was progressively downhill. Doctor Illa became increasingly concerned and ordered several T4 helper lymphocyte counts. In 1984 and early 1985, before the ELISA blood test became available, T4 lymphocyte counts were the best method to determine the status of a patient's immune response.

The T4 lymphocyte counts were consistently low. When the ELISA blood test became available, two successive blood specimens were sent to a laboratory in Southern California. Both tests came back positive. At that point Doctor Illa called in the west coast representative of the Centers for Disease Control. The representative came and talked to the husband and administered the routine CDC questionnaire to determine whether or not there was sexual contact to explain the disease. After administering the test, the CDC representative apparently concluded that this could be a case of casual transmission of AIDS.

A blood specimen was sent to the CDC to recheck the results. About this time, the children in the family became increasingly concerned about their father's failing health. They asked Doctor Illa what was wrong. Doctor Illa mentioned the possibility that their father's condition might be a case of casually spread AIDS, although he cautioned them that he was not absolutely certain of the diagnosis.

The family apparently contacted a reporter from the San Francisco

Chronicle who in turn contacted Doctor Illa and asked for information. Doctor Illa refused, saying that he wanted to have more information before making any public statement. The reporter said he was going to run the story with or without an interview and at that point, Doctor Illa foolishly agreed.

It was shortly before the interview that someone called from the Centers for Disease Control and told Dr. Illa that if he mentioned his case publicly the CDC would not stand behind him. Furthermore, he was told that the blood specimens which had been sent to Atlanta had failed to reveal evidence of antibodies to the HIV virus.

Doctor Illa went ahead and talked to the reporter and the resulting article was distributed all across the nation by wire services. It was at that point that Doctor Illa's life changed. First of all, he started getting harassing telephone calls and threats from across the country for daring to suggest that there might be such a thing as casual transmission of AIDS. Reporters came from San Francisco and sat in his office and made harassing remarks to his secretary (who happened to be his wife.) His wife became increasingly defensive and concerned about what was transpiring. Eventually, as a direct result of the harassment that she received because of the publication of the article, she left her husband.

A prominent AIDS expert came down from San Francisco General Hospital to address the staff of the hospital where Doctor Illa practiced. With no personal knowledge of the case and never having seen either the chart or medical records, this AIDS expert attacked Doctor Illa for daring to suggest there might be such a thing as casual transmission of the disease.

The effect of that attack was to discredit Doctor Illa with other physicians on his hospital staff and to seriously hurt his referral medical practice. The director of the laboratory in Southern California (where the blood tests had been performed) called Doctor Illa and apologized profusely. He said there had been some sort of terrible mistake in recording the blood test results and the virus that they had been testing for was an entirely different virus than the HTLV-III (HIV) virus. The director went on to say that he planned to publish an article on this new virus that they had discovered and Doctor Illa's name would be included in the list of credits. (Of course, the article was never published.) Then the laboratory's license was pulled by the state health department and the laboratory was not allowed to perform HIV blood testing for an extended period of time.

The most startling and revealing part of the story was the fact that the representative from the CDC who had initially worked up the case, contacted Doctor Illa and told him that he should realize that if he persisted in discussing his case "There would be serious personal consequences."

With his marriage falling apart, harassed by threatening phone calls, his referral practice badly damaged as a direct result of the presentation by the "AIDS expert" and with the threat of reprisal from an agent of the CDC, Bob Illa saw no other alternative than to put the case behind him. During the subsequent two years, as he saw the epidemic spreading and the ever-rising death toll, he must have borne a sense of frustration and guilt. Thus when I called him in January 1987, he recounted his story to me, fully realizing that our entire nation faced destruction and his continued silence did a disservice to the country that both he and I cherished. He gave me his permission to discuss the case, knowing full well that bringing up that long forgotten case could bring reprisal and retaliation. Later, he came to Santa Cruz and filmed a video interview, copies of which I took to Washington, D. C. and to Sacramento.

Now I am not saying that Doctor Illa was right and that his case was an instance of casual spread of disease. In fact, Doctor Illa kept 1/2 cc. of frozen serum from the patient for future testing. In September 1987, he sent that serum to a laboratory. The HIV test came back negative. Indeed, this suggested that Doctor Illa's case was not a case of casual transmission of HIV disease.

The significance of the story is the fact that tremendous pressure was brought to bear on him for speaking out and that an agent of the Federal Government would threaten him with reprisal and retaliation if he dared to continue talking about his case.

February 1987
The most significant event was the meeting which was held by the CDC in Atlanta, Georgia. The Centers for Disease Control invited public health experts from across our nation to come to Atlanta to discuss the use of HIV testing in doctors' offices, sexually transmitted disease clinics, drug clinics, premarital and prenatal clinics.

There were those in the CDC who realized the implications of this epidemic and wanted to try again to gather support for testing from public health officials and medical leaders. They anticipated that about 200 people would attend. Instead there were 900 attendees — mostly gay activists, gay physicians and left-wing activists. Don Berreth, a CDC spokesman was quoted as saying: "This definitely is not what we imagined. People have gone crazy over the testing issue."

Of course, he was wrong. The gay activists and the members of the AIDS Lobby had intentionally packed the meeting so that there could be no consensus and so there would be no possibility that the blood test could be used to bring the epidemic under control.

The San Francisco Sentinel, a gay publication, quoted Paul Boneberg of the Mobilization Against AIDS as saying, "I think the issue of mandatory testing is dead." He called the meeting at the CDC, "The Gettysburg of the AIDS testing issue." He went on to say, "There were certain people who advocated mandatory testing, but they were not willing to stand up in opposition to the overwhelming majority."

Indeed, there had been only two people at the meeting who had been willing to put up their hands to support mandatory premarital and prenatal testing.

Representatives of the National Gay Task Force, the National Gay Rights Advocates, the LAMBDA Legal Defense and the ARC/AIDS Vigil were there, working together to influence the conference. "We had a hell of an effect," said Boneberg. "A highly effective job was done by all the concerned groups."[4]

At that meeting, Dr. James Curran, Director of the CDC AIDS Activities Committee, stated that there were already a million and a half Americans who were believed to be infected. He went on to say that:

> One in every one hundred and sixty Americans is infected with HIV disease. Nationally, one in every eighty males is infected. In states with a high prevalence of AIDS, such as California and New York, one in every thirty men is infected. When only men between ages 30 and 39 are counted in such high prevalence states, one in nine is infected.

Yet faced with an epidemic of this proportion, the bureaucrats at the CDC bowed to the organized efforts of the militant homosexuals and their supporters who attended that February meeting in Atlanta. Although there were a few public health officers who spoke out in support of expanding the use of blood testing, most bureaucrats shrank from the vicious attack of their opponents and accepted the status quo. Screening of our population was not to be used to try to stop the spread of HIV disease.

March 1987

On March 8, an editorial appeared in the San Francisco Examiner condemning the idea that we should be using the blood test to try to stop the epidemic.

Mandatory testing before marriage makes little economic or scientific sense as it would affect few in the high risk categories of gay men and intravenous drug users. Required testing upon hospital admission would tend to keep high risk groups away. Hospital workers are not considered at risk for unknown AIDS exposure.

Of course, the writer of the editorial must have realized that premarital blood testing was not aimed at identifying gay men or intravenous drug users who were getting married. Premarital blood testing was an effort to try to stop the spread of disease into the heterosexual population. Such meaningless arguments would become increasingly commonplace in the months and years that lay ahead and serve to confuse the public as to the real issue.

Early in March, Dr. James Mason appeared before the House Energy Committee in Washington, D. C., to defend the government's policy of not requiring the reporting of people who tested positive for the AIDS virus.

There are too many examples of the wrong people finding out and taking discriminatory action against those infected with the AIDS virus.....Although reporting is desirable, until there are ways to protect confidentiality and avoid discrimination, it is irrational to call for reporting of AIDS infection.

Of course, Dr. James Mason was unable to offer any examples of people whose name had been reported to public health officers, in confidence, where that information had been made public. But Doctor Mason somehow had to defend the CDC's failure to treat HIV disease as if it was a disease. Thus, he made a totally unfounded accusation stating: "There are too many examples of the wrong people finding out and taking discriminatory action against those infected with the AIDS virus."

It would be two years after Dr. Mason made that statement in 1987 that I visited the Centers for Disease Control in Atlanta in April of 1989. At that time, I asked Dr. James Curran if he could give me **even one**

example of any person in America with HIV disease whose disease status had been reported to a public health officer in confidence where that information had been released resulting in discrimination. What was his response?

"That is a very good question. A Congressman asked that same question on the floor of the House of Representatives just a few weeks ago."

"But can you give me any examples that you know of, Doctor Curran?" I persisted.

"Well, of course, we don't monitor that sort of thing and I don't personally know of any such cases," was his response.

Doctor Mason's remarks in March of 1987 simply were not true, but so much of what has been said before congressional committees, to the media and the public has not been true. Bureaucrats must survive, and if that means that they have to distort the truth, then they will give misleading testimony. In government service, the name of the game is survival, not integrity. As a result of misinformation disseminated by public health officers, the disease continues to spread, the dying and the death continues.

✻✻✻

In every state and most communities across America, AIDS task forces have been formed. Tragically, these AIDS task forces are usually dominated by gay activists and members of the AIDS Lobby. As a result, the information released by these task forces is biased in favor of the gay position. That is why what happened in Santa Cruz, California, in early 1987 was so unusual.

Our county medical society formed its own AIDS task force made up of physicians with no homosexuals or AIDS activists as members. By early 1987, Larimore Cummins had given up his computer business and returned to the full-time practice of gastroenterology. Increasingly concerned with the course of the epidemic, he and two other physicians organized the Santa Cruz County Medical Society AIDS Task Force. The task force came up with a 3 point program which was submitted as a resolution to the March meeting of the House of Delegates. This program included:

1. Mandatory premarital and prenatal HIV testing.
2. Modifying consent and confidentiality requirements for HIV

testing so that they would be in line with blood testing for every other disease.

3. Providing sufficient funding for public health contact tracing.

In early March, 1987, I closed my office and flew to Anaheim in Southern California to attend the annual meeting of the CMA House of Delegates. However, 1987 was not to be the same as 1986. This time there was an organized plan of action. In 1986, I had been poorly informed about the implications of the HIV epidemic. By 1987, there was a legitimate AIDS task force from our medical society which was submitting a resolution. That resolution had been thoughtfully conceived to address the major issues.

In addition, I was also presenting one of my own resolutions which asked the CMA to accept HIV disease as an infectious, contagious, communicable, sexually transmitted disease. Since that had been the message of the LaRouche Initiative which the CMA, CNA, CHA, UAPD, CDA, ACLU and the CPUSA had all opposed, I felt it would be advantageous to have the CMA take a position that they looked upon HIV disease as a disease, independent of Lyndon LaRouche's quarantine rhetoric. Once HIV disease was legally accepted, standard public health techniques could be utilized to prevent its further spread.

However, the most important part of the plan had nothing to do with my actions but involved Larimore Cummins. As Chairman of the Santa Cruz County Medical Society AIDS Task Force, Larimore had gone to Sacramento and established a liaison with State Senator John Doolittle. Senator Doolittle was a bright, young, conservative Republican who was a rising star in Republican politics in the State of California. Later that year, the Senator became Chairman of the Senate Republican caucus when veteran State Senator H. L. Richardson decided to withdraw from political life.

Larimore and Dr. Leff (an internist from Santa Cruz) had been invited to testify before the Senate Health Committee the day after the CMA House of Delegates was scheduled to discuss the epidemic. It was vitally important to our plan that the House support an aggressive approach to the epidemic.

It was obvious from the way that AB3667 had been handled by CMA lobbyists in 1986 that the small clique which held the reigns of power had no intention of following the dictates of the House. They had their own agenda. But if there was someone in Sacramento who could present the positions of the House to the legislature, independent of CMA lobbyists, perhaps we could begin bringing some logic to the insanity which seemed to have engulfed our state and nation.

Two weeks preceding the meeting, I sent a personal letter to every delegate asking them to back the resolution submitted by the Santa Cruz County Medical Society AIDS Task Force.

There was an air of excitement at the House of Delegates meeting. Everyone was talking about the epidemic. Of course, in those days, most doctors looked upon the disease as "AIDS" because of the coordinated effort within the media and medical publications to confuse the issue.

Most doctors were not thinking clearly about the fact that the disease was really HIV disease and that AIDS statistics, offered to the public on a regular basis, were simply presented to give the impression that the CDC was monitoring the spread of the illness. By March 1987, the number of AIDS cases was doubling every 13 months and had increased from 14,049 in October 1985 to 28,098 by December 1986.

The initial introductory meeting of the House of Delegates was on Saturday morning. There was an air of joviality as the ruling hierarchy of the CMA went through the steps of giving the impression that the House was a democratic organization and that members would soon be voting on important issues. Of course that really wasn't true but members had to believe that — or so many physicians would not have taken a week out of their busy practices to attend the yearly meetings.

By mid-morning we had broken up and gone to our respective reference committees.

It was that morning that I heard the tragic story of Doctor Seymour Albin, an orthopedic surgeon practicing in Southern California. I have alluded to his story in Chapter 2 of Book 1. In essence, Doctor Albin was asked to examine a patient. The patient's medical condition was deteriorating and Doctor Albin assumed that it might be because the patient had AIDS. He ran a series of blood tests, including an HIV test. Because Dr. Albin's lab technician knew the patient's name, a $250,000.00 law suit was lodged which was settled out of court for $25,000.00. As Doctor Albin said in his resolution:

> WHEREAS, Section 199.21 of the Health and Safety Code absolutely forbids the disclosure of a patient's condition as AIDS antibody positive; and
>
> WHEREAS, The law established penalties of a fine of up to $10,000.00 and imprisonment of up to one year in the county jail for

disclosure to any person including a physician; and

WHEREAS, Litigants ordinarily relinquish confidentiality of past injury, disease or medical treatment, except AIDS exposure; and

WHEREAS, AIDS infection can contribute to disability; and

WHEREAS, Physicians testifying under oath as to the reason for a patient's disability are violating the present law if disclosure of a positive AIDS test is revealed; now, therefore, be it

RESOLVED: That the California Medical Association encourage the state legislature to amend Section 199.21 of the Health and Safety Code to allow physicians reporting or testifying in personal injury litigation to reveal, with immunity, the presence of a positive AIDS antibody test if it is the physician's opinion that this is a factor contributing to the patient's disability.

Doctor Albin was one of the first speakers at reference committee G on Saturday morning. His plea for a logical approach to HIV antibody testing was opposed by a series of speakers who contended that the confidentiality of HIV test results was far more important than a physician's responsibility to do what was right or proper. Each speaker, in turn, reiterated that complete confidentiality was absolutely imperative if we were going to begin addressing the epidemic and stop its spread.

Then my Resolution (704-87) was presented. It simply stated:

Be it RESOLVED: That the California Medical Association advocate handling infection with the AIDS HIV virus as with any other communicable disease.

CMA leaders placed a notation at the bottom of my resolution stating:

CMA recognizes AIDS has reached epidemic proportions...CMA...opposed the LaRouche Initiative which called for quarantine and isolation of people with AIDS or ARC related conditions and maintains that providing accurate information and educating individuals about the proven modes of transmission and the risk factors **was the only reasonable, practical way to control the spread of AIDS.** (emphasis added)

The motive behind the CMA's statement was to equate my resolution with the LaRouche Initiative and with quarantine. Furthermore, they wanted to convince the delegates that there was no place for the use of accepted public health techniques in controlling the epidemic.

An AIDS activist from Santa Clara County was one of the first speakers at the microphone. I remember his remarks quite well.

How can the California Medical Association say that HIV is a communicable disease? If we said that it is a communicable disease, we would have to treat it as we do other diseases...of course it is a communicable disease but we must not deal with it as we do with other communicable diseases because it is different from other diseases.

His arguments were really quite irrational. Yet, that same physician was at the microphones in 1988, 1989, and again in 1990 at the CMA Conventions, speaking against dealing with HIV disease as a disease. He preceded me at the microphones at the 5th International Conference on AIDS in Montreal in June 1989 — always arguing adamantly that we must not address HIV as a disease — even though it was a disease.

※※※

It was that same morning that I first encountered Dr. Mervyn Silverman. He is one of the key players in the tragic drama of this epidemic. Small in stature with graying hair and a neatly trimmed, gray beard, he has gained national notoriety as "The man who closed the gay bathhouses in San Francisco." However, public perception, many times, has little to do with what really transpired.

Doctor Silverman had been the public health director in San Francisco when the first cases of HIV disease were reported. Because of the large numbers of homosexuals living there, that city was very soon inundated with young men dying of AIDS. According to Randy Shilts, Dianne Feinstein, the Mayor of San Francisco, told Doctor Silverman in the fall of 1982 that gay bathhouses should be closed to prevent further spread of the disease, but Silverman used excuse after excuse to avoid closing them.

Silverman obviously didn't want to offend gay leaders. He suggested that bathhouses should be used as centers for education and that it would be best to keep them open so that educational material could be disseminated to the homosexual population on the dangers of rectal intercourse, fisting, rimming, oral intercourse, golden showers, water games, multiple sexual partners and the exchange of body fluids. Bathhouses in San Francisco were also to voluntarily limit "unsafe sex practices."

Responsible members of the homosexual community increasingly came to recognize that bathhouse customers were disseminating the infection. Since homosexuality is a compulsive, addictive, sexual dysfunction, education alone was not going to change the addictive nature of the condition any more than education had been able to eliminate obesity, tobacco smoking, alcoholism or the use of drugs. Indeed, after 25 years of education on the dangers of tobacco, the incidence of smoking has only been cut in half.

In 1982, we did not have 25 years to spend on education trying to stop the epidemic. In 1982, drastic action should have been taken. Time and again responsible homosexuals pleaded with the Health Director to close the bathhouses, but Doctor Silverman could always find justification for not carrying out this medically sound action.

Finally, Doctor Silverman did agree to shut down the bathhouses if there was consensus among homosexual leaders. When he was attacked by one of San Francisco's homosexual newspapers for suggesting that it might be appropriate to close the bathhouses, Dr. Silverman immediately backed down. Instead of ordering the bathhouses to shut down, he called a press conference and asked for a vote of the audience as to whether or not they favored bathhouse closure.

It wasn't until months later, in the fall of 1984, under pressure from Mayor Dianne Feinstein and homosexual Supervisor Harry Britt and a large segment of the concerned homosexual leadership that Dr. Silverman finally decided to close the bathhouses. His action was precipitated in part by a report he received from undercover agents sent to the bathhouses to see if they were actually limiting unsafe sexual practices.

The report that Dr. Silverman received described what was going on in the bathhouses in late 1984. The investigators reported that they witnessed "A man clad only in a cowboy hat and a cowboy vest, being orally copulated by two men who alternated between oral copulation and licking his thighs." A crowd of onlookers stood by and the two copulators alternated between the man wearing the cowboy hat and the crowd. At the end of the sex act, "It appeared that one of the participants swallowed the semen and then went off in search of other entertainment."[5]

Apparently that was too much for even Mervyn Silverman. He moved, shortly thereafter, to close the gay bathhouses...and then to resign from his position as health director. The tragedy was that for over two years, after the facts had become obvious that HIV disease was transmitted by sexual promiscuity among homosexuals in bathhouses, Mervyn Silverman left them open, waiting for members of the gay community to unify and ask him to close them.

During those years, hundreds, perhaps thousands, of gay young men became infected unnecessarily because a public health officer failed to carry out his assigned task to safeguard and protect the public health.

After leaving the San Francisco Department of Public Health, Mervyn Silverman became a celebrity, associating with Elizabeth Taylor and other film stars who had been friends of Rock Hudson. Doctor Silverman soon became President of the American Foundation for AIDS Research, a San Francisco based AIDS educational organization. Merv Silverman was active with public health organizations all across America, working to convince public health officials that we should turn our backs on traditional methods of approaching this epidemic and simply use education to try to stop its spread. Silverman was a member of the CMA AIDS Task Force and for years used his influence there to thwart my resolutions.

When Mervyn comes up to a microphone he usually introduces himself and lists all his titles, including his position as former health officer of San Francisco, his membership on the CMA AIDS Task Force, the fact he was President of the American Foundation for AIDS Research and a Director of the Robert Woods Johnson Foundation, etc. Such impressive credentials serve to awe the members of the reference committee and intimidate his opponents.

That morning, Dr. Silverman spoke about the importance of addressing the epidemic intelligently. He emphasized that physicians needed only two things. They needed research and education. Education was the method by which physicians were going to stop the spread of this epidemic. Education would be the key. Any efforts to use standard public health techniques, as had traditionally been used, would drive infected patients away from physicians and drive the disease underground.

I watched this short, immaculately dressed, distinguished looking man with his gray hair and beard. He was a formidable figure and obviously a formidable opponent but I knew that he was wrong. Though I was only a small-town orthopedic surgeon with no public health credentials, there was no question that Silverman was wrong.

It would be two and a half years later when many members of the public health establishment in America would stop following Mervyn Silverman's dictates and begin advocating exactly what I advocated in 1987 — that we begin addressing HIV disease as an infectious disease.

In the meantime, hundreds of thousands of Americans would become infected, unnecessarily.

When it came my turn to speak I simply stated that epidemics were traditionally controlled by identifying the people who were infected and attempting to prevent them from transmitting the disease to others. It was for that reason that HIV disease must be legally accepted as a disease.

I went on to present Resolution 735-87, the program of our county medical society task force. Members of the Gay and AIDS Lobbies were there to attack my resolutions as homophobic and to attack my motives and integrity.

Unlike any other reference committee at any meeting of the CMA before or since, the committee chairman allowed so much time for discussion from the floor that most of my other resolutions could not be addressed. The rules of the CMA stated that if no one spoke to a resolution, it could not be considered on the floor of the House. Never before nor since that day has any chairman refused to allow all the resolutions to be presented and discussed but then the issue of AIDS was not a normal issue.

As the meeting drew to a close it became obvious that I was not to be allowed to discuss my other resolutions. That would make them ineligible for presentation to the House. Therefore, at the end of the morning, I stood up and simply listed my resolutions and stated that I was speaking to all of them so that they could be brought before the House the following week.

Then we waited until Monday morning. I couldn't help but wonder how the CMA hierarchy would deal with a resolution that stated:

> Be it RESOLVED: That the California Medical Association advocate handling infection with the AIDS HIV virus as with any other communicable disease.

I had placed the CMA hierarchy in an impossible position or so I thought. They had come out savagely and deceptively against the LaRouche Initiative — which also declared HIV as an infectious disease. It was obvious that there were those within the hierarchy who opposed public health reporting and contact tracing. What would they do with my resolution?

On Monday afternoon, with reporters from all over California present, the major issue was AIDS (the HIV epidemic).

In response to my resolution the reference committee had substituted the following:

> Be it RESOLVED: That CMA policy recognize that AIDS is a communicable disease which is not casually transmitted and should be subject to the proven methods of communicable disease control which are appropriate for it: and be it further RESOLVED: That CMA continue to encourage counseling and voluntary HIV testing.

I moved to the microphone to clarify what was meant by the term, "proven methods of communicable disease control which are appropriate for it." I wanted to ask what was "appropriate" for dealing with the epidemic.

Before I could be recognized the Speaker of the House, Dr. Corlin, called upon a physician from Sacramento. It has always been accepted that a speaker on the floor would have 3 minutes to address an issue; however, in an obvious effort to limit debate and discussion on AIDS resolutions, the delegate from Sacramento said:

"We feel that because of the volume of work before the House at this time, it is in the interest of the House to limit debate to 2 minutes per member on all AIDS related issues."

Doctor Corlin immediately called for a "second" and then the vote. I moved to the microphone and called a "point of order." The following is the transcript of the exchange to show how my challenge was handled.

A Delegate: Do we have a right to talk about this? Because I think it is a very important issue. I think it is an obvious effort to limit debate on what I think is the most vital issue before our nation today.

Speaker: Thank you, very much. As many of you are in favor of the 2 minute limit on debate, say AYE. As many of you are opposed, say NO. We shall conduct the AIDS related debate based upon a 2-minute limit.

And so it was that the leadership of the CMA cleverly limited debate to 2 minutes without an opportunity for discussion. This insured that there would be no effective debate on my resolutions. Before I could move back to the microphone, Doctor Corlin called for the vote on 704-87 and it was passed. Although the amended resolution sounded very close to my original resolution, it had been subtly altered so that, in effect, it said, "The methods of communicable disease control for AIDS disease would be those which are appropriate for it."

Since the AIDS Lobby and the CMA AIDS Task Force (dominated

by Mervyn Silverman) did not feel that **any** standard public health techniques should be used in the general population, what, in effect, the House voted to support was that physicians should **not** use standard testing and contact tracing to try to stop the epidemic. Furthermore, they had changed the entire thrust of my resolution for my resolution dealt with HIV disease. The reference committee had deleted "HIV" and the House voted to consider AIDS as a disease. In 1987, AIDS was already listed as a disease under existing public health law. Of course, most of the members of the House did not realize what had happened and they certainly did not realize just how clever the opposition had been in using parliamentary techniques, deceit and sophistry to negate the will of the majority.

The next major series of resolutions dealt with consent and confidentiality requirements for testing. The original resolution dealt with deleting the written requirement for consent to testing. The resolutions committee substituted the following resolution:

> Be it RESOLVED: The CMA seek to delete legal requirements for consent to HIV testing which are more extensive than requirements generally imposed for **informed consent** to medical care...be it further
>
> RESOLVED: That CMA seek necessary legislative changes to provide that the results of a positive HIV test may be made available on a confidential basis to the physicians involved in caring for a patient; and, be it further...(emphasis added)

This resolution seemed very straightforward but you should note that the reference committee had substituted **informed consent** for **written consent**. For a physician to administer an informed consent could be far more time consuming and difficult than getting a written consent. This was simply another subtle effort on the part of the AIDS Lobby to prevent testing. Furthermore, allowing physicians to release information on test results to other physicians still left the threat of a $10,000.00 fine and a year imprisonment hanging over the head of any doctor who notified a nurse of a patient's infection.

After a rather extended debate this resolution was also passed.

The next resolution proposed that HIV disease should be reportable to public health officers as was the case with 58 other diseases in California. Doctor Mervyn Silverman responded:

"I think...what this new resolution does is totally subvert what has been passed prior to this. It means that when you have a positive antibody test you can go and report it to the Health Department. I would like to urge you to vote against this…"

And so it was that Mervyn Silverman once again came out firmly against making HIV disease reportable to public health officials.

The reference committee recommended that the majority of my other resolutions not be presented, thus preventing their discussion.

The last major issue that was brought up was the resolution by the Santa Cruz County AIDS Task Force calling for mandatory premarital and prenatal HIV antibody screening and for public health follow-up and contact tracing of patients with HIV infection. The reference committee had modified those recommendations to propose the following:

> Be it RESOLVED: The CMA encourage voluntary premarital and prenatal HIV screening; and be it further
> RESOLVED: That CMA support adequate funding so that local public health officials may carry out contact tracing for HIV infected individuals where appropriate, with attention to confidentiality and counseling. (emphasis added)

The problem with the second resolution was that the existing confidentiality restrictions of AB403 prevented physicians from reporting HIV cases to public health officials. Furthermore, the insertion of the words "where appropriate" totally emasculated the thrust of the second resolve. Did "where appropriate" mean that we were not going to try to stop spread of disease in the homosexual community? Did it mean that we were not going to try to stop spread of disease in the heterosexual community? Where was it appropriate to do contact tracing and where was it not appropriate?

With other sexually transmitted diseases, public health departments did contact tracing on all cases. With HIV disease, contact tracing was only to be done "where appropriate."

Why not have mandatory premarital HIV screening? After all, we were not going to be identifying homosexuals. What was wrong with mandatory prenatal screening? It was mandated by law in California that every newborn be tested for phenylketonuria, hypothyroidism, galactosemia and tyrosinuria and the CMA had supported mandatory neonatal blood testing despite the fact that physicians usually found only perhaps 6 cases of phenylketonuria, 16 cases of hypothyroidism and only a rare case of galactosemia or tyrosinuria in the entire state each year. No one had ever opposed mandatory testing of newborns for those rare diseases, so why object to mandatory prenatal HIV testing? After all, the objective was to save lives and try to stop the epidemic.

At the microphone, I moved to substitute the word **mandatory** for voluntary premarital screening and said:

"Premarital blood testing is well tried. It was used in the days before we had penicillin for syphilis. What we are doing is protecting the partner. We are protecting the unborn child. It is...(a)...basic fundamental of public health."

A number of delegates spoke in support of my amendment.

Initially it seemed that the house would override the reference committee. Then Dr. Silverman said:

We have said early on and voted unanimously that we want to maintain confidentiality, maintain voluntary testing and encourage that kind of testing. This is a step backward. My colleague, Monteith, has some mistakes. There is no mandatory testing anywhere in the United States, premarital or otherwise, for AIDS. The National Academy of Science, the Institute of Medicine, the CDC and the Surgeon General, all three groups and individuals have come out against mandatory testing. What you do when you do this is to drive it underground. As physicians, I think we have an obligation to encourage, and we should encourage, voluntary testing at every site: family planning; maternal and child care; premarital; prenatal; wherever we are in contact with patients who may have been **involved in high risk behavior.** The way in which we can do this is to make sure we have the trust of the patient and **confidentiality...** where we have that trust, I think we ought to maximize that. We keep eliminating the fact that we should have a very good relationship with our patients. Let's maintain that rather than bring in some obligatory type of testing which will **drive this whole thing underground.**" (emphasis added)

At that point a series of delegates rose to support Dr. Silverman, several of whom I recognized as being members of the Gay and AIDS Lobby. The subject then turned to prenatal testing.

Speakers rose to quote the position of the AMA which wanted only voluntary premarital and prenatal testing in **high risk patients.** Speakers, who on other occasions, supported mandatory wearing of seat belts, wearing of helmets for motorcycle riders, use of car seats for young children and mandatory testing and vaccination for a number of other diseases — all these speakers spoke against mandatory premarital and prenatal testing for HIV disease. One speaker attacked me personally, suggesting that I only wanted mandatory prenatal testing in order to encourage abortion because what else was there to offer an HIV-infected mother other than killing her unborn child? Of course nothing could be further from my mind, but the technique of attacking an individual is often used to draw attention away from a valid issue.

It came my turn to speak. I tried to stress that prenatal testing was necessary so that physicians could find out when the child became infected. Certainly many children were infected by transmission of disease across the placental barrier but were some of the children infected passing through the birth canal covered with their mother's blood? What percentage of children were infected from nursing? These were all questions that were unanswered in 1987. The only way physicians could discover the answers and begin to protect unborn children was to know which mothers were infected before the birth of their children.

Doctor Silverman then spoke. He said:

> I want to clarify Dr. Monteith's statements. There have been studies done. Babies that were born by C-section or vaginally showed up with seropositivity, so there seems to be no question that it is a transplacental infection that takes place. I don't really know any mother who would knowingly want to infect her unborn child. I get back to the point I made before that I think we keep losing sight of — that it is the relationship that we have with our patients and how important it is to encourage testing if we think that individual has been involved in **high risk behavior**. Mandatory testing...the only thing that this will do is possibly **drive away the very people we wish to test.**"

Dr. Silverman carried the day. Mandatory premarital and prenatal testing were voted down. The House voted in favor of voluntary testing.

✳✳✳

I moved from my seat to the back of the auditorium, feeling half sick. Admittedly, I had gotten through some of my resolutions but how many people would still contract the disease from marrying their untested sexual partner? How many more children would contract the disease from nursing? When would physicians be allowed to begin to stop this plague?

In the back of the auditorium that afternoon, several things happened.

First of all, a secretary from the San Francisco office of the CMA informed me that a local television producer had asked if I would be willing to appear the following morning. He was going to have several dignitaries and wanted me as well, since the press had reported that I was leading the drive to have HIV disease dealt with in the same manner as other diseases.

I was given the name of the producer and asked if I would call. Within 5 minutes, the secretary was back, this time somewhat flustered. She said that she had been instructed to tell me that the television producer had changed his mind and already had another guest. I thanked her for the information but had the feeling that someone in the CMA office did not want me to have an opportunity to present my views to the public.

I quickly called the television producer. He was waiting for my call and invited me to appear the following morning along with State Senator John Doolittle and Assemblyman Roos, a Democratic leader of the California State Assembly, second only to Willie Brown in power and influence.

I readily accepted the invitation, smiling to myself with the realization that someone in the CMA hierarchy would be very distressed to find that I was now going to be able to address a public forum without a two minute time limit imposed.

That incident only confirmed my conviction that there were those highly placed within the CMA, intent upon using any technique, no matter how devious, to block a free and open discussion of effective methods of controlling the epidemic.

The other important event that afternoon occurred when a neatly dressed young man approached me and introduced himself. He was an administrative assistant to Congressman William Dannemeyer and had been sent to the convention to find out what positions the CMA would take on consent, confidentiality, contact tracing, premarital and prenatal testing. It was obvious from our conversation that the Congressman was well informed and was interested in trying to stop the epidemic. Although I did not realize the significance of that meeting, many of the events that followed in the years ahead came as a direct result of our conversation that March afternoon.

❋❋❋

Monday evening I sat in my hotel room alone and dejected. I had failed. I had been unable to get through the resolution requiring mandatory premarital and prenatal testing. The House had accepted voluntary testing but that would not solve the problem. The House had voted in favor of considering AIDS as an infectious disease but my resolution dealt with HIV disease, not AIDS. AIDS was already considered a disease by state law.

In addition, the reference committee had added the proviso that physicians would deal with the disease "as appropriate"...whatever that meant. I suspected, and rightly so, that the addition was simply another delaying tactic, a clever ploy to prevent the use of public health measures.

The House had voted for contact tracing "where appropriate." Was that another clever ploy of the AIDS Lobby? We had voted to replace written consent with informed consent. Most of the members of the House did not realize that because of the legal definition of "informed consent" they had voted to make testing even more difficult.

The phone rang and a quiet, familiar voice was on the line.

"How did they vote? What did you get through?"

It was Larimore. He was calling from Sacramento where he was preparing to appear before the Senate Health Committee the following day. I told him exactly what had been accepted by the House. I also told him of my disappointment and frustration.

"You saved more lives today than you'll ever save practicing medicine," he said in his quiet, confident manner. "If the CMA accepted voluntary testing, they have accepted the concept of routine testing. I can say that the CMA has accepted the concept of voluntary, routine testing. With routine testing, anyone has the right to refuse. I can present the decision of the CMA just that way. The CMA has come out strongly in favor of testing, but wants it done voluntarily with patients having the right to decline. You did a great job."

Those may not be his exact words but that was the conversation as close as I can remember. I do remember feeling that perhaps I was not quite such a failure.

※※※

At the television studio the following morning, I had my first opportunity to meet two of the most important players in the legislative battles that were being waged in Sacramento.

Senator John Doolittle was tall, thin and youthful in appearance. His dark hair was smoothed down immaculately over the top of his head and neatly parted on one side. His boyish face was long and thin with distinctive features. His clothing was conservative. He looked every bit the part of a successful politician. Assemblyman Roos was short in stature with a full head of bushy hair. I met him in the make-up room. He seemed to be consumed with combing his hair over and over to make sure he would look just right. Whenever a young woman from the studio staff came to speak to him, he fixed her with his gaze, grinned broadly and gave her his complete attention. As soon as she was gone he was once again busy combing his hair, posing in front of the mirrors.

I shall have to admit that in speaking to him briefly, I had the feeling that he was a man who had one goal in life. That was to push forward the career of Assemblyman Roos. He probably had dreams of becoming a congressman or senator one day. Certainly, with his handsome profile and full head of hair, he had all the television attributes needed for a successful politician but I sensed a shallowness of character as I watched him fawn over each woman who spoke to him.

We were ushered into the studio. Senator Doolittle sat at the far right with Assemblyman Roos to his left. I sat to the left of the Assemblyman and a small, slightly built, public health officer sat to my left. The public health officer obviously supported the positions of the AIDS Lobby but whether or not he was a political activist, I do not know.

I don't remember all the details of the program but I do remember the discussion on HIV testing. Assemblyman Roos kept emphasizing that the HIV blood test was so inaccurate that it could not be used for widespread testing. He went on to say that ELISA testing gave almost 50% false-positive results. When I challenged him on his statistics, he drew himself tall in his seat and pontificated:

"I was in Washington, D. C. just last week talking to Surgeon General Koop. The Surgeon General assured me that the HIV antibody test was often inaccurate and that as many as half the initial positive tests were false positives."

That television broadcast was being shown live throughout Southern California and this was the area which Roos represented in the State Legislature. I am sure he was doing everything he could to appear as well informed on the subject of HIV testing as he possibly could in an effort to impress his constituents.

I looked over at Roos, then straight into the television camera and said,

"Either Surgeon General Koop doesn't understand the antibody test or you misunderstood him. The series of HIV antibody tests that we use are the single most accurate series of tests ever devised by physicians in an effort to diagnose disease. The tests are well over 99.5% accurate if properly performed. The test almost never misses a case unless the patient is in the "window" and virtually never comes up with a false positive if the full series of tests are done. That is why it is so important that we start using HIV testing to begin saving lives."

The host turned to the public health officer and asked his opinion. He stammered and more or less agreed with my statement. I could feel Roos bristling next to me, knowing that many of his constituents had heard my challenge to his irresponsible statements. However, that did not influence him. As one of the leaders of the Democrat majority he kept insisting that physicians should not be using routine testing to begin to bring the epidemic under control.

At the end of the interview, the Assemblyman glanced at me angrily, turned and stalked out of the room. It was then that I had my first opportunity to talk to Senator Doolittle.

Senator Doolittle was impressive. He was intelligent, young and aggressive. He understood the epidemic and the importance of trying to identify those who were infected in order to break the chain of transmission. It was that initial meeting with the Senator that began to move me towards the political arena, an arena in which I had no desire to be involved.

It was on Wednesday afternoon just before the House Delegates adjourned that copies of the new official CMA policy on HIV disease were distributed to the delegates. It was called the "CMA White Paper" and it outlined an effective program to begin to combat the epidemic. Although not exactly what I had hoped for, it was a tremendous stride forward in our efforts to counteract the effects of AB403.

The new program allowed physicians to tell other physicians of a patient's infection and it substituted informed consent for written consent. Tragically, most of the delegates did not recognize that substituting "informed consent" for "written consent" was designed to make testing even more difficult.

The White Paper mentioned Resolution 735-87 (from the Santa Cruz County AIDS Task Force) and stated that the CMA supported voluntary premarital, prenatal and perinatal HIV screening, as well as adequate funding "so that local public health officials may carry out contact tracing for HIV infected individuals **where appropriate...**"

The paper concluded with a reference to my Resolution 704-87 affirming that "CMA policy recognizes that AIDS is a communicable disease which is not casually transmitted and should be subject to those proven methods of communicable disease control **which are appropriate for it.**" (See Appendix IV for the full text of the CMA White Paper.)

As I left the Orange County Airport on Wednesday afternoon, I was assured by a member of the CMA Executive Committee that new legislation was already being written and that legislation would soon be introduced in Sacramento to begin to carry out the directives of the House. At last, I felt that I had finally accomplished something worthwhile, something that would begin to have an impact upon the epidemic.

As I mounted the stairs to my waiting airplane, I again had a feeling of satisfaction and accomplishment. I really believed, at that point, that the CMA was going to begin moving towards a logical approach to the epidemic. After all, the CMA White Paper outlined a program that we could all live with. But then, in 1987, I was still incredibly naive. I had forgotten the old Chinese proverb:

> If a man deceive me once, shame on him.
> If a man deceive me twice, shame on me.

I had been deceived a second time. In the days and months that lay ahead I would come to realize that the words of the leaders of the CMA had little to do with their intentions, for there were those within the hierarchy who were dedicated to preventing physicians from addressing this epidemic as a communicable, infectious, sexually transmitted disease.

In March of 1987, I did not realize that the saga of the AIDS epidemic was the story of malice and mistakes, illusion and delusion, deceit and deception, and of dying and death. I still believed that if the House of Delegates voted overwhelmingly on this issue, the CMA hierarchy would not dare to actively lobby against those positions a second time. I was soon to become increasingly disillusioned as I recognized my error.

---

1. In 1986, Doctor Mervyn Silverman, the former Public Health Director for San Francisco, was the dominant force on the CMA Committee on AIDS and sexually transmitted disease.

2. MMWR — December 12, 1986.

3. In 1988, the UAPD did allow me to present a resolution in support of the concept of the Gann Initiative and it was accepted by the representatives of the union. Thus, the UAPD was the only medical organization in California to support the Gann Initiative. Tragically, the UAPD never publicized its position.

4. San Francisco Sentinel — February 27, 1987.

5. *Private Acts, Social Consequences; AIDS and The Politics of Public Health* by Ronald Bayer (The Free Press, McMillan, Inc., p. 44)

CHAPTER THREE

March, 1987

After the ill-fated meeting at the CDC in Atlanta, in February, the CDC appointed a special 20 member panel to develop a policy on routine premarital and prenatal testing. In March, that committee reported their conclusions. The report stated that there should be no mandatory testing in our nation. They stated that voluntary use of HIV testing, accompanied by counseling and safeguards to protect confidentiality, would prevent further spread of the epidemic. They recommended that testing be done in sexually transmitted disease clinics and in clinics where patients were receiving treatments for drug dependence; women attending public prenatal clinics should be "offered" testing, but the panel **opposed** routine testing of **marriage license applicants, pregnant women** and **hospital inpatients.** The panel noted that they had heard "of a wide variety of breaches of confidentiality." They emphasized the danger of discrimination and they called for antidiscrimination laws. The panel wanted HIV testing **only in high risk groups** and actively opposed any measures to try to stop the spread of the epidemic into the heterosexual population. As a direct result of these policies, the epidemic continued its silent spread.

✳✳✳

In March 1987, the CDC reported that over 31,000 people had been diagnosed with AIDS and they predicted that within five years (by the end of 1991) 270,000 Americans would develop AIDS and 179,000 would die. In March 1987, the World Health Organization announced that there were over 100,000 AIDS cases reported world wide.

✳✳✳

In West Germany, a U. S. Army Sergeant was arrested by German authorities in Nuremberg for having intercourse with several sexual partners without warning them of the fact that he had AIDS. The man was charged under a law that prohibited causing bodily harm.[1] On the other hand, in California, a plan to place legal restrictions on people who were spreading the disease (i.e., prostitutes, IV drug users and those people who were intentionally spreading the disease) was bitterly criticized. In San Francisco, the Associate Director of Public Health said that such a plan would "give out exactly the wrong message" to the general public about AIDS and effective means of controlling it. He suggested that those spreading the disease would be better treated by "counseling." Of course, the San Francisco Public Health Officer did not comment on what society should do after a patient had been tested and counseled and continued spreading the disease.

※※※

In India, in 1987, African students were required to have HIV testing before entering the country. In South Korea, foreigners entering the country were required to have HIV tests. All throughout the world, countries moved to protect themselves from the epidemic, but not America.

※※※

A report was released in March by researchers from the Palo Alto Medical Foundation and the University of California in San Francisco, suggesting that the economic cost of the AIDS epidemic by 1991 would be 66.4 billion dollars in lost personal income due to illness and premature death.

※※※

It was late in March 1987 that the National Gay Rights Advocates (NGRA) headquartered in San Francisco issued a report condemning the policies adopted by the CMA House of Delegates. NGRA objected to the suggestion that the consent and confidentiality requirements for HIV testing were to be partially brought into line with requirements for other diseases. The NGRA report stated that modifying consent and confidentiality requirements would "turn doctors into police and would cause those people most in need of medical advice and education to avoid physicians altogether." According to Benjamin Schatz, Director of NGRA's AIDS Civil Rights project, "The fear is that less stringent controls of HIV test results would lead to blacklisting and discrimination." Furthermore, Schatz went on to say that "Any move to change consent and confidentiality requirements represented an abandonment of...doctors' responsibility to protect the public health."

※※※

April 1987
The American Medical Association announced that it was sponsoring a meeting on AIDS in Chicago. The Santa Cruz County Medical Society

Board of Governors voted to appropriate $1,000.00 to send one of our members to voice the concerns of our doctors to the physicians of the nation. Our Board of Governors picked Dr. Arnold Leff to present our concerns. Doctor Leff had impeccable credentials as a public health officer, having served on the staff in the Nixon White House, as the public health officer in Cincinnati and later, in Contra Costa County, California. In recent years, Dr. Leff had left government service and was practicing internal medicine in Santa Cruz where he sub-specialized in the care of AIDS patients. He was a member of a number of public health organizations. More than that, he was a dedicated liberal who could never be accused of being reactionary. He believed in the implementation of antidiscrimination laws and was sincerely concerned about the fears of his homosexual patients. On the other hand, he recognized the dangers posed by the spread of this disease and the necessity of beginning to utilize standard public health measures to try to stop its spread. As a result of his background and views, he was the ideal member of our medical society to attend the scheduled meeting of the American Medical Association.

Doctor Koop attended that Chicago meeting as one of the featured speakers. There were a number of other speakers who were carefully chosen by the hierarchy of the American Medical Association. Every speaker opposed routine testing. No one was allowed to speak from the podium who favored routine testing in doctors' offices and hospitals or routine premarital and prenatal testing. No one was allowed to speak from the podium who favored using standard public health techniques to try to stop the epidemic. Rather, the speakers stressed the necessity of requiring special consent to perform the blood test, the importance of confidentiality and counseling and, of course...condoms.

During the question and answer period at one of the sessions, Doctor Leff stepped to the microphone and spoke to an audience made up of physicians and concerned citizens from across America. He outlined the program of the Santa Cruz Medical Society AIDS Task Force and suggested that physicians start testing to identify those who were infected and stop the chain of transmission. The response to his remarks was one of overwhelming support. Indeed, Doctor Leff's remarks were greeted with far more enthusiasm than those of the scheduled speakers, because the assembled doctors in the audience recognized the enormity of the problem and wanted a logical response. Yet, no one was allowed to speak from the podium who favored the use of standard public health techniques to stop the epidemic.

※※※

Doctor Otis Bowen, Secretary of Health and Human Services, gave a talk to the National Governors' Association in Washington, D. C., early in 1987. Referring to AIDS as "a public health problem of awesome proportions" he said:
"It can involve millions and millions of people who are going to die as a result...AIDS could well become one of the worst health problems in the history of the world."
Pointing to the fact that we must begin to do testing over the objection of those who stated that testing would infringe on the rights of the individual, Doctor Bowen declared, "We may have to sacrifice a few of these individual rights if we are going to conquer this epidemic."[2]

※※※

In Arizona a U. S. Army Private was charged with assaulting three other soldiers with a biological weapon. PVT. Adrian Morris was cited with four counts of aggravated assault and three counts of criminal misconduct and discrediting the military because he had had sexual relations with three partners without informing them that he carried the AIDS virus. Since the Army had tested all military personnel and had informed those who were infected as to their responsibility, the actions of this soldier showed a total disregard toward those he might infect and ultimately kill. The Army held that anyone who showed such callous disregard for their fellows should be punished.

On the other hand, all across America, no effort was being made to identify those who were infected and were infecting others. Even if people were infected and were knowingly spreading the disease, no legal action was being taken to protect the public. It was apparent that public health efforts were aimed at protecting the rights of the infected. The uninfected segment of our population had no right to protection.

※※※

During the spring of 1987, Larimore was maintaining a close liaison with Senator Doolittle's office in Sacramento. The Senator had submitted ten separate bills dealing with various aspects of the epidemic to the state legislature. There was SB (Senate Bill) 1000 which advocated changing consent and confidentiality requirements for HIV testing to bring them in line with requirements for all other diseases.

Senator Doolittle had a bill requiring mandatory premarital testing (SB1001) and a bill requiring mandatory prenatal testing. There were bills dealing with individuals who were knowingly spreading the disease, bills dealing with those who were giving blood when they knew they were infected, etc. Larimore suggested to the Senator that several of his key bills should be amended to bring them in line with the CMA White Paper. Thus, instead of SB1001 requiring mandatory premarital HIV testing, the bill was amended to require that doctors doing premarital health examinations offer a voluntary, premarital HIV blood test. In a similar manner, another bill was amended to require doctors to offer voluntary prenatal blood testing to all pregnant women.

Since the California Medical Association had consistently supported legislation requiring mandatory blood testing bills for newborn infants and had supported many other mandatory health measures (including premarital syphilis testing), it seemed unthinkable that the CMA would oppose bills requiring physicians to offer voluntary premarital and prenatal blood tests. Never for one minute did Larimore or the Senator imagine that CMA Lobbyists and officials would dare to actively oppose both voluntary premarital and prenatal testing. Yet that is exactly what occurred.

❊❊❊

On May 22, 1987, the MMWR reported three cases of female HCW's who had become infected as a result of blood coming in contact with their intact skin. These three cases came to be known as the "Splash Cases."

The first instance was a woman who got a small spot of infected blood on her finger and had it there for 20 minutes before washing her hands. She was discovered to be HIV positive when she went to a **blood bank** to donate blood.

The second case was a woman phlebotomist who was drawing a blood specimen. The top of the tube flew off and blood splattered onto her face and into her mouth. She washed immediately. She was discovered to be HIV positive when she went to **give a blood transfusion** nine months later.

The third case was a worker who spilled blood on her hands from a machine that separated blood components. Despite washing within a few minutes, her blood test converted from negative to positive within three months.

Thus, by May of 1987 physicians recognized that infected blood on a person's skin could lead to fatal infection.

It is interesting to note that two of these three cases were only picked up at **blood banks** when the patients went to donate blood. Why? Because the CDC has repeatedly said that routine testing of HCW's was unnecessary.

---

1. AMA News — March 13, 1987; p. 34.
2. AMA News — March 6, 1987; p. 47.

CHAPTER FOUR

AIDS is surreptitiously spreading throughout our population and yet we have no accurate measure of its scope. It is time we knew exactly what we are facing.
— President Ronald Reagan, Addressing AMFAR, May 31, 1987

The 3rd International Conference on AIDS was held in Washington, D. C., from June 1 through June 5, 1987. The night before the conference started, the American Foundation for AIDS Research (AMFAR) held a gala, black tie, fund raising event at the Potomac Restaurant in the 3000 block of K Street, N.W. in Washington, D. C. Elizabeth Taylor was there. She had founded AMFAR two years previously. Doctor Mervyn Silverman, the President of AMFAR, was there, his graying hair and beard glistening in the bright lights. Dignitaries, celebrities and prominent physicians from across America were at the event. Media representatives and television camera crews were there to record the President's first public policy statement on the AIDS epidemic.

In preparation for President Reagan's talk, his Domestic Policy Council had spent weeks thoroughly debating various programs that could be instituted to try to stop the epidemic. The presidential advisors felt strongly that the time had come to stop playing politics and start trying to control the disease. Their recommendation was for widespread HIV antibody testing and the use of contact tracing. The President was to call for mandatory testing of federal prisoners and immigrants. The presidential advisors suggested that state governments should require (mandate) premarital testing and expand routine testing as rapidly as possible. Secretary of Education, William Bennett, strongly supported this program. The lone dissenter at the Domestic Policy meetings was...C. Everett Koop.[1]

And so it was that President Reagan gave his keynote address to the assembled dignitaries at the AMFAR meeting on the evening of May 31, 1987.

America faces a disease that is fatal and is spreading. This calls for urgency not panic. It calls for compassion not blame. It calls for understanding not ignorance...We must not allow those with the AIDS virus to suffer discrimination. The public health service has stated that there is no medical reason for barring a person with the virus from any routine school or working activities...There is no reason for those who carry the AIDS virus to wear a scarlet 'A'.

Mr. Reagan called for the Department of Health and Human Services to add AIDS to the list of contagious diseases for immigrants and for aliens seeking to live in America. He asked the Justice Department to start testing all federal prisoners and asked the individual states to start testing their prisoners as well. He advocated "testing of patients in veterans' hospitals" and he urged the various states to "offer routine testing for those who seek marriage licenses and for those who visit sexually transmitted disease or drug abuse clinics."

Not only will testing give us more information from which to make decisions, but in the case of marriage licenses, it may prevent at least some babies from being born with AIDS.

He went on to say, "Any effort at education must stress values." (i.e., moral values)

He called on the Department of Health and Human Services to try to find out how far the disease had spread in our society. In May of 1987, almost six years into the epidemic, Americans had no idea how widely the epidemic was disseminated. The President stressed the need for routine testing and widespread testing and concluded his remarks by saying:

No one knows to what extent the virus has infected our entire society...AIDS is surreptitiously spreading throughout our population and yet we have no accurate measure of its scope. It is time we knew exactly what we are facing. And that is why I support routine testing.

The President's remarks were met with hisses and boos from the gay and AIDS activists in the audience.

Outside the Potomac Restaurant, demonstrators paraded with signs demanding: "IMPEACH REAGAN." Along the Potomac River, there was a candlelight vigil made up of people who suffered from AIDS. The leader of the vigil condemned Ronald Reagan for perpetuating the epidemic and demanded more federal funding for AIDS research.[2]

It was on the following day, June 1, 1987, that Vice President Bush addressed the opening session of the 3rd International Conference on AIDS. He advocated broader HIV testing at both the state and federal level to determine who those individuals were who were infected with the AIDS virus so that our nation could begin to bring the epidemic under control. His remarks were met with jeers, boos, and hisses from the audience. When he stressed the importance of strict confidentiality of HIV test results, his remarks were met with cheers and applause. Any time he veered from the AIDS and gay agenda, he was attacked. When he followed their agenda, the applause was widespread.[3]

The meeting of the 3rd International Conference on AIDS was held at the Washington Hilton which had an auditorium capable of seating 4200. There were over 6000 attendees. Many people had journeyed from across the world to that meeting because of their deep concern about the epidemic. However, a large component of those in attendance were homosexuals and AIDS activists, intent upon manipulating AIDS policy to follow their program rather than a logical, sound, medical approach to the epidemic. That is how it was in June of 1987 in Washington, D. C. at the 3rd International Conference on AIDS. That is how it was in June of 1989 in Montreal at the 5th International Conference on AIDS and at the 6th International Conference in San Francisco in 1990 and that is how it still is today.

The demonstrators paraded around the convention, carrying signs saying: "MR. REAGAN, YOUR APATHY IS KILLING US" and "REAGAN, REAGAN, STOP THE CHARADE, TESTING IS NOT A CURE FOR AIDS."

Police wearing yellow rubber gloves arrested 64 demonstrators who were blocking traffic in front of the White House. It was announced at that meeting that the Burroughs Wellcome drug, AZT, was showing the possibility of favorable results in the treatment of patients with AIDS and there might be some hope of altering the course of the disease, although AZT would certainly not bring about a cure. Discussing the possibility of a vaccine, it was suggested that by late 1987 there might be some early trials using vaccines which had already been developed, but there was no possibility of a vaccine being generally available until the mid 1990's or later.

At the meeting, the subject of routine HIV testing was mentioned only to be condemned. Although there were many people at the conference who supported testing and contact tracing, few dared to speak out for fear of being physically attacked by angry demonstrators. In one instance, the exhibit booth set up by Dr. Paul Cameron of the Family Research Institute was physically attacked by an angry gay activist who smashed the television set and knocked over card tables because he objected to material being presented. Police arrested the demonstrator, then promptly released him without bringing charges, under pressure from powerful political figures in Washington, D. C. (Senator Edward

Kennedy).

※※※

June 2, 1987

The New York Times announced that two New York City welfare and hospital agencies had stated that they were overburdened with the rising AIDS caseload. At city hospitals, there were over 340 AIDS patients every day — and they were only allowed to stay for a few days, then moved on because of the shortage of beds.

Robert Haynes, Chairman of the Council of the Coalition for the Homeless in New York City stated:

"Hundreds of people with AIDS are living in barrack shelters. To my mind there is no question that a year from now, AIDS will be the primary cause of homelessness."

※※※

It was during this same period that Larimore Cummins and Arnold Leff were making regular trips to Sacramento trying to implement the programs laid out in the CMA White Paper. Amazingly, CMA lobbyists and CMA spokesmen were actively opposing the policies which the House of Delegates had embraced. SB1000 was a bill that would have changed consent and confidentiality requirements for HIV disease to those used for every other disease. Liberal Democratic State Senator, Diane Watson, asked Senator Doolittle to alter his bill to stipulate that if a patient declined testing, that he/she would be required to sign a statement to that effect. Senator Doolittle realized that every legislative vote was going to be important so he agreed to Diane Watson's request. What was the result? Senator Watson still refused to vote for his bill, but the California Medical Association was able to use that addition to SB1000 to justify their opposition. Senator Doolittle promptly agreed to delete the addition, yet the CMA kept using Senator Diane Watson's amendment as justification for opposing SB1000.

The CMA actively opposed Senator Doolittle's bill SB1001 for voluntary premarital blood testing. Furthermore, the CMA opposed the voluntary prenatal testing bill. It soon became obvious that, once again, the leaders of organized medicine were intent upon circumventing the policies established by the House of Delegates in March.

※※※

June 5, 1987

This was a watershed day in my life. Just as June 5, 1981 marked the watershed for our society with the report of the first cases of AIDS in the MMWR, so June 5, 1987 changed my life forever.

The first event occurred when I read an article published in the People's Daily World, the official publication of the CPUSA. That newspaper was a conduit for Soviet propaganda; it's goal was to influence American policy decisions. On page 16A, the writer discussed President Reagan's speech six days earlier. After condemning the President's position favoring HIV testing and contact tracing, the article went on to say:

"A major complaint about the Administration's policy is the focus on testing instead of (on) funding research and public education on AIDS."

How strange it was that the CPUSA objected to HIV testing in America but did not object to the use of widespread mandatory testing in the Soviet Union and Cuba. That indeed was a strange paradox.

The second event that was destined to influence my future occurred late in the evening on June 5. It was a television program. It was not the average, everyday program aimed at the mindless masses. This was a very unusual program and it contained a message aimed at the American public. The message?

"We as a nation were not to try to stop the epidemic with testing."

Furthermore, for the first time, I was to see a highly placed official from the U. S. Public Health Department intentionally attempt to mislead the public.

It was somewhere after 11:30 p.m. on the west coast when Ted Koppel hosted a four hour "Television Town Meeting of the Air." There was a large panel of guests assembled in Los Angeles with direct television links to New York, Washington, D. C. and Tokyo, Japan. The staff of ABC's Nightline had recruited most of the key players in the drama of the AIDS epidemic, the people who had played decisive roles in establishing our failed public health policy. I was destined to encounter many of them as the tragedy of the epidemic unfolded. The guests that evening included:

1. Doctor Jonathan Mann, Director of the Global AIDS Project of the World Health Organization.

2. Gary Bauer, Chief Advisor to President Reagan on domestic policy issues.

3. Jeff Levi, Director of the National Gay and Lesbian Task Force.

194 AIDS: The Unnecessary Epidemic

4. Carol Leigh, the red haired prostitute representing COYOTE, (Call Off Your Old Tired Ethics) who I encountered in Montreal in June of 1989.
5. Dianne Feinstein, at that time the Mayor of San Francisco, the city with the second highest number of AIDS patients per capita in the nation.
6. Paul Volberding, Chief of the AIDS Clinic at San Francisco General Hospital and a bitter critic of routine HIV testing and mandatory reporting.
7. Doctor Anthony Fauci, coordinator of AIDS research at the NIAID Division of the National Institute of Health.
8. Leonard Matlovich, a former Air Force Lieutenant who had been discharged because of his homosexuality. He was infected with the HIV virus.
9. Morgan Fairchild, the actress.
10. Doctor Stephen Joseph, the Chief Public Health Officer of New York City.
11. Congressman William Dannemeyer.

With the exception of Gary Bauer, the presidential advisor, the lone spokesman for a rational approach to the epidemic was Congressman William Dannemeyer. That television program was my first exposure to the outspoken conservative from Southern California. I had met his assistant at the CMA convention in March and I had heard of Bill Dannemeyer for many years and knew that he was a staunch anti-Communist, a conservative and a professing Christian, but beyond that, I knew very little about him.

Bill Dannemeyer had a distinctly masculine, craggy face, a large nose, prominent jaw and an infectious smile that would flash across his features even when he was under bitter attack from members of the AIDS and Gay Lobbies. The Congressman's points were always clear, concise, organized, and spoken with compassion and sincerity.

Ted Koppel did a superb job of moderating the four hour marathon. He made it appear that both sides of the issues were equally presented, but as I later analyzed the video tape of the program, I could see that the message being presented was the message of the gay activists, carefully disguised to give the appearance of fairness and impartiality. Whenever Congressman Dannemeyer spoke, he was immediately countered by Jeff Levi of the Gay and Lesbian Task Force or by Doctor Anthony Fauci. As a result, Bill Dannemeyer was unable to influence the majority of those in the television audience that evening or to convince them of the validity of his statements. But for those of us who understood the epidemic, his words rang true.

Ted Koppel started out with a beautiful cliche:

"AIDS...we don't know how to cure it...we have to learn how to live with it."

Mr. Koppel's opening remarks were characteristic of the cliches that were heard for many hours — eloquent, misleading statements. Yes, we do not know how to cure the disease but we did not have to live with it. We should have started to control it in April of 1982 at the beginning of the second stage of the epidemic...but we did not. In 1987, we might still have controlled the epidemic and limited the death toll but television programs such as that four hour "Television Town Meeting of the Air" served only to confuse the issues and give the American public the feeling that the use of standard public health efforts to control the epidemic would serve only to infringe upon civil rights and drive the disease underground.

The entire thrust of the program was to engender sympathy on the part of the audience for the tragic victims of the disease. Certainly we should all be sympathetic toward them but we should also be sympathetic towards the uninfected. They have rights as well. The most tragic victims are those who are contracting this disease unnecessarily because society has not used those tools which were readily available in 1982 and 1985 to begin to bring the epidemic under control.

Doctor Anthony Fauci of the National Institute of Health is a man of short stature. His short hair is carefully plastered down over the top of his head. He wears rimmed glasses and speaks clearly and convincingly. Tragically, he consistently used convincing arguments to deceive the audience. Doctor Fauci started out by telling the audience how HIV disease wiped out the immune system and how it was primarily spread by blood and blood products, from mothers to children or by sexual contact. He went on to say that kissing was safe, even kissing on the lips was safe and that there was no danger of the spread of this disease within household contacts or by closeness or by contact with people who were infected. Certainly, as a key researcher, he must know of the instances of spread among health care workers and within families, like the case of Craig Stenger in Pennsylvania. It was just that he did not want the public to know of those instances.

Ted Koppel then called on Congressman Dannemeyer. Bill Danne-

meyer attempted to bring out the fact that testing for HIV disease was important. He pointed out that there were three reasons why we should do testing:
1. To have some idea of the incidence of the disease.
2. So that we could do contact tracing and find out who had the virus, who had given the virus to the infected patient and to whom the infected patient might have given the infection in order to break the chain of transmission.
3. So we could get patients under treatment.

Before Dannemeyer could elaborate further, Jeff Levi of the National Gay and Lesbian Task Force interrupted, saying:

"AIDS is a different disease."

Levi insisted that Americans didn't need testing and if we wanted to know the incidence of the disease we should do seroprevalence studies. He went on to suggest that public health officers could simply go into the general community and interview a small number of people and test them to determine the overall incidence of the disease in the nation. He insisted that there was no need for routine testing and reporting of cases to public health officers. He insisted that HIV test results would only mislead people. He reiterated the "AIDS Lobby Line" that counseling was far more important than testing.

Ted Koppel then brought up President Reagan's speech of May 31 when the President asked the Department of Health and Human Services to determine how far AIDS had penetrated into our society. The question was then raised, "Could we protect confidentiality?"

Quickly, some nameless commentator flashed onto the screen from Florida. He said that HIV test results were incorrect 25 to 30% of the time. Then the commentator went on to say that 7 people had recently committed suicide in Florida when they learned that they were HIV positive. The obvious message being conveyed to the public was that HIV testing was inaccurate and people with false positive tests often commit suicide.

This video sequence was followed with another interview with a man who had just lost his job when his employer found out that he had AIDS. The message? Get tested and you will lose your job.

The scene switched to Gary Bauer, the presidential advisor on domestic policy issues. When Ted Koppel asked Bauer how doctors could possibly protect confidentiality and keep people from losing their jobs and being discriminated against, Mr. Bauer simply said:

"There is no evidence that America's medical system isn't working or that confidentiality is being broken."

Koppel immediately replied: "How can AIDS be treated like any other disease? After all, are there any other diseases like AIDS?" He then went on to challenge the idea that people immigrating into America should be tested. His line of reasoning (sophistry) was this:

Should we test immigrants in America or should we test them in their own countries before they come to America? If they come to America and are found to be HIV positive, would we send them back home, infected and sick with their illness? And if we did test them in their home country and they were found to be negative, they could still be in that window of infectiousness where the antibody test has not yet turned positive. The immigrants could have the infection when they arrived on our shores without our knowing. So why bother to test immigrants at all since test results could sometimes be inaccurate?

Bauer responded. He pointed out, first of all, that we test immigrants for tuberculosis, syphilis and other communicable diseases, in holding areas, before they are admitted to this country. If they are found to be infected, they are sent home so that their illness will not become the burden of American taxpayers. Furthermore, although agreeing that there was a window of infectiousness, Gary Bauer stated, quite correctly, that testing would pick up the vast majority of those who were infected. Furthermore, just because a few people would be missed was no reason to discontinue testing. His points were well made but completely ignored by Mr. Koppel.

Carol Leigh, the prostitute from COYOTE, was presented to the audience as a "sex worker." She immediately quoted some rather questionable statistics — but then statistics always are impressive to those who are uninformed. She insisted that prostitutes were known to pass on less than 5% of all venereal disease in America and that prostitutes, for the most part, used condoms and were active in sex education. Carol Leigh expressed tremendous concern over laws being presented to State Legislatures all across the country mandating that prostitutes be tested. Furthermore, she pointed out that Senator John Doolittle of California wanted to have a law passed that would make it a felony for an infected prostitute to continue plying her trade. Carol Leigh thought that such a law was terribly unjust and she objected to prostitutes being made "scapegoats."

It was at that point that Congressman Dannemeyer spoke up. He pointed out that the epidemic was directly related to perversion and promiscuous sexual activity and that the union of one man and one woman was the foundation of the family and the family was the cornerstone of our society.

Before he could go on, Koppel quickly interrupted to bring on Dianne Feinstein, the Mayor of San Francisco, who stated that testing for HIV disease would not stop the epidemic. Speaker after speaker pointed out that HIV testing confused the issue and would bring about fear and uncertainty. Financially, we couldn't afford to do testing and contact tracing. It was far too expensive to try to stop the spread of this disease as we had all other illnesses. What was needed was more money to take care of the tragic victims of the epidemic.

The entire thrust of the television program that night was to downplay the necessity for HIV testing. Testing was not the answer. The answer to the epidemic was education. Education should begin in the lowest grades in school. Education would remove embarrassment from discussions of sexual matters. Education was aimed at **desensitizing** our children. The word **"desensitize"** was actually used by a sex educator in the audience to describe the program that was planned for our schools. Yes, the thrust of sex education was to **desensitize** the children of America to sex, to remove modesty and embarrassment, to take away the mystery and the anticipation from sex. Sex education was the key to stopping the epidemic...

Congressman Dannemeyer spoke to that issue as well. He pointed out that with the massive expenditure of federal funds for sex education and family planning there had been a 50% increase in teenage abortions and 100% increase in teenage pregnancies. He was quickly cut off by Koppel and the subject was dropped.

Doctor Stephen Joseph, the Health Director of New York City was introduced. He spoke of the importance of expanding testing but only in the context of requiring consent, confidentiality and extensive counseling before testing was done, and then only in high risk groups.

Time and again, gay speakers rose in the audience to speak about their program to influence the course of the epidemic. They had a program which should be followed. It was a program of consent, confidentiality, counseling, sex education and condoms. That is how we were going to stop the epidemic.

Harvey Firestone, a New York homosexual playwright was interviewed. He emphasized what a terrible thing it was to talk about mandatory testing and stated that if we ever have mandatory testing, he would be the first to go to jail. He went on to talk about how you could have 1000 sexual contacts and you wouldn't get AIDS. The important thing was what you did with those 1000 sexual contacts. You could be in danger from having just one sexual contact and doing the wrong thing. You could have 1000 sexual contacts and if you used safe masturbatory techniques you would have nothing to fear.

A nurse in the audience rose to ask if there was the possibility of getting the disease by casual contact. The question was referred to Doctor Anthony Fauci from the National Institute of Allergy and Infectious Diseases (NIAID). Doctor Fauci insisted that there were relatively few health care workers with unexplained AIDS and that the chance of getting the disease from a needle-stick injury was only a fraction of a percent. Therefore, according to Dr. Fauci, health care workers were not in a high risk group. He then went on to discuss the case of a dentist who had been found to have been infected with the virus from working in his patients' mouths. Doctor Fauci pointed out that there had been 1200 dentists who had filled out questionnaires and given blood samples and only one of them was found to carry the virus without identifiable risk factors. He then emphasized that dentists very often stuck themselves with needles and it was possible that this one infected dentist might have stuck himself with an infected needle. Of course, there was no evidence that the dentist had stuck himself with an infected needle, but that was unimportant. It was obvious, from the presentation, that Dr. Fauci had to establish the fact in the audience's mind that the dentist had gotten the disease from a needle stick, because the only other possibility was that the dentist had gotten the disease by the respiratory route — and that possibility would be too frightening to reveal to the public. It was at this point that Ted Koppel mentioned the case of the three women who had developed HIV infection after having blood splashed on their skin.

Doctor Fauci quickly pointed out that it was important to understand that these women did not have AIDS. They had simply seroconverted and had become infected with the virus — as if somehow being infected with the virus was all right as long as the disease had not yet progressed to AIDS. By making his point so cleverly, Dr. Fauci was able to allay fear and intimate that HIV seroconversion and infection were somehow different from AIDS.

At another point in the evening, the question of casual transmission of disease was brought up. Dr. Paul Volberding from San Francisco emphatically stated that there was absolutely no possibility of casual transmission of the disease. At this point, Congressman Dannemeyer agreed but raised the question of the 3% of AIDS cases that are consistently reported by the CDC where there are no identifiable risk factors. This 3% had been reported by the CDC year after year, after year, and Congressman Dannemeyer simply raised the question, "If there is no such thing as casual transmission of disease, how do you explain the constant 3% of unexplained cases which have been reported by the CDC?"

Doctor Fauci was quick to reply. He stated that some of those cases represented patients who had not yet been worked up by the Centers for Disease Control and some of the others represented people who had died before being interviewed. He emphasized that people should not dwell on the 3% of cases which are unexplained. Why? Because that tended to detract from the fact that we knew that the disease was primarily spread by sexual contact, from mothers to children and by transfer of blood or blood products in the other 97% of cases. Therefore, it was inappropriate to discuss that 3% of the cases in which we did not know the means of transmission.

At another point, Dr. Paul Volberding mentioned that the virus could not survive outside the body and that people did not have to worry about the spread of the virus except by intimate sexual contact. Congressman Dannemeyer promptly referred to the report in the Lancet showing that the virus could live for seven days in dry form and ten days in liquid form outside the human body.

Immediately Doctor Fauci was called upon to dispute the Congressman. Of course he couldn't dispute the report from the Pasteur Institute. His reply was to the effect that we need not talk about the virus living outside the human body because that would detract from the modes of transmission that we knew were important...such as sexual transmission, transmission from mothers to their children and transfer of blood or blood products.

There were telephone operators in the studio taking calls from across the nation. When a telephone caller mentioned that health care workers should be tested, a gay activist in the audience rose to say that if we tested health care workers "we would drive them underground and once they were underground they would be far more dangerous." Yes, the message was clear. Trying to test health care workers or anyone else would simply drive the disease underground and increase the chance of the disease being spread. Therefore, we should not try to identify those who had the virus; we should not try to stop the spread of disease.

One of the major thrusts of the program was to push the necessity for a national health insurance program. Jeffrey Levi of the National Gay and Lesbian Task Force stressed the need for national health insurance. Leonard Matlovich, the gay activist retired from the Air Force, stressed the need for national health insurance. Doctor Stephen Joseph, Health Director of New York, had spoken out in favor of national health insurance.

Somehow it seemed that national health insurance would bring an end to the problem of AIDS. With socialized medicine, everybody who had the disease would have adequate funding and treatment.

The problem with that line of reasoning is that they have a national health insurance program in Cuba — and in Cuba those who are infected are quarantined. They have a national health insurance program in the Soviet Union and are doing mandatory testing of large segments of their population. They have national health insurance programs in nations of Africa — but their socialist programs have resulted in the bankruptcy of their economies and a total breakdown of all public health programs. Yet the theme of many of the gay activists is that America needs socialized medicine — as if somehow that is going to solve the problem of the AIDS epidemic.

I was up until 4:00 a.m. the following morning. I recorded the program and watched it again and again. It was so obvious that Dr. Fauci of the NIH was misleading the public. Doctor Fauci had reassured the American public that "You didn't get AIDS by getting blood splashed on your skin — you just got infected with the virus." He kept telling the public not to be concerned about the 3% of cases for which the means of transmission was unknown. Instead, they should consider those cases where the means of transmission was definitely proven. They were not to be concerned about the fact that the virus can exist outside the body, but rather emphasize the known facts about the disease. He assured the public that it was perfectly safe to kiss. He inferred that the dentist who had the disease probably got it by sticking himself with an infected needle. The dentist must have acquired the disease by that means, because to suggest that there was respiratory spread of the disease might cause the public to panic and then the government would have to admit that their entire program for controlling the epidemic was a failure.[4]

There had been one man who had been willing to stand against the rest of the panel. There was one man who had been willing to challenge the audience and the callers. His name was William Dannemeyer. He could smile when he was attacked; he could present his position clearly and concisely. He wasn't afraid to speak out on marriage, morality and God's plan for society. Here was a man I could follow, a politician who was obviously a man of principle and integrity...in a nation of equivocal men.

I determined that I would, somehow, meet Bill Dannemeyer and, perhaps with his help, I could play some small part in bringing a measure of sanity to the madness that seemed to have engulfed our society — a madness which might soon lead to the destruction of our freedoms and our nation.

※※※

A few days later, I called Congressman Dannemeyer's office in Southern California and made an appointment to meet him in Anaheim. It was obvious, when talking to his staff, that they knew who I was. The following day I received a call from the Congressman's office. Mr. Dannemeyer was not going to be in Orange County on the day that had been arranged but he was going to be flying into San Francisco on Saturday morning. Could I meet him at the airport? I assured the caller that I would be there.

※※※

It was reported early in June that a New Hampshire bill had gone before the State Legislature. The purpose of the legislation was to appropriate over one-half million dollars to be used for HIV education and for establishing AIDS clinics but because a mandatory premarital testing bill had been amended onto the bill by the State Senate, the New Hampshire House killed the legislation. Liberal politicians did not want mandatory testing of any sort for HIV disease — despite the fact that they supported mandatory blood testing for many other diseases. No, there was to be no mandatory testing in America — no matter how many lives it might save.[5]

※※※

A report published in the AMA Medical News in June of 1987 reported that knowledge of a positive HIV test did not seem to influence high risk behavior among gay men. The report revealed that "although many participants in the study of gay and bisexual men had switched to safer sexual practices, those who learned that they were infected were no more likely to switch than men who did not learn of their antibody status." The article went on to note that many of the infected men became depressed, anxious and suicidal once they learned of their positive test results.

The message of the article was clear. Testing of homosexuals was not beneficial. Since testing of this group was not beneficial, why should testing be carried out on a wide scale in our nation? The obvious rationale of this argument is similar to the sophist who argues that, since all Chinese are men and since all Caucasians are men, therefore, all Chinese are obviously Caucasians. Just because some homosexuals are reported to be irresponsible it does not mean that the vast majority of the population of our nation will not act responsibly when told of their infection. Tragically, many physicians reading this article and similar articles in medical journals published across our nation eventually became convinced that it was unwise to use testing to stop the spread of disease in the heterosexual population.

***

June 12, 1987

Halfdan Mahlar, Director General of the World Health Organization, warned against the use of a "racist and fascist approach to stop the spread of AIDS." and against "discrimination and fear." The WHO had come out in opposition to the use of routine HIV testing in America and had embraced the use of **consent, confidentiality, counseling** and **condoms** to stop the epidemic in western nations. Strangely, while the WHO opposed the use of widespread testing in the West, they did not oppose the use of widespread HIV testing behind the Iron Curtain and in Cuba. It seemed that there were to be two diametrically opposite approaches to controlling this epidemic. There was to be restricted testing in the West and extensive testing in Eastern bloc countries. (By 1990, the Soviet Union had performed over 50 million blood tests, screening its population). Amazingly, no one in America commented on this discrepancy.

***

It was in the latter part of June of 1987 that Larimore and I drove to

San Francisco to meet Congressman Dannemeyer. We both recognized that the Congressman appeared to be the only national figure willing to take an unpopular stand in order to try to save our nation from the ravages of the epidemic.

We were to meet at the VIP Room at the San Francisco International Airport. When Bill Dannemeyer entered the meeting room, I knew I was in the presence of an unusual human being. His wrinkled face frequently broke into a grin. His questions were pointed and his grasp of the HIV crisis was thorough. What impressed me most was the fact that he took notes on our entire conversation. I sensed that our meeting was not simply a passing interview, given in an effort to impress potential supporters. Here was a man who was personally involved in the battle to save our nation and he was recording any and all information that he could glean which might be helpful in the fight. As we talked, he told us:

"The tragedy is that there are only five Congressmen on the Hill who really understand the epidemic, and two of them are on the other side."

He was referring to Congressmen Dan Burton from Indiana, Robert Dornan from Southern California and himself on our side and to Henry Waxman and one other liberal Democrat on the other side.

The details of what we discussed that afternoon have long since faded from my memory. What I do remember were the strong, masculine qualities that Bill Dannemeyer manifested. Here was a man of integrity; here was a man of principle; here was a man willing to speak out in favor of God, family and country. Here was a man who had the courage to stand against the vicious attacks of the AIDS and Gay Lobbies. His deeply-lined face reminded me of the face of John Wayne during his latter years. Indeed, Bill Dannemeyer seemed to represent all those features of strength and character which Americans had come to identify with the image that John Wayne portrayed. But here was a real man who had real qualities — not the product of Hollywood producers and publicity managers. Here was the man I had seen on ABC's "Television Town Meeting Of The Air" who was willing to stand and proclaim the truth over the jeers of the audience.

Bill Dannemeyer roared with laughter when we told him of some of Merv Silverman's statements and Larimore gave the Congressman copies of clippings from the San Francisco Chronicle showing how Mervyn Silverman had delayed the closing of the bathhouses in San Francisco for almost two years because he wanted the bathhouses to be used as "centers for distributing educational material."

When Congressman Dannemeyer left us that afternoon, I knew that somehow, in some way, things were going to be different. That meeting was the beginning of a new adventure and that encounter with Bill Dannemeyer would one day inspire me to take one of the greatest gambles of my life. But, once again, I am getting far ahead of my story.

✻✻✻

In June 1987, a young cardiologist from Johns Hopkins Hospital sued the hospital administration. Apparently the 32-year-old physician contracted the HIV virus in 1983 when a blood-filled vial exploded and cut his hand. Since he was an employee at the hospital when the injury occurred, he wanted the hospital to provide for his medical care and for financial assistance to his wife and child when he died. There was some question as to when the doctor contracted the disease.

Since the Centers for Disease Control has consistently discouraged doctors and health care personnel from being tested, the doctor had no way of actually proving when his infection occurred. Furthermore, had he been tested, he could have cut down the risk of transmitting the disease to his wife during that latent period between the time of his infection in 1983 and the time when he was diagnosed with AIDS in December of 1986. (The blood test was available for over one and a half years during that period).

However, the CDC has consistently maintained that health care workers were not to be routinely tested. They were not to know if they were HIV positive so they could protect their families or be placed under treatment or so they could establish whether or not they had become infected on the job. Thus this young doctor was forced into the embarrassing position of having to sue his employer in the hope that he could obtain financial help to cover his medical expenses and compensation to care for his family after his inevitable death.

✻✻✻

It was late in June 1987, when Surgeon General C. Everett Koop gave an exclusive interview to the American Medical News. He stated that he felt that doctors should start doing routine testing on all patients going into hospitals for major surgery. Doctor Koop went on to say that..."If the testing were implemented, then every member of the surgical team can know when they are at risk and take the proper precautions."

Obviously the Surgeon General knew that health care workers and physicians were at risk. Yet the Centers for Disease Control has continued to discourage surgeons from doing routine testing on patients being admitted for surgery. That was the case in 1987. It is still the case in the 1990's.

✳✳✳

It was also late in June when the AMA Board of Trustees released their report on HIV testing. Tragically, the entire emphasis of their report was on using HIV testing **only in high risk groups** and in **high risk areas.** The AMA report showed no interest in testing in low risk areas or in low risk groups. The entire thrust of their HIV testing program was to try to stop the epidemic in homosexuals and IV drug users. The spread of disease into the heterosexual population was not to be addressed.

✳✳✳

On June 25, the Senate of the State of California approved SB1000, Senator John Doolittle's bill which had been modified to bring it into line with the CMA White Paper. The CMA actively opposed the legislation stating, "The result of (SB1000) would be to discourage people from being voluntarily tested for the disease." Commenting on SB1000, California State Assemblyman, Art Agnos said:
"It's a very bad bill and would damage our efforts to combat AIDS in California. That is why every public health group is against it."[6]
SB1000 never got out of the Assembly Subcommittee because of CMA opposition. The bill was effectively killed.
On July 10, 1987, the People's Daily World (page 5A) noted that:
"Civil libertarians and health experts are concerned over the bills authored by Senator John Doolittle. Doolittle's bills would cut the state's confidentiality law, allow testing...without a patient's consent and widespread disclosure of those results. Critics warn that such measures would drive away those most in need of testing and hurt efforts to limit the spread of AIDS."[7]
Of course, SB1000 did not remove consent requirements for HIV testing. The bill simply would have brought consent requirements for HIV disease in line with consent requirements for all other blood testing. Tragically, the special consent requirements for HIV testing have continued to act as a barrier to routine HIV testing in our state.

July 1987

Reverend Lou Sheldon invited me to give a talk on AIDS in Sacramento before the Coalition for Traditional Values. There were a number of State Senators and Assemblymen in attendance. I was able to point out the monumental problems confronting our nation as a result of the HIV epidemic as well as the official CMA policy as outlined in the CMA White Paper. Amazingly, none of the legislators had ever seen or heard of the CMA White Paper nor had they any idea as to its content. It appeared that CMA lobbyists and CMA leaders had been very effective in their efforts to keep the contents of the CMA White Paper one of the best-kept secrets in Sacramento.

❋❋❋

In mid-July, a report was released from Johns Hopkins in Baltimore, Maryland. Routine testing had been performed on large numbers of patients coming into the University Hospital Emergency Room. The investigators found that **if testing was limited only to those who had risk factors** (i.e., homosexual and bisexual men, IV drug users and those who admitted to having sexual contact with any of the above) **over half of the HIV-infected cases would have been missed.** Thus, by limiting testing to those in risk groups, it was obvious that the disease would continue to spread through the community.

It was on July 31 and August 1 that the Council of the CMA met. I was later told that the discussion on AIDS was put off until the very end of the meeting when the majority of the responsible members of the Council had left. In any event, a document did come out of that meeting which reaffirmed the position of the CMA White Paper but also endorsed the position taken by the AMA. This policy guaranteed that HIV testing was to be limited to those in high risk groups and assured that no effort would be made to try to stop the spread of the epidemic in the heterosexual population of our nation.

❋❋❋

Despite the official CMA position taken in March and confirmed again on August 1, 1987, CMA lobbyists and the President-elect of the California Medical Association, Dr. Laurens White, actively lobbied against legislation supporting both voluntary premarital and prenatal testing. Using any possible excuse they could to justify their position, they were successful in blocking the majority of Senator Doolittle's legislation. But one bill did get out of committee over CMA's objection.

When SB1001, Senator Doolittle's bill on voluntary premarital blood testing, came up for discussion before the legislative health committee, Larimore Cummins and Arnold Leff attended the hearing under the auspices of the Santa Cruz County Medical Society. Doctor White was there to lobby against the bill. During the discussion, Doctor Cummins pointed out that voluntary premarital testing was official CMA policy and he used the CMA White Paper to justify his position.

Assemblyman Bill Filante is a physician from Northern California. Ordinarily he follows CMA policy positions; however, on this occasion, having been in attendance at the CMA meeting in March and realizing that premarital blood testing was the cornerstone of any effective public health policy, he cast the swing vote in support of the bill. As a result of his vote, SB1001 passed out of the committee and onto the floor where it passed by an overwhelming vote.

You must understand that members of the California State Legislature would never dare to publicly oppose sound public health policy. The AIDS and Gay Lobby had to use the committee structure to block legislation. Assemblyman Willie Brown controlled that committee structure with an iron fist. Few Democratic legislators had the courage to oppose him. If they did, they knew they would be repudiated by their party leadership at the next election. For years Willie Brown worked to keep effective AIDS legislation bottled up in legislative committees. Despite the fact that Brown is black and he knew that the epidemic was decimating the black youth of our nation, he favored the gay position over the interests of blacks. Fortunately SB1001 passed out of committee without Willie Brown's knowledge and once on the floor of the Assembly he was unable to prevent its passage.

※※※

The reaction to Doctor Cummins' and Doctor Leff's appearance before the Assembly Health Committee was swift and predictable. The response was aimed at silencing dissent by representatives of our county medical society and forcing us to accept the policies of the CMA hierarchy. As pointed out earlier, virtually every AIDS Task Force in the entire nation was under gay domination — except for the Santa Cruz County Medical Society Task Force.

On August 3, 1987, Doctor Rodney Lowe, President of our medical society, received the following letter from Dr. White.

"I had the rare privilege of listening to Dr. Larimore Cummins from your medical society, claim that the leadership of the CMA does not represent the doctors in California and that Dr. Cummins does. Both Dr. Cummins and you and the Santa Cruz County Medical Society are performing a grave disservice to the CMA and to medicine.

"You have not even considered the possibility you may be wrong or that your interpretation of the actions of the House of Delegates might be incorrect...We would also point out that every other reputable medical group has agreed with our position or was, in fact, more adamant in restricting the doctors ability to practice medicine. To have you publicly cloud the issue or pretend that you, in fact, understand the will of the CMA members, I find repugnant...

"We would prefer a unified front and, through the CMA, are trying to arrive at a consensus position. None of us gets everything out of a consensus that we want, but your actions weaken medicine and embarrass me, personally."

On September 8, Dr. Laurens White came to the monthly meeting of our Board of Governors. Fortunately our secretary recorded the events of that meeting. What follows is a transcript of what was actually said. Doctor White started out with an angry attack on Larimore and Arnie Leff saying,

"You do not represent the physicians of California. You represent the Santa Cruz County physicians — don't make that statement again. I won't let you get away with it again."

Doctor Rodney Lowe is a gentle, quiet mannered, plastic surgeon. I was surprised when Rodney abruptly interrupted Doctor White's tirade and announced, emphatically, that he would not tolerate any further angry outbursts or condemnation at our meeting. Doctor White then changed his tactic.

"A study of the Western Journal of Medicine points out that only 1 out of 6 California physicians knows how to diagnose AIDS. Most of us don't know enough about AIDS to have strenuous feelings about what should be done. The study points out that a great part of the problem is dislike for homosexuals. The point of my being here is — doctors here are no better and no worse than elsewhere. Almost all of Doolittle's bills and Agnos' bills are related to testing for antibodies, not diagnosing AIDS. All of these issues have nothing to do with diagnosing the disease but focuses on the antibody status."

Doctor White's statement only served to confuse the issue. HIV disease and AIDS were diagnosed by the HIV antibody status. AIDS was simply the terminal stage of HIV disease. Was this a conscious effort to confuse the physicians on our Board as to the true nature of the problem or did it represent a lack of understanding on Doctor White's part?

LARIMORE CUMMINS: "We voted in March that we want doctors to be able to act like doctors. We want the requirements for doing the HIV test to be no different from the requirements for general testing of blood in similar situations."

DOCTOR WHITE: "We (also) want to relax the confidentiality requirements. The goal of the CMA is to allow doctors to test where appropriate and report the status to appropriate persons. The Doolittle Bill had a couple of things in it that we couldn't support. The chain of information was too broad. We don't believe that lab technicians, for instance, should be included — they should be careful of all specimens. Doolittle's bill allowed information for transmittal too far down the chain. We objected to the wording, (in the bill) 'Licensed medical personnel' as too broad."

DOCTOR MONTEITH: "In 1986, the CMA House passed a resolution to change consent and confidentiality requirements. The Council called this an assault on our patients and refused to act. Isn't the Council answerable to the House? How can you justify this?"

DOCTOR WHITE: "We supported a bill, last year, to do that. The Governor vetoed it."

(I could not let Laurens White get away with distorting what had really happened.)

DOCTOR MONTEITH: "Agnos' bill, last year, (AB3667) did not do away with written consent. It was the Gay Bill of Rights bill. It was not what we wanted...Why did we (CMA) oppose premarital testing?"

DOCTOR WHITE: "Because it was mandatory. After we opposed it, they took (it) out..."

DOCTOR CUMMINS: "You are on record opposing that bill despite amendment (the premarital testing bill)."

The discussion at the meeting went on and on and it was pointed out that the State Public Health Officers Association **opposed all current legislation** until antidiscrimination legislation was passed. Several of the members of our medical society asked why the CMA didn't simply write a law which included antidiscrimination legislation and then allow doctors to begin treating the epidemic as an infectious disease.

Dr. Sean Murphy, a family practitioner from Watsonville, summed up the issue clearly when he stated:

"The basic issue is an individual's right to not be tested versus the danger of spreading the disease. Does a person have a right to spread the disease? There is a double standard on HIV (disease) and other STDs." (Sexually transmitted diseases).

We talked on about the necessity of doing testing to identify those who were infected so that infected people could be educated and so there could be the threat of action against those who were infected and were knowingly spreading the disease.

DOCTOR LARIMORE CUMMINS: "I believe that those who know they are infected will not spread it (HIV disease). The purpose of testing is prevention and behavioral modification."

DOCTOR WHITE: "I disagree. There is no evidence that people will change their behavior if they know...(they are infected). (Besides) some antibody negative people are infectious."

And there it was. The President-elect of the CMA opposed testing because he felt that many people who were infected would not change their behavior. He did not believe that education of those who were infected was worthwhile. Furthermore, he used the fact that there are rare instances when people do not develop a positive antibody test as a justification for not doing general testing. It was obvious from Dr. White's statements that we would make no headway with the CMA hierarchy. They had their own agenda and it did not include using HIV testing to try to stop the epidemic.

That meeting strengthened the resolve of our Board of Governors. Shortly thereafter our Board of Governors sent out a letter to all members of the House of Delegates asking if they supported Senator Doolittle's bill to change consent and confidentiality requirements. The response to that letter was surprising, both to our Board and to the hierarchy of the CMA.

❋❋❋

In August 1987, a frightening article appeared in the Journal of the American Medical Association. This article suggested that as many as 1 in every 200 heterosexual women without risk factors on the West Coast already carried the virus. Based upon studies done in Alameda County in California, 2 out of 337 women in premarital clinics and 2 out of 299 women in the sexually transmitted disease clinics were found to be infected. That suggested .53% and .67% respectively, or over 1 in 200 women carried the virus. Despite this frightening new information demonstrating the spread of disease into the heterosexual community in the West, no effective steps were taken to stop the epidemic. After all, what could be done? The testing in the clinics in Alameda County had been done anonymously.

※※※

September 1987

Reports from Uganda were released which revealed that 1 in 10 Ugandans living in Kampala were infected with the virus. In Malaba and Busi, two eastern Ugandan towns near the Kenyan border, 80% of the women and 30% of the men had clinical AIDS. Ugandan physicians blamed the high rate of disease on the prostitutes who lived among the major truck routes and serviced the truck drivers.

In Africa, health authorities recognized that prostitutes were spreading the disease but in America and in western nations, public health authorities proclaimed that prostitutes were educating their customers on the danger of AIDS and on safe sex techniques. Anyone who talked about trying to prevent infected prostitutes from spreading the disease was accused of "scapegoating" and infringing on the prostitutes' "human and civil rights."[8]

※※※

During September 1987, President Reagan began appointing members to the Presidential AIDS Commission. This commission was to hold meetings during the ensuing 9 months to try to develop a program to combat the epidemic. The Gay and AIDS Lobbies feared that members of the committee might not follow their agenda and that the commission report might advocate treating HIV disease like all other infectious diseases.

According to the People's Daily World of September 12, 1987, (page 5A):

"Two groups asked President Reagan...to add people to his AIDS Commission who would be more representative of those...affected by the disease and to balance the extreme views of four panel members. The Public Health Citizens Research Group and the ACLU made the request...and said that 'the 13 member commission is illegally constituted and lacks mainstream views.'"

Thus began the efforts of the AIDS and Gay Lobbies to destroy the effectiveness and the credibility of the Presidential AIDS Commission.

The AIDS and Gay Lobbies set out initially to control the information that was considered by the committee, hoping that the commission would favor a program that would deal with the epidemic as a civil rights issue rather than a medical issue. This was to be a difficult task because there were people on that commission who were truly impartial.

The means by which the Presidential AIDS Commission Report was eventually captured by the forces of the left is one of the most amazing segments of the story of this epidemic and involved Admiral Watkins, soon to be appointed as Chairman of the Commission.

✳✳✳

Cliff and Louise Ray, whose home had been burned down in Arcadia, Florida, on August 28, 1987, were brought to Washington, D. C. to tell their story before the Senate Labor and Human Resources Committee. The People's Daily World of Wednesday, September 16, 1987, (page 5A), quoted Mrs. Ray as saying:

"We hope that what we've gone through is going to help America to open its eyes and say, 'This family could have been us.'"

Senator Kennedy reflected on the discrimination against the Ray family, saying, "You have to ask yourself what kind of society we are when you have this kind of reaction" (to HIV disease).

All across America there was a reaction of shock, guilt and repugnance at the thought of burning down the home of three infected children. But no one ever asked the most important question:

"Who really benefited from that tragedy? Who would use that tragedy for their own political purposes?"

✳✳✳

Articles began appearing across America about that time alluding to the work of Doctor Robert Strecker, a gastroenterologist and internist from Pasadena, California. Doctor Strecker suggested that the AIDS virus had been created by genetic engineering under the auspices of the World Health Organization. Furthermore, he alleged that the virus had probably been introduced into Africa via the WHO's smallpox vaccination program and into America in the hepatitis vaccine used for clinical trials among homosexuals. Although Doctor Strecker's work had received only limited coverage in the United States up to that time, his theories had been widely circulated throughout Europe and Africa and were being used by the KGB in an effort to confirm the fact that America was the origin of the disease which was devastating Africa.

I really had never heard of Doctor Strecker up until that time. As events unfolded, I am sure that he came to regret that I ever did hear about him. But once again I am getting ahead of my story.

❋❋❋

In early September, an HIV-infected male prostitute was arrested in Los Angeles and indicted for having sex with a client. The client, in turn, became infected. In addition, the infected prostitute attempted to sell his blood to a blood bank.[8]

Tragically, there were increasing numbers of infected homosexuals and prostitutes who were acting irresponsibly and spreading the disease across the land but any suggestion that the nation should take steps to control such activity was met with accusations of "homophobia" and "bigotry." In instance after instance, the ACLU came to the defense of those who were intentionally spreading the disease. The ACLU repeatedly justified their action proclaiming that they were "protecting the civil rights of the diseased."

❋❋❋

September, 1987 marked the first reported case in which a laboratory worker (at the National Institute of Health) became infected while working with the virus. Apparently the worker had been infected a year earlier while handling a concentrated sample of a viral strain, the same identical strain that was found in the worker's blood. The information had been suppressed for a year by NIH. Why? Despite the fact that the laboratory used rigid protective techniques and specialized equipment and there had been no break in technique, the employee had become infected. There was an obvious implication that the disease had been spread by the respiratory route. Jim Brown, a spokesman for the U. S. Public Health Service, stated:

"Nothing has changed on how AIDS is passed from person to person...We do not know how this individual became infected but we believe (that) lab workers are safe..."[9]

❋❋❋

On September 3, the Washington Times reported a survey of students at the University of Maryland. Ninety-five percent of them knew all about the factors involved in the transmission of AIDS (i.e., transmission by sexual means or sharing needles). Although 77% of the students polled said that they recognized that condoms should be used...only 30% of them had ever used condoms and then they used them only occasionally. Although the overwhelming majority of the students interviewed believed that heterosexuals were at risk for contracting HIV disease, less than 10% believed that they personally were at risk. The vast majority of the students interviewed had not changed their sexual habits, despite the fact that they all had received AIDS education.

Surveys at Tulane and Stanford universities were similar to those at the University of Maryland. The knowledge rate among students was high but behavior modification was low. It was suggested by public health officers that there were probably already hundreds of infected students on university campuses across our nation. At that point, public health authorities should have started routine testing of all students admitted to colleges and universities. However, nothing was done to try to stop the spread of the disease. By 1989 anonymous testing of college students revealed some campuses with almost a 1% incidence of infection but since testing was always anonymous there were no means of identifying those who were infected.[10]

On September 30, 1987 the New York Times reported that inner city women at high risk for AIDS infection were now well informed of risk factors but few had changed or modified their activity.

In 1987, the entire public health program in America was based on education and behavioral modification rather than attempting to introduce those techniques of testing and contact tracing which were used for all other sexually transmitted diseases. In the 1990's, education and behavioral modification were still being used almost exclusively and the epidemic continued to spread — and the dying and death continued.

1. *Private Acts, Social Consequences — AIDS and the Politics of Public Health* by Ronald Bayer, The Free Press; pp. 163-164.
2. Washington Times — June 1, 1987.
3. New York Times — Tuesday, June 2, 1987.
4. *And The Band Played On* — Randy Shilts, St. Martin's Press; Reference to CDC policy of avoiding public panic; p. 107.
5. Refer to the Manifesto of Montreal, Chapter I, which states there was to be no mandatory HIV testing in America.
6. AMA Medical News — July 17, 1987.
7. People's Daily World, July 10, 1987; p. 5A.
8. AMA Medical News — August 7, 1987, p. 32.
9. San Francisco Chronicle — September 5, 1987, p. 2.
10. Washington Times — September 3, 1987, p. 5.

CHAPTER FIVE

Knowledge is better than ignorance.
Knowing is better than not knowing.

— Lt. Col. Robert Redfield, Chief of the AIDS Service,
Walter Reed Hospital

When the letter arrived from Congressman Dannemeyer's office asking me to come to Washington, D. C. on September 21 to testify before the Congressional Subcommittee on Health and the Environment, I promptly contacted the Congressman's office. I learned that a number of concerned Americans would be going to Washington to appear before this Subcommittee to speak in opposition to Congressman Waxman's AIDS legislation (HR3071) and in support of Congressman Dannemeyer's bills. I managed to convince the Congressman's office that they should invite Larimore as well, since I recognized that he would be an important witness.

At our own expense, Larimore and I flew to Washington to meet with the Congressman and to testify. That meeting and subsequent events started a cascade of events that would soon lead both Larimore and me into ever increasing prominent positions in the battle to address the HIV epidemic. It was at this point that I came to recognize that some people in high positions at the Centers for Disease Control had no intention of carrying out President Reagan's HIV policies or following the Presidential directive to determine the incidence of HIV disease. At that time, we had no idea how far it had spread. Still, in the 1990's all efforts to determine the true incidence of the disease in the general population have been effectively thwarted. To demonstrate the tactics that were used, I would like to record here the testimony before the Subcommittee on Health and the Environment on September 21. Doctor James Mason, who is quoted, was the Director of the CDC at that time. By 1989, he had become Assistant Secretary of Health at HHS.

Congressman Dannemeyer was addressing Doctor Otis Bowen, Secretary of the Department of Health and Human Services.

CONGRESSMAN DANNEMEYER: "Mr. Secretary, I think President Reagan issued an order recently that required HHS to establish guidelines for testing a requisite sample of the population of America for the virus for AIDS. It is my understanding that there was a requirement that HHS establish these guidelines by July 18, 1987. Could you tell me what the status of the guidelines is and when we can expect this testing to take place in this country."

SECRETARY BOWEN: "May I refer that to Dr. Mason?"

MR. DANNEMEYER: "Thank you."

DOCTOR MASON: "Immediately after the President's request that this kind of information be provided with dispatch, the CDC invited a group of national consultants, including The Census Bureau, The National Center for Health Statistics and people in the academic field to consult on doing a national random seroprevalence survey.

"It was the general feeling of the group we brought together that because of the difficulties inherent in getting responses on a household survey where you were actually going to the household and drawing blood, there would have to be a series of events that took place prior to the actual sampling on a national basis. We are working as rapidly as we can through all of these problems."

MR. DANNEMEYER: "We have limited time. Are the guidelines in existence right now?"

DR. MASON: "Guidelines for what?"

MR. DANNEMEYER: "For testing this requisite group of people in America for the presence of the virus."

DR. MASON: "National experts are developing these right now."

MR. DANNEMEYER: "When can we expect to have them?"

DR. MASON: "As soon as they are through."

MR. DANNEMEYER: "Do you have any idea when that is going to be?"

DR. MASON: "It's a little like pregnancy, nine women cannot produce a baby in one month..."

Faced with an epidemic that threatens to destroy our nation, faced with an epidemic that had already killed tens of thousands of Americans and would soon kill millions more, Dr. James Mason of the CDC was talking about "9 women cannot produce a baby in one month." He was playing word games. As of the writing of this book, almost four years after the President called for immediate surveillance testing, HHS and the CDC still have not carried out the extensive seroprevalence studies in the general population ordered by President Reagan in May of 1987.

I testified that same day before the committee and told the story of Dr.

Robert Illa and the fact that he had been threatened by an official from the CDC if he dared to speak further about the case which he thought represented casual transmission of HIV disease. Before going to Washington, I had made a copy of a video tape of Dr. Illa's story and had taken that copy with me. I offered the tape to the committee. Interestingly, no one besides Congressman Dannemeyer showed any interest in that interview.

There were four events that were associated with our trip to Washington. The first event was the opportunity to meet Shepherd Smith, a businessman who had given up his livelihood and mortgaged his home in order to finance an organization called Americans for a Sound AIDS Policy (ASAP). This organization served as a rallying point for those of us who were concerned about the epidemic. Meeting Shepherd Smith gave us access to that small cadre of concerned and courageous Americans who were anxious to do something to try to stop the dying and unnecessary death.

The second event was the opportunity to meet Judy Weltin and her husband from Brodheadsville, Pennsylvania. They told me the story of Craig Stenger, the boy who had presumably contracted the disease while living in the same household with his infected mother and father. I referred to their story in Chapter 3. As you will recall, Craig's mother had gotten the infection from a contaminated blood transfusion when Craig was four years old. As a result of that meeting with the Weltin's, I was able to check out their story further and to confirm the apparent casual transmission of HIV disease, thus disproving the official line of the Surgeon General, the CDC and the AIDS and Gay Lobbies that there has never been a case of casual transmission of the disease. Once again, I would reiterate that casual spread of the disease is uncommon and only occurs with prolonged, intimate contact in families, with deep kissing and the exchange of saliva or among health care workers, but it does occur.

The third event was our meeting with Congressman Dannemeyer. The Congressman took Larimore and me to lunch and asked us to read an initiative that he had written which he hoped to place on the ballot in California in 1988. He gave us each a copy of his handwritten notes and asked for our comments.

The fourth event was Larimore's invitation to go to the White House. Working through Missy Hancock, one of Congressman Dannemeyer's administrative assistants, Larimore was able to get an invitation to meet one of Gary Bauer's assistants. As mentioned earlier, Bauer was President Reagan's chief advisor on domestic and public policy issues. I had seen him on Ted Koppel's "Television Town Meeting of the Air" in June. Bauer had a small staff of dedicated conservatives who had ready access to the President and who could relay information on important issues.

Larimore's opportunity to have that audience at the White House would ultimately lead to numerous contacts during the ensuing months, contacts by which Senator Jesse Helms would receive information from Santa Cruz that the Senator used in debates on the floor of the Senate. Other information that Larimore provided was used by presidential advisors in forming national policy. It is amazing how our little town of Santa Cruz began to have an influence far beyond its boundaries and how Larimore, in his quiet, unassuming way, was beginning to influence both state and national policy. Certainly he has never asked for notoriety and is strongly opposed to my telling his story, but some of the facts that he was able to glean from his White House contacts are vitally important to your understanding of the subsequent course of the epidemic. It is vitally important that you know the background of the sources of information which I will describe...as I tell you how the President of the United States and his staff tried to use the power of the Presidency to influence the handling of the epidemic — but were thwarted by even more powerful forces intent on blocking the use of logical measures to halt the spread of this disease.

✳✳✳

In September the State Legislature in Louisiana passed a law requiring (mandatory) routine premarital blood testing. The Louisiana State Medical Society immediately came out in opposition to the new law and was joined by the American Civil Liberties Union. According to the report in the AMA News, the attorney for the ACLU in New Orleans said:

"This law is asking for trouble since in low risk groups the rate of false positives is very high. We may see people killing themselves."

✳✳✳

It was also in the fall of 1987 that the CDC issued a directive mandating that health care workers treat every patient in the hospital as if they were infected with HIV disease and hepatitis. Health care workers were told that "they should take universal precautions with all hospital patients to protect themselves from the possibility of infection." Universal precautions included wearing gloves when coming in contact with blood or infected secretions.

Health care workers in hospitals were told that there was no danger from saliva since saliva was not infectious. On the other hand, dentists and dental technicians were told that they must use universal precautions when working in the mouth with saliva. I believe that wearing gloves on the ward is important — but the idea of using universal precautions in an operating suite is totally ridiculous and the CDC knew it. For 50 years surgeons have worn gloves, masks and gowns in surgery and, yet this is the only policy that the CDC recommended to protect surgical personnel.

The problem is that wearing masks, gloves and gowns will not protect a surgeon or his nurse from the HIV virus. Surgical personnel often get needle sticks and surgical gloves will not protect them from such injuries. Surgical masks transmit fine aerosolized matter to the surgeon's mucous membranes and blood is often splattered onto a surgeon's face. In 1987, it was important for surgeons to order routine blood tests on all surgical patients so that doctors could know who was infected in order to protect medical personnel from acquiring the infection. But surgeons were not encouraged to test patients routinely. Indeed, everything was done to discourage doctors from testing patients preoperatively. Despite the fact that even Surgeon General Koop had suggested that all patients going into the hospital for major surgery should be tested, the CDC has continued to actively discourage presurgical testing. There is little question from reading CDC reports that the basic thrust of CDC policy has been to discourage doctors from doing routine hospital admission testing or from testing health care personnel.

❋❋❋

In September, the California State Senate was considering new legislation (AB87) which had been introduced by Assemblyman Art Agnos of San Francisco. AB87 included an antidiscrimination law. It mandated sex education in all California schools and included a section requiring "informed consent before HIV testing." The informed consent provision of this legislation mandated that physicians must tell their patients that the HIV test was inaccurate, that they might lose their jobs, their insurance policies and homes if confidentiality was breached. Passage of AB87 would have meant a virtual end to HIV testing in physicians' offices in California. Initially the bill had been supported by the CMA. Then the CMA Council took a position of "no position." Finally the CMA Council came out and took a position of "oppose unless amended." According to the AMA News, the President-elect of the CMA, Doctor Laurens White, said publicly that "the position (of the CMA Council) had not been officially upgraded (to support) because the CMA Council had not had a scheduled meeting." According to the AMA News, Doctor White supported AB87 in Sacramento (despite the position taken by the CMA Council).

Although the bill passed the legislature, it was ultimately vetoed by the Governor.[1]

***

In Washington, D. C. at the first public meeting of the Presidential AIDS Commission on September 9 and 10, the Commission was met by a "loud and often jeering crowd of gay rights activists and people with AIDS.[2]

***

Doctor Warren Bosdick had been President of the California Medical Association in 1961. By 1987, he was the former Dean of the College of Medicine at the University of California in Irvine. Still practicing, although in his 70's, Dr. Bosdick appeared before Congressman Waxman's Subcommittee to **speak against** the concepts of **anonymous testing** for HIV disease. He stated that anonymous HIV testing was "very, very dangerous." He went on to say that anonymous testing for the HIV virus gave "a person with AIDS a sanctioned right to hide and escape from all procedures necessary to control the spread of the disease and would serve as a direct threat to the survival rights of the uninfected majority of the population." Doctor Bosdick pointed out that anonymous testing prevented the reporting of the disease to the public health officer, contact tracing and efforts to break the chain of transmission.[3]

***

October 1987
In October, a Dallas pediatrician announced that he was selling his

practice because his case load had fallen off when his patients learned that he had tested positive for HIV disease. Information about his infection became public knowledge when the doctor filed a lawsuit and obtained a restraining order against a former roommate who had threatened to inform the doctor's patients and local professional groups that Dr. Robert Huse had AIDS. The doctor complained that he was being discriminated against simply because he was infected. An article appeared in the AMA News discussing this event and went on to discuss the tragedy that had befallen this physician. The message relayed to the reader by that article was clear: our society needed antidiscrimination laws to keep people from discriminating against those who were infected. Furthermore, the inference of the article (though not stated) is that testing leads directly to discrimination. On the other hand, knowledge of the doctor's disease status would never have been made public had the doctor not told his roommate and then filed a lawsuit against him. It was only after that lawsuit was filed that information became public knowledge. As with so many articles being published in newspapers during this period, the entire emphasis of the article was on the dangers of discrimination and the tragedy that befell victims of discrimination. There was never any mention of the large numbers of people, both homosexual and heterosexual, who were acquiring the disease unnecessarily because public health officials were not addressing the epidemic as an epidemic and not trying to stop its spread.

❋❋❋

In October, newspapers reported that the Ray family had moved from Arcadia to Sarasota, Florida and that the children had entered school. Of course, the family could have stayed in Arcadia where the children had been admitted to school under a court order and had started attending classes, but the family elected to move to Sarasota after going to Washington to testify before Senator Kennedy's committee. By October, the Ray family had received a million dollar judgment against the school district in Arcadia. They had received substantial financial donations from across the country after their home burned and the family had brought suit against the company that supplied the anti-hemophiliac preparation that led to the infection of their three children.

❋❋❋

Probably the most significant event of October 1987 occurred in San

Francisco, a city where gay activists wielded immense political power. San Francisco had the highest incidence of gay infection anywhere in our nation. The significant event was the seroconversion of one nurse at San Francisco General Hospital after a single needle stick with an HIV-infected needle. It is strange how God or destiny or fate will influence events. Like the "shot heard around the world" that began the battle at the bridge at Concord in 1775 and set in place a chain of events that culminated in America's Revolutionary War, so the tragedy of that one nurse's seroconversion led to a chain of events that motivated another woman to become involved in this battle. That one woman has probably had more of an influence on the course of this epidemic than any other person in America except perhaps Bill Dannemeyer. Her dedication to truth and her personal sacrifices put the male physicians of this nation (including myself) to shame. If this epidemic is ever brought under control and America survives as a free nation, it will be in large part because of the efforts of this one woman.

In April of 1989, I was in Atlanta at the Centers for Disease Control talking to Dr. James Curran. I asked him why he didn't openly support testing to control the epidemic.

"I'm caught in the middle," he protested. "Between Congressman Waxman on one side and Bill Dannemeyer and Lorraine Day on the other."

Gay activists have threatened to kill her. They have threatened to throw acid in her face and to kill her family. During the fall of 1988 when she was actively campaigning for Proposition 102, Doctor Day had to travel with a bodyguard because of the numerous threats made against her life, yet she has persisted in her efforts to awaken physicians to the dangers that face the medical profession and our nation.

Her awareness of the epidemic came about when that one health care worker at San Francisco General Hospital became infected. It was at that point that Dr. Day, Chief of Orthopedic Surgery at San Francisco General Hospital and an internationally known and respected surgeon, started a one-woman crusade to address the epidemic.

She went to the Infection Control staff at her hospital and asked how this infection could have occurred since infectious disease specialists had repeatedly assured surgeons that there was absolutely no possibility of health care workers acquiring HIV disease from needle-stick injuries. It readily became apparent that infectious disease physicians at San

Francisco General Hospital had been intentionally downplaying the risk of infection.

Dr. Day then asked to be tested in order to protect her surgeon husband and her family. No one seemed to know how to go about getting HIV testing for the house staff although the hospital had supposedly been performing routine HIV testing on all those who routinely worked on the AIDS Ward.

Dr. Day had blood specimens drawn on herself and her staff and took them to the Administration. The Administration waited two weeks to inform her that all the blood specimens had been left out and gotten moldy. Apparently there were those at the hospital who actively opposed routine blood testing of the house staff. After submitting new blood specimens, it took seven more weeks to get the blood test results.

At meetings of the staff surgeons at the hospital, Dr. Day brought up the necessity of doing routine testing on all patients being admitted for surgery. At that time it was thought that as many as 30% of the patients on her service were in one or another high risk group — either homosexuals, bisexuals or IV drug users. Testing later revealed that on one occasion on one of her services 90% of her patients were HIV infected.

Initially, almost all the chiefs of the various surgical subspecialties agreed that it was only logical and rational to try to identify patients who were infected and might have an altered immune system — not only for the patient's protection but for the protection of the hospital staff. The surgeons recognized that the danger of a needle stick was very real but few of them realized that the incidence of seroconversion was 1 in 200 from an HIV-infected needle-stick injury. To rational physicians it was only logical to try to find out if a patient carried the virus. That's what doctors have always done — even though many of the diseases they diagnose were incurable. After all, to most doctors, knowledge was better than ignorance; knowing was better than not knowing. As soon as information got out that Lorraine Day was recommending routine HIV testing on patients admitted to her surgical service, the AIDS and Gay Lobbies began bringing political pressure to bear. Virtually all the other chiefs of the surgical services at the hospital backed away from doing what was obviously medically sound. Many months later when I was talking to Dr. Day she said,

"The trouble with those fellows is that they just didn't have any guts."

And that was really true. Faced with demonstrations, angry denunciations and threats, most doctors would rather compromise than fight. When representatives from ABC's Nightline came to San Francisco to interview Dr. Day for Ted Koppel's evening program, the Administrator at San Francisco General Hospital informed her that she could not be interviewed on the hospital grounds but would have to go outside. Then she was called into the administrator's office and told that she must stop suggesting that it was a sound medical practice to do routine HIV testing. In response to the obvious threat to her university appointed position, Dr. Day announced that she would persist in testing and furthermore she intended to carry out studies to determine whether there was danger to medical personnel in the operating room from the vaporization of blood or bone particles which occurs with the use of a drill, saw or a Bovie (an electric knife). It was already known that doctors could disseminate the papilloma virus by vaporization using a Bovie. Was it possible to disseminate the HIV retrovirus in a similar manner? Was there potential danger of infection of health care personnel working in the operating room? Certainly the CDC had shown no concern. They had made no effort to determine the danger of spreading the HIV virus via the respiratory route in surgery. Indeed, almost all published studies on the spread of HIV in HCW's had **excluded surgeons,** as was done with the HIV studies published from San Francisco General Hospital.

At this point, Lorraine Day was told that she would not be allowed to carry out these studies.

As a result of this confrontation one of the vice-chancellors of the University of California went to see Dr. William Murray who was the Professor of Orthopedic Surgery at the Medical School in San Francisco. The vice-chancellor notified Dr. Murray that,

"If you don't bring that woman under control, we'll cut off all your funds for research."

In response to this very obvious threat, Dr. Murray is reported to have replied,

"Not only will I not bring her under control, I will use our own orthopedic department funds to help her."[4]

That is just what happened. At last, the AIDS Lobby and the Gay Lobby had found someone that they could not intimidate. When Lorraine Day was invited to attend a meeting of the American College of Surgeons to discuss the epidemic, someone purporting to represent the CMA called the American College and told them not to allow her to speak.

City lawyers called her and announced that they intended to cancel her surgical malpractice coverage so that if she were sued, she would have no coverage. Every effort was made to silence her; however, because she was attractive, articulate and convincing in her presentation, she was invited to more and more medical meetings across the nation and was able to penetrate the conspiracy of silence and misinformation that had been disseminated by medical journals and the media. More and more, she began to make doctors realize the dangers that they face.

Described in the San Francisco Chronicle as a "brassy, bossy blond," she is all of those. But I say this with no disrespect. She is an intelligent and articulate woman. To survive in a man's specialty as the chief of a busy orthopedic service, one has to be bossy and forceful. To be willing to stand up to the administration of San Francisco General Hospital and risk her position as a tenured professor, she had to be brassy. As an attractive blonde who has the respect of every orthopedist in Northern California who I know, she is one of the few women in orthopedics who has maintained her femininity while working successfully in a profession dominated by males. Her personal impact and her spreading of information about this epidemic has awakened many physicians to the very real possibility that their lives and the lives of their staff and families are endangered. As a result of her lectures many doctors throughout this nation have changed their surgical technique and begun wearing the equipment that is necessary to protect their lives in the era of HIV disease.

❋❋❋

In October, the Board of Education in New York City announced that it would supply teachers and all public school employees with one and a half million pairs of rubber gloves to be used in case it was necessary to clean up blood from HIV-infected children on the schoolground or give assistance to an infected student who was bleeding. Although teachers and students were reassured that there was absolutely no reason to worry about children attending school with HIV disease, gloves were made available to all employees in the New York City school system.[5]

In New York, the State Health Commissioner, Dr. David Axelrod, announced that HIV testing could no longer be performed in public laboratories. Henceforth, all testing for HIV disease would only be allowed in special laboratories. These laboratories included "blood and tissue banks, state, city or county laboratories, laboratories located in hospitals affiliated with medical schools, the American Red Cross or New York blood programs or research laboratories doing public health work under contract." This directive from the State Health Commissioner prevented all private laboratories from doing HIV blood testing. Doctors could not do the test in their own offices. Thus it became virtually impossible for physicians in the State of New York to carry out routine HIV testing in their private practices. This was simply one more barrier that Dr. Axelrod and the AIDS and Gay Lobbies intentionally placed in the way of physicians to keep them from using the blood test to stop the spread of HIV disease. In the 1990's the epidemic is out of control in New York City — in large part because of the actions of Dr. Axelrod, the AIDS Lobby and the Gay Lobby and their success in blocking the effective use of HIV testing.

❋❋❋

There were only two states that adopted mandatory premarital testing. One was Illinois, the other was Louisiana. It took six months before the AIDS and Gay Lobbies were able to get the law reversed in Louisiana, but in the State of Illinois, routine premarital blood testing was voted in by the State Legislature. The premarital testing bill was guided through the legislature by another courageous woman — State Representative Penny Pullen. The governor signed the law. Surgeon General C. Everett Koop went to Chicago shortly thereafter to attack the concept of premarital HIV testing.

"I can't think of any worse way to spend your money," he said.

"Homosexuals and IV drug users, those groups at high risk, are unlikely to apply for marriage licenses and most couples today have probably had sexual relations before applying for a marriage license."

Doctor Koop certainly should have known that you could have sexual relations a dozen times and not contract the disease. But if one were to enter into a life-long sexual relationship with someone who was infected, in all probability, the uninfected marital partner would contract the disease within one or two years and ultimately die. Furthermore, premarital testing was not aimed at high risk groups. It was aimed at trying to stop the third epidemic — the spread of the disease in the heterosexual population. By ridiculing premarital testing, Dr. Koop gave credence to the positions of the AIDS and Gay Lobbies which were intent upon blocking the use of routine premarital testing to stop the spread of the epidemic in the heterosexual community.[6]

※※※

On Saturday, October 10, 1987, the People's Daily World criticized President Reagan and his AIDS Panel, stating that,

"Reagan has not been reluctant to express support for...HIV testing...but it's fraught with **danger to constitutional rights.**" (emphasis added) The article concluded with the statement "No one is immune from the effects of the AIDS crisis. As the disease grows, it will take a toll not only of its victims and their families but on the fabric of our society...Millions of lives are at stake."

Yes, the Communists understood that this epidemic could destroy America just as efficiently as a nuclear attack. Yet they were intent on blocking the use of testing in America, while condoning testing in Cuba, Russia and other Communist countries.[7]

※※※

It was also in October 1987 when hundreds of thousands of AIDS demonstrators marched on the White House under the auspices of "The National March on Washington for Gay and Lesbian Rights." Signs proclaimed, FIGHT AIDS — NOT PEOPLE WITH AIDS and MONEY FOR AIDS — NOT WAR. During the speeches that followed, President Reagan was vilified and deprecated for not working to bring the epidemic under control, for not spending vast sums of money for education and the care of the infected and for refusing to support antidiscrimination and confidentiality laws.

The demonstrators brought out the AIDS quilt with one thousand nine hundred and twenty patches on it representing the 25,000 people who had already died of AIDS.

It was at that march in October of 1987 when the parade organizers passed out a list of their demands. These demands were quite similar to those that were passed out in Montreal at the 5th International Conference on AIDS almost two years later, except that in Washington in 1987, they demanded the overthrow of the South African government, the end to apartheid, and freedom and democracy for South Africa. Their list of demands in 1987 proclaimed that there was to be no mandatory HIV testing in America for any reason. Furthermore, they demanded a massive program of redistribution of the wealth of the nation to overcome our social ills. There was a demand for lesbian rights and gay rights; they demanded that all anti-sodomy laws be done away with and that all forms of discrimination against gays and lesbians be outlawed.

❋❋❋

During the same month, New York State announced that they were going to start a program of widespread **anonymous** testing. A hundred thousand blood samples were to be collected from hospitals and clinics all across the state to try to determine the incidence of the disease. Of course, the patient's name was to be removed from the specimen so that there would be no way of telling which patients were infected. New York State Health Commissioner, Dr. David Axelrod was quoted as saying:

"We need more accurate information about the number and distribution of individuals already infected with the virus to plan necessary medical services and to target AIDS prevention efforts."

Tragically, no efforts were made to try to identify those who carried the virus so that they could be enrolled in treatment programs or modify their sexual activity to break the chain of transmission and death. Instead, New York State announced it was spending over three million dollars to do extensive **anonymous** testing, to gather statistics...but not to try to stop the epidemic[8]

❋❋❋

In late October 1987, the Santa Cruz Coalition for Traditional Values held a public meeting to discuss the problems of the AIDS epidemic. Paul Gann was there. Now, for those outside California, the name "Paul Gann" may not be well known, but to those within California, Paul Gann was a living legend. An old-line conservative, for years he had fought the State Legislature to cut back on taxation, regulation and regimentation of the individual. Along with Howard Jarvis, he sponsored Proposition 13 which limited spiralling property taxes in California. Year after year, he worked to limit governmental power over the lives of the individual. Then it happened. Over a period of several months, Paul Gann became increasingly ill. In the months that followed, his physician could not determine what was wrong with him. He grew progressively weaker, lost weight, ran a fever and became susceptible to recurrent infections. His lymph nodes began to swell. It was his wife who insisted that he have an HIV antibody test because of the blood transfusions that he had received several years earlier. The test was positive. Paul Gann had ARC, a prelude to AIDS and death. Paul Gann did not sit back and bemoan his fate, nor did he demand an antidiscrimination law to protect HIV carriers. Instead, he became embroiled in the AIDS issue and an outspoken proponent of using HIV testing in an effort to bring the epidemic under control.

Paul Gann was seventy-five years old. He wore dark, horn-rimmed glasses, his forehead was well over the top of his head and there was a band of gray hair around the sides of his head. His clothes hung limply from his frail body and he moved slowly when he walked. Yet this aging, HIV-infected patriot still had the drive, determination and ambition to be involved. In October of 1987, he was already a leading spokesman for using HIV testing to stop further spread of the disease. In the months that lay ahead, Paul Gann became the leading proponent of a new State initiative—Proposition 102—which would have declared HIV disease a legal disease in California and finally allowed doctors to begin addressing the epidemic and stop the unnecessary dying and death.

"There is only one way to stop the spread of AIDS and that's to find out who has it and to stop them from spreading it to others," Gann told the audience that night. Civil rights was not the issue. This was a medical issue and had to be addressed as such. People were becoming infected because other people did not know that they had the virus and were, in many instances, unintentionally giving it to others. "Who had the right to sentence me to death?" Gann asked. "Nobody."[9]

✳✳✳

On October 15, a lawsuit was filed against the President of the United States by a number of left-wing groups including "The Public Health Citizen's Research Organization," "The People With AIDS Coalition," "The National Minority AIDS Council," "The American Public Health Association," "The Gay Men's Health Crisis" and several individuals. The suit asked for a preliminary injunction halting the Presidential AIDS Commission's work until the President appointed members to the commission who would be more favorable to the left-wing position.

The suit charged that "The White House had violated the Federal Advisory Committee Act which requires the membership of an advisory committee to be fairly balanced in terms of point of view."

The situation of the Presidential AIDS Commission, at that time, was that the AIDS and Gay Lobbies could count on only a minority of the 13 members to represent their position. The groups filing the lawsuit wanted a dependable majority to assure that the committee's report would come out favorable to their position — a position which would oppose testing and the use of public health measures to stop the spread of HIV disease. The lawsuit was eventually dropped but it demonstrated the importance that the AIDS activists placed on the report that would be forthcoming from the Commission.

✼✼✼

During 1987, a number of articles were published in medical journals and in the liberal media across America. The recurrent theme of these articles was that physicians should not use HIV testing to try to stop this epidemic, physicians should not use testing to identify those in the general population who were infected.

An article was published in the prestigious New England Journal of Medicine on July 23, 1987 pointing out the potential dangers of widespread testing and the high incidence of false-positive test results that could be expected when screening low risk populations for evidence of infection.

Suddenly, for no apparent reason, article after article began appearing in medical journals, reinforcing the idea that widespread use of the HIV blood test to control the epidemic would be counterproductive and would falsely identify large numbers of people as being infected.

In October 1987, a similar article appeared in the Journal of the American Medical Association, reporting that HIV testing in low risk populations would lead to an unacceptable incidence of false-positive test results. Utilizing a statistical analysis based upon what would happen if poorly supervised laboratories did poor and inaccurate blood testing in low risk populations, the article showed a high incidence of false positive blood tests. Totally ignoring the U. S. Army report documenting their experience in testing low risk populations with a carefully monitored laboratory, this article in JAMA from Harvard University by Cleary, et.al., purported to show the futility of attempting to stop the epidemic using HIV testing in the general population.

Larimore wrote an article in JAMA refuting the statistics in the Harvard article. Using his own statistical analysis, he demonstrated the fallacy of the Harvard presumption. The editors of The Journal refused his article but did publish his letter to the editor. There were several other letters critical of the Harvard study. The Harvard authors answered every letter but Larimore's. Quite obviously they were unable to challenge his refutation of their work.[10]

Another article appeared in the October 16 issue of The Journal of the American Medical Association. It was a "Letter to the Editor" describing the case of a 58-year-old black man who had been inaccurately diagnosed as having AIDS by bronchoscopic washings which were reported to show evidence of Pneumocystis carinii pneumonia. Furthermore, his HIV blood test had been reported as being positive. The patient resigned his position as a school teacher, anticipating he had a terminal illness and would soon die. Later, re-evaluation of the slides from his bronchial washings and rechecking of his blood test at another institution showed that there was no evidence of HIV disease and that the original diagnosis had been incorrect. The article stressed the social and psychological consequences of the misdiagnosis of AIDS.[11]

On October 6, in the Wall Street Journal, there was a discussion of an article that had been published in the British medical journal, Lancet. The article stated that people could carry the virus for long periods of time before their HIV test turned positive. The Lancet article was a report from socialist Finland, discussing a number of infected Finnish homosexuals who had been followed for three years. Initially, their blood tests were consistently negative and, in some instances, it took two to three years for their HIV test to turn positive. Going back over their blood specimens, however, Finnish investigation verified that the homosexuals had the infection for years before their blood test turned positive. Based upon this new information, it appeared that it really wasn't worthwhile doing widespread blood testing of our general population because many people could harbor the virus, yet their blood test would not reveal it. Was this a valid observation? The blood test was accurate enough for the Army to use to screen military recruits. The blood test was accurate enough to protect our blood supply. The blood test could be used in other countries for general screening, but the blood test was not accurate enough to screen America's population to try to stop the spread of the epidemic in our land.

It was the following month, in November 1987, when the New York Times published their editorial (to which I referred in Book One,

Chapter Three) pointing out the dangers of widespread testing of the American population and cautioning the Presidential AIDS Commission that they should not recommend general testing of the population because of the high incidence of false-positive test results in low risk populations. (See Appendix VI)

Within five short months, a series of articles was presented to the medical profession and the public giving reason after reason as to why physicians should not start using the blood test to stop the epidemic. As a result, the disease, the dying and death continued.

※※※

In October the Secretary of Education, William Bennett, released a handbook for educators suggesting that teaching about AIDS should be carried out in a moral context and should stress moral issues. The handbook even suggested that education should "teach restraint as a virtue." The handbook suggested that "the safest way to prevent infection with the deadly AIDS virus was to avoid premarital sex and illegal drugs." Representative Tom Weiss (Democrat from New York), the Chairman of the House Human Resources and Intergovernmental Relations Committee, condemned the handbook stating that the message of Secretary Bennett's handbook was "terribly misguided" for focusing almost exclusively on "the moral message of abstinence." Although acknowledging that abstinence was the only safe way to avoid the disease, Representative Weiss felt that more stress should be placed on the role of condoms in preventing transmission of the disease.

※※※

In the fall of 1987, the Department of Health and Human Services was preparing a pamphlet to be distributed to every home in our nation under the auspices of the U. S. Public Health Service. They were planning on distributing 45 million copies of that pamphlet which would discuss sodomy and various forms of sexual perversion and the part that these activities played in spreading the epidemic. Officials highly placed in the White House felt that much of the information contained in this booklet was inappropriate. As a result, the initial distribution of the publication was delayed while the White House, representatives from the CDC, HHS and the U. S. Public Health Service ironed out the information which was to be presented so that it would not be offensive to the general population. The eight page pamphlet was eventually released in mid-1988 and is reproduced in Appendix II. Surgeon General Koop's picture appears on the cover of that pamphlet along with his statement. Certainly, Secretary of Education William Bennett had no input into that public health pamphlet, because there was not one mention of the words "morality" or "marriage" in the entire publication. It was in this pamphlet that the U. S. Public Health Service recommended their novel, scientific approach to stopping the epidemic. That approach did not include testing. Rather, they suggested that —

"If you know someone well enough to have sex, then you should be able to talk about AIDS. If someone is unwilling to talk, you shouldn't have sex."

I couldn't help but wonder what the scientific rationale was for that profound recommendation. Repeated surveys of the public had shown that men would lie to their sexual partners to gain sexual favors, yet faced with this epidemic threatening the very survival of our nation, public health officials suggested that, "If someone is unwilling to talk, you shouldn't have sex." (See Appendix II for the full text of the report).

❋❋❋

On October 9, 1987 it was reported that a second laboratory worker had been infected with the AIDS virus after handling a highly concentrated viral solution and apparently cutting his hand. Information about the infection had again been withheld (suppressed) for over one year by governmental officials. The patient had been contaminated in late 1985 and the infectious disease status was first detected in May of 1986. However it was not until October 9, 1987 that the National Institute of Health saw fit to release the information to the general public. As one analyzes the pattern of suppression of information by governmental officials during this epidemic, it becomes increasingly obvious that vital information is often repressed for prolonged periods of time for fear of alarming the public.[12]

❋❋❋

In the Santa Cruz Sentinel, the local newspaper in my hometown, an article appeared in October criticizing Doctor Larimore Cummins and our County Medical Society Task Force for daring to suggest that routine hospital admission HIV testing should be performed. A local psychiatrist was interviewed. He pointed out that, "It was stressful for patients to go into the hospital" and he felt that "HIV testing would simply add to the emotional stress and might lead to a number of severe emotional disorders." He went on to point out the dangers of the risk of a breach of hospital confidentiality and the false sense of security that hospital personnel would experience if a patient had a negative blood test and yet was still in the latent period of infectiousness. The article suggested that the Centers for Disease Control guidelines did not require routine testing of patients being admitted to the hospital and concluded with the statement that, "The risks involved in routine testing are so great that no one should have to undergo that risk unnecessarily."

❈❈❈

In the months that followed, a number of efforts were made to discredit the Santa Cruz County Medical Society AIDS Task Force. Leaders of the California Medical Association were openly critical of our medical society for daring to speak out about the CMA Executive Committee's position opposing premarital and prenatal blood testing and SB1000. We were told that our medical society should not criticize the position of our leaders. Letters were sent to members of our medical society demanding that we stop our criticism of CMA policy. It appeared that the CMA Executive Committee had their own plan. The epidemic would be stopped by education and behavioral modification and testing was not to be used routinely in the general population.

❈❈❈

November 1987
November was an exciting month. I had the opportunity to journey to Washington, D. C. and be interviewed in the White House.

There were a number of events which had transpired since my trip to Washington in September. First, I had read through Congressman Dannemeyer's handwritten notes on the initiative which he hoped to submit to the voters in November 1988. Bill Dannemeyer is one of the most courageous legislators in this nation but there were flaws in his initiative which would have perpetuated the problems that physicians faced in trying to address the epidemic. I wrote to him and diplomatically suggested certain changes in his initiative. Apparently Larimore did the same because the next thing I heard, Congressman Dannemeyer had gone to Senator Doolittle's office in Sacramento, put the initiative on the Senator's desk and said, "You write it." At that point, Senator Doolittle assigned the task to his administrative assistant, Ted Blanchard and, Ted, along with Larimore, hammered out what came to be known initially as "The Dannemeyer Initiative," then "The Dannemeyer-Doolittle Initiative," then "The Dannemeyer-Doolittle-Gann Initiative" and ultimately, "The Gann Initiative — Proposition 102." I was asked for my input in writing the initiative, but because of the pressures of work and a number of other projects, I declined. It is just as well that I did. As events unfolded, an organized, statewide program developed to try to discredit me and to discredit Proposition 102 as well. When that occurred, I could honestly tell reporters that I had had nothing to do with the writing of the initiative.

❋❋❋

When the final history of the HIV epidemic is written, and if our nation survives, there will be a dozen names of men and women of courage and integrity who worked and sacrificed, risking all to awaken our nation to its peril. Close to the top of that list will be the name of a quiet, unassuming man named Shepherd Smith. I had met him two months previously in Congressman Dannemeyer's office. Shepherd had no medical background. He was a Christian businessman trying to make a living like most Americans. Unlike most Americans, however, he was willing to become personally involved. Realizing the significance of the epidemic, he had given up his livelihood and set out to put together an organization to coordinate those people across our nation who felt strongly that HIV disease should be treated as a medical condition and not as a civil rights issue.

Centering his organization in Washington, D. C., he managed to obtain support from various sources (i.e., insurance and pharmaceutical companies). His organization always operated on a shoestring and eventually he had to mortgage his home to pay expenses and keep his organization functioning. But function it did and it still exists today. "Americans For A Sound AIDS Policy" is known by the acronym ASAP (which can also stand for "as soon as possible"). Working closely with Major Robert Redfield (later to become Lt. Col. Redfield) and Colonel Donald Burke — both of Walter Reed Hospital — and a handful of other concerned citizens across the nation, Shepherd acted as a clearing house for the dissemination of information on what was happening.

On one side of the battle you had hundreds of gay organizations and hundreds of gay publications, all coordinated to effectively block HIV

testing. They were funded with countless millions of dollars of taxpayers' money. Then there was the entire gamut of organizations on the left
— from the ACLU to NOW to the National Lawyers Guild (the legal
arm of the Communist Party). There was the CMA, the CNA, the AMA,
the AHA (American Hospital Association), the CDA and the CHA.
There were literally hundreds of organizations which were working
with the Gay and AIDS Lobbies to block testing. On our side, there were
only a few organizations. One was the National AIDS Prevention
Institute (P. O. Box 2500, Culpeper, Virginia 22701) headed by Doctor
Ed Rowe, a fundamentalist minister who created his AIDS organization
as an outgrowth of an old line anti-Communist organization, the Church
League of America.

Gene Antonio, author of *The AIDS Cover-Up*, published an AIDS
newsletter and spoke across the nation but he had no organization. His
life had been threatened repeatedly.

Doctor Paul Cameron was a psychologist in Washington, D. C. He
headed the Family Research Institute. He spoke across the nation and
circulated a newsletter. Paul's life was threatened repeatedly and acts of
physical violence were used to intimidate him. He had done a great deal
of work on the psychology of homosexuality and its origins. Although
he supported testing and contact tracing, he had unfortunately alienated
most of the responsible leaders on our side of the battle because of his
insistence on placing a tattoo or mark on all those who were infected,
reminiscent of the tattooing of concentration camp inmates by the Nazis
during World War II.

Another spokesman for testing was Dr. Bill O'Connor, a family
physician from Northern California who openly advocated confining all
those who were infected in quarantine camps — also reminiscent of the
Nazi treatment of homosexuals. Both Paul Cameron and Bill O'Connor
held positions which inflamed the fears of homosexuals and their
positions were both medically unsound and politically counterproductive.

Reverend Lou Sheldon heads the Coalition for Traditional Values in
California. He openly supported testing and contact tracing in his
newsletter sent to Evangelical Christians in California. Both he and his
wife have been repeatedly harassed with bomb threats.

Unfortunately, none of these small groups were effective on a
national level. Thus the only national force on our side of the ideologic

battle was Shepherd Smith's organization, ASAP.

※※※

In November of 1987, ASAP held the First International Conference on HIV Disease in Washington, D. C. I decided to attend and, furthermore, I decided that the time had come to try to reach people in high places in government to make sure they had a grasp of the issues involved and the barriers that had been utilized to prevent physicians from addressing the epidemic. Larimore had gotten into the White House and had a conference with one of Gary Bauer's assistants. If Larimore could get in to see Gary Bauer's assistant, I was determined to see Gary Bauer. I wrote a letter to Mr. Bauer asking for an audience. A few days before departing for Washington I received a confirmatory telephone call and the appointment was arranged.

The keynote speaker the first evening at the First International HIV Conference was Dr. Robert Gallo. Dr. Gallo is the father of retrovirology and internationally acclaimed as one of the world's leading cancer researchers. Having discovered HTLV-I and HTLV-II, the retroviruses which produce T-cell leukemia and Hairy Cell leukemia, it was his fundamental work in retrovirology which laid the foundation for the work of Dr. Luc Montagnier at the Pasteur Institute in isolating the HIV virus in 1983. Although the French had been the first to identify the virus in one patient, it was Gallo's team which identified the virus in literally dozens of other patients and confirmed beyond any shadow of a doubt that clinical AIDS was produced by the Pasteur Institute retrovirus.

Dr. Gallo had called the virus HTLV-III, linking it to his two previous retroviral discoveries. The French had called their virus, the LAV virus. An international team of scientists determined that a more appropriate name would be the HIV virus (Human Immunodeficiency Virus) since it was a lentivirus (an animal virus) quite different from the HTLV strain of retroviruses initially discovered by Robert Gallo.

Dr. Gallo and Luc Montagnier then agreed to share equally in credit for discovery of the virus. There were some who were extremely critical of Robert Gallo and suggested that he had "stolen" the virus from Luc Montagnier. Of course, there were certain jealousies between the leaders of the American and French researchers — but both men had risen above petty jealousies and acknowledged that each was dependent upon the other for their success in one of the greatest scientific accomplishments of all time — the isolation of the retrovirus responsible for HIV disease within two years of the first reported cases of AIDS.

Dr. Gallo addressed the audience at the HIV conference in Washington that first evening in November, 1987. Dr. Gallo has a reputation for having an extremely volatile temper that can be set off with the slightest provocation. If you have not read Randy Shilts' book, *And The Band Played On,* I suggest that you read the section on Dr. Robert Gallo. Perhaps overly dramatic and perhaps overly critical of Dr. Gallo, the book certainly paints the picture of a scientist who few would want to cross or challenge in a scientific forum, and that was what made the events of that evening so unforgettable.

Dr. Gallo, the world famous scientist, father of retrovirology and co-discoverer of the HIV virus, stood at the podium making his introductory remarks. There were perhaps 150 to 200 attendees at the conference that evening. Suddenly in the center of the auditorium, a tall, gaunt, blonde-haired young man stood up and shouted a series of challenges at Gallo.

"You stole the virus from Luc Montagnier. He discovered the virus and you stole his discovery," he shouted.

I sat in my seat in shocked disbelief. The rude young man went on to identify himself as a member of the Lavender Hill Club and the LAMBDA Legal Defense and Education Fund — both gay activist groups intent upon blocking the use of HIV testing and also intent upon disrupting any meeting held by those who favored testing. The young man then proceeded to attack Dr. Gallo for being responsible for suppressing drugs which could be beneficial to those dying of AIDS.

I could not take my eyes off Dr. Gallo. He grasped the podium with both hands. His face reddened; his body tensed. I waited for the explosion of Dr. Gallo's famous temper. The rude, young man continued his litany of vilification. When he paused for a moment, Dr. Gallo spoke quietly into the microphone. He spoke politely and authoritatively. He outlined the background behind his agreement with Luc Montagnier to share jointly in credit for discovery of the HIV virus. He pointed out his extensive research work on various AIDS drugs, trying to determine whether or not they were safe so that lives would not be lost unnecessarily. He pointed out the dangers of taking drugs of little or no proven value and the possibility of toxic or lethal side effects. Faced with a vicious, angry, hostile young man, Dr. Gallo presented his points clearly, concisely and with a quiet dignity that made me realize that I was in the presence of a truly great and remarkable man. Instead of exploding angrily, and denouncing the rudeness of his antagonist, Robert Gallo answered his charges thoroughly. There was another speaker that evening from the government laboratory in Los Alamos, New Mexico. Most of the details of what he said have been forgotten but I do remember his remarks on the amazing mutability of the HIV virus. He pointed out that his RNA virus mutated a million times faster than an ordinary DNA virus. The Los Alamos Laboratory had been able to analyze the biochemical changes that were occurring in the virus as it altered its chemical structure. He pointed out that if you took two identical viruses and placed them side by side and allowed them to replicate separately, they would each differ from the original by 1-1/2% at the end of one year. That meant that at the end of one year, the two viruses would be 3% different, chemically, from one another. At the end of ten years, they would each differ from their original status by 15%, so that the two viruses would differ biochemically from one another by 30% in their chemical make-up. This rapid mutation would make vaccine production difficult if not impossible. The researcher was careful to reassure us that in its current state, the virus was not communicable by insect vectors (mosquitos, bedbugs, flies, etc.) as were so many other lenti-retrovirus. He was in agreement with the commonly accepted facts that this disease was transmitted primarily by sexual contact and by blood transmission but he voiced his concern that the rapid mutation of this virus could alter its chemical make-up and change its means of communicability. If this should occur the results would be devastating. In each individual who was infected the virus was continuing to mutate and change. The more people who were infected, the more chance that some disastrous form of mutation would occur.

It was the next day that Dr. Theresa Crenshaw addressed our meeting. Dr. Crenshaw was a tall, attractive, blonde sex therapist. Sex therapists deal with all sorts of strange sexual behavior and sexual dysfunction. From what I have read I have often wondered if some of their therapies might border on the immoral. As Dr. Crenshaw spoke that morning, many of the subjects she covered were personally embarrassing, even after having been a physician for 35 years. But Theresa Crenshaw is another unusual and courageous woman. She had been in the practice of sex therapy in Southern California for many years. Because of her concern over the epidemic, she had closed her practice and was spending her time trying to awaken the American public to the dangers of the HIV epidemic. Recognizing the fact that testing was necessary, she had spoken on the subject at many meetings. As a result of her remarks, she had encountered numerous threats to her life and a constant pattern of harassment...for daring to suggest that physicians should begin addressing the disease as a medical issue.

At the time of that meeting, she had already been appointed to the Presidential AIDS Commission and would spend the following seven months working full-time without compensation because of her deep concern over what was happening to our society. Writing articles for magazines across the nation, addressing audiences and standing up to the attacks of gay activists, she was one of those rare people of conviction who put principle ahead of personal safety.

I am somewhat saddened to see how many courageous women have taken a stand...and how few men. In an article written for the monthly publication of The National Association for AIDS Prevention some months later, she alluded to the dangers of promiscuity of our youth and the nation's unreasonable reliance upon condoms as a means of stopping the spread of disease. Pointing to the well known fact that condoms fail 10% of the time in preventing pregnancy, when a woman was only fertile two or three days a month (while the HIV virus was lethal every day of the month), she expressed her concern over the frightening implications for the spread of disease among our youth.

Colonel Donald Burke spoke that morning. Prematurely gray, strikingly handsome with an athletic build, he cut an impressive figure in his military uniform. Speaking from his vast experiences as the officer in charge of supervising extensive HIV testing carried out by the Army, he was able to point out the reliability of HIV testing and the fact that the frequent reference to false positive blood tests was nothing more than a myth. In 1987, he felt that the incidence of false-positive HIV tests was about 1 in 130,000, based on studies which the Army had done in the Midwest where the incidence of disease was 1 positive HIV test in every 10,000 military applicants.

Going back over the 13 positive blood specimens that had been reported in 130,000 military applicants, he had sent the frozen blood specimens to several other laboratories for confirmatory analysis. Only

1 of their positive tests was a false-positive, giving an incidence of 1 false-positive in 130,000 military recruits. By 1989, by improving the techniques for testing, the Army had reduced the incidence of false-positives to far less than 1 in 1 million.

Major Redfield was there. Bob Redfield is one of those unusual, humble human beings whom fate has placed in a key position at a crucial time in history. Wearing rimless glasses, prematurely bald with a rim of brown hair on the sides of his head, his appearance was in marked contrast to his friend, Colonel Burke. When Redfield talks casually, he uses his hands and gesticulates freely. He had gone into medicine because he wanted to take care of people, not because he wanted to become rich or prosperous. He had gone into the Army because he felt that there would be an opportunity to do scientific research. He had tried to get into several cancer research programs but had been unsuccessful. Destiny had placed him on the medical service at Walter Reed Hospital when the first cases of AIDS began to appear.

Working with Robert Gallo, Redfield had identified the virus in 18 or more of his cases on the wards at Walter Reed Hospital and by March of 1984, he was using the HIV blood test routinely — one year before the test was available for general use in this country. There were several important things that he found. First, he found that the disease was readily spread from males to females and females to males. Although the heterosexual spread of AIDS was known to occur in Africa, it was not recognized in America in 1984 because we were not making the diagnosis of HIV disease until people passed into the terminal stage of the illness and developed AIDS. Bob Redfield, using the HIV blood test, was able to show that the wives of infected men were regularly becoming infected. Secondly, he made one of the most important and fundamental observations concerning HIV disease. By following the course of patients who were infected with the retrovirus, he recognized the fact that HIV disease was a chronic, progressive illness. The disease often started with a mild flu-like syndrome. The patient could then be totally asymptomatic for a prolonged period of time but all during that period the patient's T4 helper lymphocytes were gradually declining. The illness would go through a series of stages. The patient would first develop swollen lymph nodes, then a significant alteration in immune response; later patients would develop ARC (AIDS Related Complex) and finally AIDS. Redfield was the first physician to recognize that HIV

disease is a chronic, progressive and ultimately fatal, sexually
transmitted disease. He devised the Walter Reed staging of the disease
— starting with a Walter Reed Stage 0 and progressing to Walter Reed
Stage 6, which was the terminal stage of AIDS before death.

Redfield made one point over and over. He stated that physicians
should try to determine whether or not patients had the disease. The line
of reasoning promulgated by the Gay and AIDS Lobbies was that
doctors should not try to find out who had the disease because you
couldn't cure it — so why bother to try to find out who was infected?
You would find this sophistic argument repeated over and over in
medical journals and at medical meetings, until many good people
began to repeat the lie, but Major Redfield rebuffed that argument with
the simple statement:

"Knowing is better than not knowing. Knowledge is better than
ignorance."

He repeated that statement over and over. That statement is absolutely
true. It is one of the most profound statements made concerning this
epidemic. Doctors need to know if a patient has the infection to protect
that patient, to get that patient under treatment and keep him/her from
giving the disease to others. The message of the AIDS Lobby was
exactly the opposite. "Don't find out who has the disease because if you
find out it will lead to discrimination and the violation of the patient's
civil rights."

Dr. Vernon Marx, an Associate Professor of Neurosurgery at Harvard
Medical School, was one of the speakers. He went into great detail
covering the progressive neurologic changes that one sees with HIV
disease. Not only was there an AIDS dementia directly related to the
virus but there were a number of other diseases and conditions involving
the central nervous system which could lead to progressive dementia.
Lymphomas of the brain were a very common condition associated with
the terminal stages of AIDS. Cryptococcosis, toxoplasmosis, herpes
encephalitis and a myriad of other progressive brain diseases could
result. But the amazing part of his lecture was his statement that **AIDS
dementia was a reversible condition** when treated with AZT. Even in
1987, **HIV disease was treatable.** It was important to know who was
infected so that patients could be treated, yet doctors were being actively
discouraged from doing testing and getting patients under treatment.

I left the conference on the second morning and took a taxi to the White House on Pennsylvania Avenue. People in sleeping bags were lying on the sidewalks in front of the White House or leaning up against lampposts along the street. This was an obvious effort to demonstrate the existence of poverty in America. Here in the shadow of the White House were the poor and homeless of our society. What was obviously needed were more governmental programs (such as existed in Socialist countries) to eliminate poverty and homelessness.

Across from the White House there is a public park. There were tiers of posters in the park calling for the disarmament of America and condemning our nation as a militaristic, fascist society. The park was littered with signs and placards — just left there as a constant reminder of the fact that, in our society, any excess will be tolerated in the name of "freedom."

I shall never forget walking alone through the grounds of the White House. There was a small annex building to the right where I was to meet Mr. Bauer. As I entered the building nestled beside the White House, I passed tiers of television cameras and cameramen, all waiting expectantly for some important person to pass by. I looked over at them and waved. I am sure that some of them wondered who the tall, gray-haired man was and if he was anyone of importance. I could have assured them that he was not.

The waiting room of the annex to the White House is the size of an average living room. The heavy wooden molding separating the walls from the ceiling gave the room an air of age and elegance. Large paintings adorned the walls. One of the paintings caught my eye. It was the classic picture of George Washington crossing the Delaware. Unfortunately, it was only a print of the original, but still impressive in its portrayal. That picture gave the visitor a feeling of being one with the history of the United States.

When I was ushered into Gary Bauer's small but neatly kept office, I was somewhat taken back. Gary Bauer is extremely small in stature. If you passed him on the street you might think he was in his early thirties. His hands are delicate, his features youthful. He stands little over 5' 3" tall. Certainly his physical characteristics are not the least bit impressive but I have interviewed ambassadors, generals, senators and congressmen, and only a very few times have I really been impressed. I had not been with Mr. Bauer for more than a few moments when I realized that I was in the presence of a very unusual person. Holding the degree of Doctor of Laws, having moved from one key position to another in Washington, now holding one of the highest nonelected positions in the country, Gary Bauer had a keen intellect and certainly a grasp of the problems that faced our nation as far as the epidemic was concerned.

"The President and I do not understand why no one out there is concerned about the epidemic," he said. "The President is very concerned but we don't seem to be getting any response from the public. We are not receiving any mail supporting the President's position."

Mr. Bauer went on to tell me how President Reagan had been contacting Republican governors throughout the country since his speech on May 31, trying to get them to support state legislation to begin addressing the epidemic. It was the President's belief that health matters were something that individual states should deal with, not the federal government. The President had appointed his Presidential AIDS Commission to act in an advisory role but then he recognized that, according to our constitutional system of government, health matters were to be dealt with on the state level. As a result of his conviction, the President had contacted the governors of New Hampshire and Illinois and other Republican governors throughout the country. But whenever the governors publicly spoke of encouraging legislation to begin addressing the epidemic, there would be demonstrations.

Then there were other officials from the federal government who would contact the governors to tell them that using standard public health techniques was not appropriate for this disease because AIDS was different. And so it was that in many instances the governors would not abide by the President's recommendations. If the governors did try to support responsible State Legislation they could be assured that there would be heavy political pressure brought to bear to discourage them from trying to bring the HIV epidemic under control.

I told Gary Bauer of my concern about the policies of the Centers for Disease Control. I expressed my concern with Doctor James Mason's obvious deceptive reply to Congressman Dannemeyer during his testimony before the Waxman Committee in September which I spoke of in Book II, Chapter 4. I pointed out that it was obvious that Dr. Mason had no intention of carrying out the President's orders to determine the prevalence of HIV disease in our nation. Instead, he had avoided the question with evasive answers — such as his reply, "It's like pregnancy — nine women cannot produce a baby in one month"...I expressed my deep concern that a high government official would intentionally play word games to evade a direct question when our nation faces an epidemic of unparalleled magnitude. I remember, very well, Gary Bauer's reply:

"I don't understand the Centers for Disease Control and I don't understand Dr. James Mason. He is a good family man and a good Mormon, yet the Centers for Disease Control has refused to recommend sound public health policy. They have started doing limited surveillance testing in the Midwest where they know the incidence of the disease is limited. I have heard that they are going to come up with a report that is going to tell us that the incidence of the disease is falling. We know that isn't true."

I left Gary Bauer's office with mixed emotions. I realized that this presidential advisor was a man of unusual perception. He was knowledgeable about the epidemic and was committed to trying to do whatever was necessary to bring it under control. On the other hand, it appeared that even the President of the United States was unable to significantly influence federal or state policies. It appeared that the President, with his position and all his powers of persuasion, had been thwarted in his efforts to bring some sanity to current public health policy.

How true my observation was that day became apparent one year later. After the defeat of Proposition 102 in November of 1988, Larimore got in touch with his friend on the White House staff. Larimore expressed his deep concern over the fact that Proposition 102 had been an effort to carry out President Reagan's program to encourage routine testing at the state level but Proposition 102 had been overwhelmingly defeated. At that time the presidential advisor told Larimore that during the preceding months President Reagan had repeatedly sent directives to the U. S. Public Health Service and the Centers for Disease Control to try to get them to follow his policies. In each instance the agencies ignored the directives and in some instances they had done just the opposite. Surgeon General Koop had gone about the country speaking against premarital testing...as he had done in Illinois. The White House advisor expressed the frustration of the administration at the fact that they had been consistently blocked in their efforts to direct an intelligent, responsible approach to the epidemic. Furthermore, they had no means of getting information to the public — and the epidemic continued to spread, the dying and the death continued.

It was the following morning at the meeting of the "Americans For A Sound AIDS Policy" that Gary Bauer came to discuss the epidemic. I remember relatively little about his talk other than the fact that he suggested a comprehensive approach to the epidemic but what I do remember was the gaunt, young homosexual from the Lavender Hill Club and the LAMBDA Legal Defense and Education Fund. This young man had been a disruptive influence at the meeting since that first evening when he challenged and insulted Doctor Robert Gallo.

During Bauer's talk this gaunt young man moved to the front of the auditorium with his flashbulb-equipped camera in hand. He sat in the first row and kept flashing his flashbulb — obviously not taking pictures — but simply trying to disrupt Mr. Bauer's talk. I counted the flashes — at least 18 of them — used in an intentional, disruptive manner to temporarily blind the speaker. If you have ever given a talk and had somebody taking flash pictures you realize that there is a momentary period of blindness that follows each flash. When one or two flash pictures are taken it may be a little irritating but eighteen successive flashes coming every minute can completely disorient a speaker. That was the technique which was used that morning against Gary Bauer — the representative of the President that the homosexuals hated. What was even more disconcerting was that no one in the audience had the courage to ask him to leave. Instead, the rude young man was offered an opportunity to give a talk to the assembled delegates so he could vent his anger, hatred and frustration on the audience, an audience he perceived as being responsible for the spread of disease in the homosexual community.

1. AMA News — September 18, 1987; p. 25.
2. AMA News — September 25, 1987; p. 20.
3. AMA News — October 9, 1987; p. 6.
4. Personal Communication with Lorraine Day, M.D.
5. AMA News — October 23/30, 1987; p. 27.
6. AMA News — November 6, 1987; p. 25.
7. People's Daily World — Saturday, October 10, 1986.
8. AMA News — November 6, 1987; p. 27.
9. Santa Cruz Sentinel, October 28, 1987; p. A6.
10. JAMA, 1987; Vol. 258; p. 1757-1761.
11. JAMA, October 16, 1987; Vol. 258; p. 2063.
12. Wall Street Journal — October 9, 1987; p. 5.

CHAPTER SIX

Still, if you will not fight for the right when you can
easily win without bloodshed, if you will not fight
when your victory will be sure and not too costly, you
may come to the moment when you will have to fight
with all odds against you and only a perilous chance
for survival. Indeed, there may be a worse case. You
may have to fight when there is no hope for victory,
for it would be better to perish than to live as slaves.

— Sir Winston Churchill

By late November 1987, I was firmly convinced that the epidemic was
going to be allowed to run its course. Gary Bauer had given me a glimpse
of the impotence of the President of the United States in his efforts to
address the epidemic and if the President could not influence the
epidemic, who could?

The Congress of the United States was under the control of liberal
Democrats. For 34 years, since the Democrat sweep of Congress in
1954, the House of Representatives has been under the control of a
political party committed to a Socialist America. In 1986, over 98% of
Congressional incumbents running for re-election were elected. It was
almost impossible to vote out an incumbent congressman. The American public had lost control of their government. In 1987 there was a
massive bureaucracy that was running our nation, hell-bent upon
blocking a logical public health program to try to stop the unnecessary
suffering and death.

It was also quite obvious that a small clique within the hierarchy of the
CMA was intent upon blocking the will of the physicians of our state.
In 1986, they refused to carry out the directive of the House of
Delegates. In 1987, they had not only refused to support the official
CMA White Paper, they had actively lobbied against many of the
positions which had been embraced by members of the House.

The left-wing media in America kept clamoring about the need for
confidentiality and the dangers of discrimination parroting the lie that
the only way to stop the epidemic was to pass new antidiscrimination
laws (handicapped laws) and give those who were infected special

privileges and protections. Almost no one ever talked about the moral implications of the epidemic, about teaching our young people ideas of chastity and sexual responsibility or the fact that many of them would die as a result of promiscuity, despite the fact they used condoms. More and more children were being born infected with the virus. More and more of our adolescents and youth were found to be infected.

By late 1987, there were only three states in the nation where HIV was actually being treated as an infectious, contagious disease. Although there were a few other states with some form of reporting, many of the states were simply doing anonymous reporting to public health officers and little public health follow-up was used to try to stem the spread of the plague into the heterosexual community.

It was this situation and my frustration and impotence that led me to write **that letter.** It was **that letter** which was stolen and would have such a profound effect on Proposition 102. It was the intentional misrepresentation of what **that letter** said which would ultimately be responsible for the deaths of tens of thousands of people and the prolongation of the epidemic. To understand why I wrote **that letter,** you must understand my state of mind and my thought process. Knowing that the very survival of our nation as a free society was at stake, totally frustrated by my inability and the inability of the President of the United States to influence the course of the epidemic and realizing that the CMA hierarchy would not follow the dictates of the House, I decided to write **that letter. That letter** was a personal communication between myself and Charles Armour, a friend whom I had known for 25 years — going back to the time I had been actively involved in the conservative movement trying to awaken our nation as to the dangers of America's drift towards socialism. That letter was a plea for help, a plea to try to disseminate information on an epidemic that threatened to kill millions of Americans. **That letter** was mailed in Santa Cruz and sent to Massachusetts. Somewhere between my office and Massachusetts, a copy of **that letter** was intercepted by those within the "Brotherhood of the left" or the "Brotherhood of promiscuity." The letter was held for almost a year and then sent to every major newspaper in the State of California in October of 1988, just before the November election. The letter was then **intentionally** misquoted by virtually **every** major newspaper in the state in an effort to defeat Proposition 102. The Gay and AIDS Lobbies have extensive organizations with tens of thousands of dedicated activists. Tragically, on our side, there were only a few people who really cared enough to be involved.

By October of 1988, a year later, I was involved in a Congressional race against one of the most powerful men in the House of Representatives. The intentional distortion of what I said in **that letter** very effectively discredited me in the minds of most of the voters in my Congressional district and profoundly influenced the fate of the Gann Initiative. When the Gann Initiative (Proposition 102) was defeated it assured that the use of responsible public health programs would be delayed across the land for years and that tens of thousands — perhaps hundreds of thousands — of our countrymen would die unnecessarily. (See Appendix IV for the full text of **that letter**).

※※※

In November 1987, I was actively engaged in writing my resolutions to be presented to the House of Delegates in March of 1988. I planned to present one resolution which stated that the CMA should accept HIV disease as a communicable, sexually transmitted disease and that the disease should be listed as a disease under state law so there would be routine testing and reporting as physicians did with other sexually transmitted diseases.

Furthermore, I recognized the homosexuals' fears about the issue of confidentiality. It appeared that there was no way we were going to be able to change current law requiring fines and imprisonment for physicians who released information about a patient's HIV status. One of the factors which was mentioned again and again by those on the left was their concern that contact tracing, by its very nature, would mean that a public health officer would go to a patient's sexual partner and tell them that there was information that they might have contracted HIV disease. The individual who was contacted might surmise who the primary infected party was — the so-called "Index Patient" — and as a result, theoretically, he/she might tell others of the Index Patient's infectious status. In an effort to circumvent that danger, I submitted a second resolution stating that current confidentiality restrictions (which had been placed on physicians and medical personnel) should be extended to those contacted by public health officers. Thus when sexual partners were notified of their possible infection, they would also be notified that they were not allowed to communicate this information to others without being in violation of state confidentiality laws. I felt that if confidentiality was **really** a factor and the fear of exposure was **really** the driving force behind the homosexuals' reluctance to allow testing, then this new concept would expand protection of confidentiality and alleviate their fears. I was not in the least bit convinced that confidentiality was the real issue. I felt that the confidentiality issue was simply one of the smoke screens used to confuse the issue. But if there was any basis for the fears of the AIDS and Gay Lobbies because of the possibility of a breach of confidentiality during contact tracing, then my resolution would have addressed and corrected that situation.

What happened to that resolution in Reno at the CMA Convention in March of 1988 came as no real surprise.

❊❊❊

November 20, 1987

The Journal of the American Medical Association reported on testing of umbilical cord blood from 602 women who had delivered children in a Brooklyn hospital. The testing showed that 2% of the blood tests were positive for HIV disease. That meant that 2% of the mothers were infected with the virus and were going to die. Of the 12 women who were found to be HIV positive, 7 of them had risk factors and 5 of them did not. That meant, if doctors followed CDC guidelines for testing, they would miss almost 50% of those infected. The editorial in the Journal of the AMA called the results of the study "sobering."

The article went on to state: "We need to recognize that HIV infection in women and the resultant cases of pediatric AIDS will likely unfold in...selected urban populations throughout the United States." The CDC reported, at that time, there were already 516 children who had contracted AIDS from their mothers.

❊❊❊

On November 24, the President of the AMA, Dr. Allen Nelson, testified before the Presidential AIDS Commission. Doctor Nelson stated:

"HIV testing and counseling should be made available across America...(but) testing of low incidence populations would divert finite testing and counseling resources from high risk individuals who volunteered for testing." He went on to say: "The cost to uncover one case of infection in a low incidence population is extremely high...(and) the danger of false-positive tests could result, frequently, in irreparable adverse results to innocent parties...(since)...the incidence of false positives would be 1 in 20,000 tests."[1]

***

December 1987
It was obvious that the epidemic would soon spread into the promiscuous youth of our nation, yet nothing was being done to stop it. By December of 1987, it was obvious that the incidence of syphilis was rising rapidly after its decline during the early part of the decade. The steady increase in both syphilis and congenital syphilis demonstrated conclusively that education and behavioral modification had failed to alter patterns of sexual promiscuity. Yet public health professionals led by the Surgeon General reiterated that we had no means of fighting the epidemic other than to use education and behavioral modification.

***

On December 16, Army Sergeant Vincent Stuart at Fort Sill, Oklahoma pleaded guilty before a court-martial to having sex with a female soldier without notifying her that he carried the virus or without using any protective device. The woman had become infected. The sergeant was given two years imprisonment for what was termed "aggravated assault." However, all across America infected citizens continued infecting their unsuspecting sexual partners — and no measures were taken to slow the spread of disease in the general population.

***

Admiral Watson, Chairman of the Presidential AIDS Commission warned that the spread of the disease into the heterosexual population would increase dramatically during the next ten years. He pointed out that people looked at the AIDS statistics and felt that there was little danger of heterosexual spread of AIDS. In December 1987 only 4% of the 48,574 reported AIDS cases had been acquired by heterosexual transmission. Tragically, people were still reading AIDS statistics and believing that they represented what was happening with the epidemic. The media never told the public that there were no statistics on HIV disease to determine how far the disease had spread into the heterosexual community. The only reliable figures were the Army statistics which showed that 1 out of every 4 infected military applicants was a woman.[2]

In December, the AMA News carried a cover article on Dr. Lorraine Day. Dr. Day was quoted as saying that she wanted to be able to test anyone she thought needed to be tested and that she felt that a physician had the right to test his/her patients.

The article quoted Dr. Russel Patterson, Jr., the Vice-Chairman of the AMA's Council on Ethics and Judicial Affairs, Dr. Paul Volberding who heads the AIDS Clinic at San Francisco General Hospital and Doctor Lesley Anderson who practiced at Pacific Presbyterian Medical Center. According to the article, all three doctors questioned Lorraine's position supporting routine HIV testing of hospital patients. Despite the fact that 90% of the orthopedic surgeons in the State of California would agree with Dr. Day's statement, the only physicians who were interviewed were those who disagreed with her position. All through the article, Dr. Day's position was attacked and discredited, suggesting that her major reason for wanting to identify those who were infected was so that she could discriminate against them and withhold medical care.[3]

***

For over two years, a small group of AIDS patients and their supporters had been camping on a grassy area outside the United Nations Plaza in San Francisco to protest the fact that the Reagan Administration was not giving more money for AIDS research and the care of AIDS patients. Angela Davis, one of the directors of the Central Committee of the American Communist Party, addressed the group on several occasions. On other occasions, members of other revolutionary groups picketed and helped to raise financial assistance for the demonstrators. It was in mid-December of 1987 when three members of the group chained themselves to the door of the government office building at the United Nations Plaza in an effort to dramatize their frustration with the Reagan Administration and the fact that the President was doing nothing to try to stop the epidemic.[4]

***

A report prepared by the American Medical Association Board of Trustees came out firmly against any effort to routinely test either hospital patients or HCW's. The report stated that hospital employees should work out a program to try to prevent the occupational spread of disease but routine testing was not to be used to identify infected patients or those within the health care profession who were infected. The special report further stated: "The value of routine antibody testing of either health care workers or patients is not known...Transmission in the health care environment has occurred only through accidental needle sticks and blood splashing." The report also said that there was no evidence to show that if a hospital worker knew that someone was infected they would be more careful. Of course, the report did not point out that no one had ever done a study to determine whether or not this statement was true. Common sense and any health care worker would tell you that HCW's needed to know who was infected in order to protect themselves.

By December of 1987, there were already several thousand health care workers dead or dying from AIDS. How many more were infected with the virus and spreading it to their families or sexual partners? No one knew because the AMA and the CDC opposed testing of HCW's to find out. HCW's lives were quite obviously expendable.

✳✳✳

The House Select Committee on **Children, Youth and the Family** released a report stating that "The nation's health care and foster care systems were overburdened and ill-equipped to deal with the expected increase in pediatric AIDS cases by the year 1991." The report further stated: "Of the estimated 270,000 individuals who are expected to contract the Acquired Immune Deficiency Syndrome by the year 1991, 3,000 of them will be infants and children under the age of 13."

✳✳✳

The AIDS quilt was a patchwork of 2,176 panels, each 3X6 feet in size. It was being shown in communities across the nation to dramatize the deaths of those who had succumbed to the epidemic. Each panel symbolized a headstone. Those who transported the quilt from city to city claimed that the quilt showed the necessity of facing the epidemic. They proclaimed that America was at last doing something definitive about the epidemic. America was creating a gigantic quilt and sending it from community to community to draw attention to the fact that people were dying of AIDS.

✳✳✳

It is rare that one reads a magazine article that sets off a chain of events that leads to a confrontation with 40 angry demonstrators, yet that is exactly what happened.

It was early in December when I picked up my copy of the November issue of Commentary magazine, a publication of the American-Jewish Committee. The lead article was entitled, "AIDS: Are Heterosexuals At Risk?" and was written by Michael Fumento. The article alleged there was really very little risk of acquiring AIDS from heterosexual contact in America. Pointing out that there were only 18 heterosexually transmitted cases of AIDS in San Francisco (out of some 3,361 reported cases) and similar small numbers in Los Angeles and Houston, the author set out to convince the reader that the specter of the heterosexual epidemic was created by homosexual activists in an effort to frighten the general population into supporting government funding for research and the care of AIDS patients. He went on to suggest that women acted as a "firebreak" to the spread of the virus and reported one study that showed only a 20% incidence per year of transmission of the disease from an infected man to his noninfected wife. The author totally ignored a number of other studies which showed how readily the disease was spread from one infected marital partner to the other. He went on to suggest that the heterosexual spread of the epidemic in Africa was really caused by the use of "contaminated needles, blood transfusions and ritual scarification." Then he inferred that there might be a hidden incidence of bisexuality in Africa responsible for the devastating spread of disease into the heterosexual population. The article was full of cliches and what I felt were frank distortions. I was fairly well read in HIV literature at that time and there was no question that this article was misleading. I did not know the motivation of the author but I knew that he had taken selective studies to prove his point — a point which I believed to be totally invalid.

I jotted down a few notes and then dictated a hurried rebuttal which I forwarded to the editor of Commentary. Month after month, I scanned the "Letters To The Editor" section looking for the publication of my reply. It was not until months later that I would learn the fate of my correspondence.

✻✻✻

As of December 1987, only two states, Colorado and Idaho, were using contact tracing. Six states, (California, Colorado, Illinois, Massachusetts, Maine and Wisconsin) had passed laws on confidentiality. Ten states had passed laws barring discrimination against those infected with the HIV virus. Four states and the District of Columbia had passed laws preventing insurance companies from testing for HIV status before issuing life and health insurance policies. State legislatures across the country were dealing with bills to address the epidemic, however, in state after state, efforts to deal with the epidemic from a medical point of view were effectively blocked by demonstrations, threats, and intimidation.

※※※

On December 10, the People's Daily World commented on the new LaRouche AIDS Initiative — Proposition 69 — stating:

"The initiative would require doctors and local health officials to report the names of AIDS patients...who would then be subject to quarantine laws. Opponents of the initiative consider that the new LaRouche initiative is a thinly veiled attack on gays and said it would hurt efforts to find an AIDS cure."

※※※

A special task force report prepared by the Massachusetts Hospital Association predicted that the cost of taking care of AIDS patients in Massachusetts would rise from 20 million dollars in 1987 to one-quarter of a billion dollars within a ten year period. The financial implications of the epidemic threatened to bankrupt the state within a decade. But this would not be just in Massachusetts. All state governments and the entire health care industry would be facing financial ruin by the late 1990's as hundreds of thousands of people already infected with the virus began coming down with clinical AIDS.

※※※

December 1987 marked the end of my second year in the battle against the epidemic. Since the California Legislature had failed to enact laws to change consent and confidentiality requirements and since HIV disease was still not considered an infectious disease in the State of California, there were now three state initiatives being presented to the voters. The first initiative was Proposition 69 which was to be on the ballot in June. Lyndon LaRouche had spent almost one-quarter of a million dollars a year and a half previously to qualify Proposition 64. Now he was back with essentially the same initiative. Once again his initiative stated that "HIV disease was an infectious, contagious, communicable disease and the condition of being a carrier of HIV disease is an infectious, contagious, communicable condition and both should be (considered)...on the list of reportable diseases." But once again LaRouche and his supporters brought up the necessity of quarantine...which served only to inflame the fears of the homosexuals and insure the defeat of his initiative.

The second state initiative was the Gann Initiative, Proposition 102. Petitions were being circulated throughout the state in December to qualify that initiative for the ballot in November 1988. Written in large part by Larimore and Ted Blanchard from Senator Doolittle's office, the initiative attempted to modify existing public health law so physicians could begin addressing the epidemic as a disease rather than as a civil rights issue.

❈❈❈

Doctor Larry McNamee, a radiologist from Whittier, California, organized a group of some 300 physicians which came to be known as "California Physicians For A Logical AIDS Response." Larimore was on the Board of Governors; I was listed on the letterhead as a supporter. This small group of doctors then tried to rally public support for Proposition 102. By November of 1988, several thousand physicians had joined Doctor McNamee's organization to support the Gann Initiative in opposition to the position taken by the CMA. Tragically, few voters in California learned that large numbers of physicians had broken ranks with organized medicine to support a sound, logical HIV policy. The blackout of news concerning Proposition 102 by the liberal media was effective and few voters really understood the Gann Initiative.

The third initiative was the Block Initiative, put forward by Sheriff Sherman Block of Los Angeles County. This initiative (which came to be known as Proposition 96) stipulated that if anyone attacked a police officer and there was an exchange of body fluids (i.e., blood or saliva) or if someone raped a woman, that person could be forced to have an HIV test by court order.

A representative of the San Francisco AIDS Foundation belittled the Block Initiative saying, "The way the Block Initiative is worded, anyone charged with a crime...where there is any exchange of body fluids, would have to be tested. I could be walking down the street...perspiring, and be arrested for jay-walking. If my sweat got on the officer, I would have to be tested. This is absurd."

Articles began appearing regularly in newspapers across our land in December questioning whether HIV disease was really the cause of AIDS. Doctor Peter Duesberg, a University of California virologist, raised that question and suggested that there might be another etiology for the disease. He stated that he did not believe that a retrovirus ever caused cancer and specifically rejected the belief that AIDS was produced by the HIV virus.

As I read his material, I reflected on the numerous side issues which were being raised in reference to the epidemic (i.e., (1) Doctor Strecker's suggestion that HIV disease had actually been produced by the World Health Organization; (2) the KGB's allegation that the disease was produced by the Central Intelligence Agency; (3) other writers suggesting that the epidemic had been created by the KGB; and (4) now Doctor Duesberg was contending that AIDS was not produced by the HIV virus).

I had a feeling that, intentionally or not, there were a number of irrelevant issues being introduced, designed only to confuse the public and expend a great deal of energy arguing and discussing matters which were of no real consequence. The real issue was "Why aren't we using standard public health techniques to try to stop the further spread of this disease?" Did anyone really believe that there would have been so many efforts to block the use of standard, accepted public health techniques if this disease had not initially developed in the homosexual population? Yet, the homosexuals were the ones who were dying because public health officers had not used accepted techniques early in the epidemic to stop its spread. Now our society was wasting time and effort, arguing about how the virus originated instead of addressing the real problem and identifying those who were infected in order to stop further spreading.

※※※

In December, I went to Los Angeles to tape a television interview — this time with an anchorman and anchorwoman from one of the networks and a left wing AIDS activist. The AIDS activist was adamant in insisting that physicians should not be allowed to use testing on the general population or use public health follow-up in an effort to control the epidemic. I was amazed to find that the program producer, the anchorman and anchorwoman were all firmly committed to my position. The interview went very well. The only problem was that, to my knowledge, the program was never aired. The regularly scheduled time when it was to be shown was cancelled. I had a friend in Southern California who called the station to find out when the program was to be shown. He was informed that it was to be aired at 5:30 one morning (when most people would be asleep). My friend got up early to watch the program but once again it was not shown. When he called the station again he was told that they had no further plans to air the interview.

This experience was just one of a number of times that I encountered frank censorship. Despite the fact that a number of people at the television station were supportive of my position, someone at the station suppressed the broadcasting of that debate.

***

By December, our county medical society was under constant attack by the hierarchy of the CMA for daring to interfere in the legislative process. Larimore received a number of letters from Dr. John Tupper, Chairman of the Legislative Committee of the Council. Doctor Tupper was critical of our medical society for daring to challenge CMA leadership. The general thrust of his letters was to tell us to get back in line and that doctors must stand together: there was no place for a renegade medical society that was trying to influence legislation. When Larimore pointed out that CMA leadership had consistently refused to follow positions taken in the CMA White Paper, Dr. Tupper reiterated that medicine could not be effective if any one individual medical society took their own positions in opposition to that of CMA leadership.

***

By early December, the Santa Cruz County Medical Society had received replies to its poll of the House of Delegates. The vast majority of those who replied were solidly behind our position in support of SB1000 and in opposition to the position of CMA leadership. It was obvious that the hierarchy was deeply concerned. Thus it was that Dr. Fred Armstrong, the President of the CMA, requested a special meeting with our medical society's Board of Governors to plead with us to stop having our representatives speak before legislative committees in Sacramento.

Fred Armstrong was a member of the Seventh District Delegation, the delegation to which I belong. He was an internist practicing in Santa

Clara County and, in my opinion, a committed liberal. I had watched him operate within our delegation for years. At times, I would be able to rally every member of the Seventh District Delegation behind my position — with one exception. That exception was invariably Fred Armstrong. At other times he was able to rally the whole delegation behind his position — that is, everyone but me. Although I consistently disagreed with him and everything he stood for, I had to respect him. At least he stood for **something** and was willing to fight for his beliefs in contrast to so many physicians who didn't understand the political or philosophic issues that medicine faced in the 1980's. Of medium height — perhaps 5' 7" or 5' 8" tall, with slicked down, graying hair, thick glasses and striking blue eyes, Fred Armstrong was an effective spokesman for the liberal position. Addressing our Board of Governors in December, he took a number of tacks.

First, he pointed out that Santa Cruz was the only medical society in the entire state which had expressed concern with the way the CMA hierarchy was handling the epidemic. When I pointed out that the Orange County Medical Society was also upset with the hierarchy, Fred then argued that physicians must stick together if we hoped to be effective. He stressed that it was necessary that the members trust the leaders just as the leaders must carry out the wishes of the members. He went on to offer our medical society key positions in the policy-making bodies of the CMA. He promised that a member of our medical society would be appointed to the CMA AIDS Task Force. In addition, the president of our medical society would be allowed to address the next meeting of the Council to express our concerns. All that Fred wanted was a written statement from our Board of Governors in support of the efforts of the CMA as they worked to come up with laws that would change consent and confidentiality requirements. All he wanted was an agreement that our medical society would no longer try to influence state legislation.

Armstrong's talk was effective and swung many of the naive and unsophisticated members of our governing board to his position. I pointed out to Dr. Armstrong and the Board that our poll of delegates showed that the vast majority of the delegates supported our position over the position taken by CMA leadership. Fred shrugged off the poll as unimportant.

When it came time to vote, the majority of our Board agreed to issue the requested letter. As the vote was taken, I looked across the room at Larimore. I could see him sadly shaking his head. Too many of the members of our Board were awestruck by the President of the powerful CMA coming to our small county and pleading for our support. To refuse his request would indicate mistrust of the CMA President. Most doctors could not truly believe that our leaders would really betray medicine and the public.

From that moment on, I realized that whatever I did I would have to do alone. Tragically, good men, such as those on our Board could be so readily swayed. However, I had been deceived before and I again remembered that time-proven Chinese proverb:

"If a man deceive me once, shame on him.

If a man deceive me twice, shame on me."

Within several weeks, Larimore was in Sacramento as a private physician, no longer representing the Santa Cruz County Medical Society. He was there to support Senator Doolittle's bill which required that a voluntary HIV antibody test be offered to every pregnant mother in the state. Such testing would allow us to begin to identify those mothers who were infected with the hope that we might be able to protect their unborn children from contracting the disease by nursing. As expected, the CMA lobbyist was there and steadfastly refused to speak in support of that legislation despite the fact that voluntary prenatal testing had been one of the basic thrusts of the CMA White Paper.

Larimore later told me how the CMA lobbyist sat opposite him at the legislative meeting and fixed him with an intense stare — keeping that fixed stare on him all during the afternoon. That was his childish way of attempting to embarrass Larimore. Not a word was spoken. The lobbyist refused to respond to Larimore's greetings. There was just the intense, angry, hostile stare from the paid lobbyist of the CMA, a man intent upon carrying out the policies of the CMA hierarchy.

※※※

It was in mid-December when I went to Sacramento to confer with Governor George Deukmejian's Administrative Assistant. This gave me an opportunity to relay information indirectly to the governor in an effort to convince him that the hierarchy was not speaking for the doctors of California. I was able to give the governor's representative a copy of the CMA White Paper. He was amazed to see the official policy position of the CMA and exclaimed that he had no idea that the doctors of the state supported the use of HIV testing. Though I have no way of knowing whether or not my revelations were actually relayed to the governor, I would like to think that the information presented may have played some part in convincing the governor to take his most courageous stand.

Ten months later, in October of 1988, the governor publicly came out and supported Proposition 102 which declared HIV disease to be a disease. That stand brought the wrath of the Gay Lobby, the AIDS Lobby and the entire liberal establishment down on the governor. It was one of the most costly stands of his career. Tragically, the results of that stand will have far-reaching consequences for him, the California Republican Party and ultimately the State of California. Why? Because the defeat of Proposition 102 demonstrated to the governor and Republican leaders that **the gay and AIDS activists are apparently the most formidable political force in California** and Governor Deukmejian, Senator Pete Wilson and the entire hierarchy of the Republican Party subsequently acquiesced to the demands of the Homosexual Lobby. The Republican leaders accepted the position that they would oppose the use of accepted public health measures to control the epidemic. That tragic decision will have far-reaching implications for the survival of our nation.

❊❊❊

January 1988.
It was in January that I made one of the most impulsive and foolish decisions of my life. That decision was motivated in part by Congressman Dannemeyer's remark the previous June at the San Francisco Airport when he said, "There are only five members of the House who really understand the epidemic — and two of them are on the other side."

After Dannemeyer's comment I kept thinking that if I were in Washington, I might somehow be able to convince members of Congress of the magnitude of the epidemic.

My Congressional District is the 16th District and is represented by Congressman Leon Panetta. He had run essentially unchallenged for a number of years and has cleverly managed to cultivate support from both Republicans and Democrats in the district. Despite the fact that he is a radical leftist with a 90% Americans for Democratic Action (ADA-Socialist) voting record and an ACLU voting record of over 90%, he has been able to create the image of being a political moderate. Leon consistently supported Congressman Henry Waxman in his efforts to pass AIDS legislation which would mandate a federal antidiscrimination law as well as federal consent and confidentiality requirements. If those laws had passed they would have prevented doctors from ever addressing HIV disease as a medical issue.

Panetta consistently voted for higher taxes. He supported the Halloween Tax Bill of October 1987 giving members of Congress (including himself) a third salary raise during 1987. He consistently voted against the Strategic Defense Initiative and a strong defense for America. He had been on the committee of 14 members of the House of Representatives which had volunteered to raise funds for the **Institute for policy Studies in April of 1983.** The Institute (IPS) is an organization which interlocks directly with the World Peace Council which is funded by the KGB. The background of the IPS is described in the book *The Covert Cadre—Inside the Institute for Policy Studies.* David Horowitz, former editor of Ramparts magazine and long associated with Communist activities before his conversion to Americanism, wrote the forward to that book and pointed out that the purpose of the IPS was,

"To lay siege to democracy's defense and to cripple its resistance to totalitarian advance."

Leon Panetta's true character was best demonstrated by the part he played in stealing a congressional election in Indiana in 1982 in the celebrated race between the Republican candidate McIntyre and the Democrat candidate McClosky. In that race, McIntyre won the election by 300 votes and was certified the winner by the Secretary of State of Indiana. The Congressional Democrats led by Leon's good friend Jim Wright challenged the election results. Legally, Jim Wright did not have that prerogative since certifying winners in an election is a state matter. In addition, at that time the Democrats already had a 50 vote majority in Congress. The recount demanded by Jim Wright gave the election to McIntyre a second time. Jim Wright then demanded a third count of the votes. The third count again gave the election to McIntyre. Not to be dissuaded by the election results, Jim Wright sent his dependable henchman, Leon Panetta, to Indiana to supervise a fourth count. With two Democrats and one Republican (Bill Thomas, R-C), Panetta proceeded to recount the votes until the Democrat candidate was ahead by four votes. Then he refused to count the remainder of the votes.

With dozens of votes left to be counted, Leon Panetta announced that the Democrat candidate, McClosky, had won.

Even the liberal New York Times challenged Panetta's handling of that recount. When McClosky was sworn into Congress, Republican members of the House walked out to demonstrate their disgust. For years thereafter, few Republicans would speak to Leon Panetta for they recognized him as a man devoid of integrity.

Tragically, because five of the six major newspapers in the 16th Congressional District are hard core leftist publications, the average citizen in the district had no idea that their elected representative was an unprincipled scoundrel committed to the policies of the far left.

As I mentioned earlier, in the Congressional election of 1986, over 98% of all incumbent congressmen in America were re-elected. It should have been obvious that the American people had lost control of the House of Representatives. For 34 consecutive years, prior to 1988, the Democrat Party had controlled the House of Representatives as America moved progressively toward socialism, financial insolvency and the centralization of all power in a paternalistic, regulatory government. During those 34 years the very fabric of American society had been eroded. Our faith, our families and our freedoms had been progressively undermined and destroyed. God had been taken out of our schools and replaced with instruction in atheism. Morality had been removed from our educational institutions and replaced with values-neutral sex education. Our nation faced a skyrocketing national debt, rising crime, an educational system that had graduated 27 million illiterates and the threat of the fall of Central America to Communist Imperialism.

Recognizing the problems that faced our society, realizing that our nation faced an epidemic that threatened to undermine the very structure of our society and seeing Leon Panetta re-elected again and again, I was intrigued with the thought of running for the Republican Congressional nomination in the primary election scheduled for June of 1988.

In January, Congress was scheduled to vote on continuing aid to the Freedom Fighters in Nicaragua. President Reagan asked all three major networks (CBS, NBC and ABC) if they would allow him to address the nation on the evening before the congressional vote. All three networks informed the President that since he had nothing new to say, they would not allow him television time. It was obvious that the television networks were intent upon the defeat of the anti-Communist Nicaraguan forces.

The following day when the congressional vote was taken, Leon Panetta joined the majority in voting to cut off **all funds** to the Contras. It was at that point that I made my decision. I decided to run in the Republican primary with the hope that I could challenge Panetta in November.

I am not a politician. I am a physician and an amateur historian. I had no knowledge as to how a political campaign is run. I had no funding and I had no organization behind me. My decision was ill-conceived. I should have realized that if 98% of congressional incumbents had been re-elected in 1986, the chances were slim to none that I could defeat a well-entrenched incumbent who had managed to deceive the public so effectively for so many years. How ridiculous my decision to run for political office was would not become obvious until the votes were counted in November.

✳✳✳

In February 1988, I filed my petition with the Secretary of State and became a candidate for the Republican nomination. When I signed that application I agreed to

"Uphold the Constitution of the United States and to defend it against **all enemies foreign and domestic.**"

As I read that statement, I realized that we did have domestic enemies — enemies who were dedicated to preventing physicians from stopping this epidemic, enemies who were intent upon destroying our nation, enemies who realized that this epidemic would destroy America far more effectively than a nuclear attack.

✳✳✳

February 1988.

In early February, the California State Republican Central Committee held its convention in Santa Clara. Representatives from county central committees all across the state were in attendance. This was my first state-wide political meeting and my first glimpse of how the political process really works.

Larry McNamee was there selling copies of his new book, *AIDS — The First Politically Protected Disease.* As mentioned earlier, Larry was a practicing radiologist from Whittier. He was studying for a law degree and was also President of "California Physicians for a Logical AIDS Response." By November of 1988, his life would have been threatened repeatedly because he dared to oppose the AIDS Lobby's agenda. He was one of those rare people who seemed to be able to do a dozen things at once and do all of them well. Of medium height with blonde, short–cropped hair, a stocky build, a slight limp and a quiet manner of speaking, he gave the impression of intelligence and confidence. He was there at that Republican meeting primarily to address the convention and gain their support for Proposition 102 (the Gann Initiative).

Congressman Dannemeyer was there as well, hoping that he too would be allowed to address the convention. Dannemeyer had already contributed over $100,000.00 of his own money to finance the collecting of signatures to qualify Proposition 102 for the November ballot. How many other politicians do you know who would risk large sums of **their own money** to save millions of lives? Would you? I can tell you that Bill Dannemeyer never got repaid a significant portion of his contribution — but he has never mentioned that fact publicly. It is rare to find a man of integrity in a world of equivocal men. Even at that time, Bill Dannemeyer's life had been threatened repeatedly because of his efforts to introduce legislation to try to stop the epidemic. He had to take special precautions whenever he traveled or attended public functions, yet he persisted in his efforts to awaken our population, a population which seems indifferent to the danger that we face.

It was on the first day of that convention that I had an opportunity to see how effectively the homosexual and AIDS Lobbies had been in placing their people into positions of power within the Republican Party. At that convention there were a number of responsible Republican leaders who were concerned because the homosexuals had established a Gay Republican Club within the Republican Party, an organization referred to as "The Log Cabin Club."

These Republican legislators wanted to have the gay Republican unit decertified, feeling that it was totally inappropriate that self-proclaimed homosexuals should be allowed to use the Republican Party to advance the gay political agenda. After all, the Democrat Party had traditionally been the party of the homosexuals, the radicals, the leftists and various ethnic minorities. The homosexual contingent had been able to gain control of the Democrat Party platform and to get that party's acceptance of: (1) homosexuality as a legitimate alternative lifestyle; (2) the homosexual program for values-neutral sex education; (3) the homosexual program for HIV disease; (4) the homosexual program for anti-handicap and antidiscrimination legislation. In 1988, the homosexuals were organizing to take over the traditionally conservative Republican Party.

It was obvious that it was their intent to control both political parties and to use their political power to destroy the traditional pro-family and moral positions espoused by Republicans. Homosexuals supported abortion, they had an alliance with Planned Parenthood, the ACLU and the radical left. By taking control of the Republican Party, they could use the platform to oppose any use of accepted public health techniques and testing to control the epidemic. Tragically, the Republican legislators who wanted to decertify the Log Cabin Club were never allowed to bring up the issue. Why? Because the leaders of that Republican convention were effectively under gay control.

The most important meeting on the first afternoon was the committee on Health and Human Services. That committee was assigned the task of dealing with three AIDS initiatives...the LaRouche Initiative (Proposition 69), the Gann Initiative (Proposition 102) and the Block Initiative (Proposition 96).

The meeting was chaired by Assemblyman Bill Filante, a legislator who usually supported the homosexual position and who attended the meeting of The Log Cabin Club in Palm Springs in 1990.

Doctor Gladden Elliott, former President of the CMA was there. He was the first speaker of the afternoon and stated that the CMA opposed all three AIDS initiatives (despite the fact that the House of Delegates had yet to convene in 1988).

The first initiative discussed was the LaRouche Initiative. I sat next to Congressman Dannemeyer who leaned over and whispered:

"There's no sense backing LaRouche, even if what it says is right — I did that a year and a half ago and it served no useful purpose."

There was a number of speakers who rose to denounce Lyndon LaRouche and his radical policies. Then I went to the microphone and stated that HIV disease should be considered as an infectious, contagious and communicable disease just as the initiative stated. I pointed out my dislike for LaRouche and everything he stood for but reiterated that we were dealing with an epidemic and what the LaRouche Initiative

said was only logical since the initiative did not advocate quarantine or
the isolation of HIV carriers.

My remarks were countered by a rather small, balding, obviously gay
young man who moved to the front of the room and in a trembling voice
and with a quivering finger pointed in my direction, shouted:

"We know all about you. My friends in Washington have told me all
about you. You want to send us all to Molokai!"

As so often happens, all attacks are directed at condemning the
speaker rather than addressing the subject. If you can destroy the
credibility of the speaker, you can discredit what he has said — even if
what he has said is true. When the little, balding man paused for a
moment, I spoke from the rear of the room,

"I have a hundred dollars in my wallet right now which I will leave
with anyone in this room if you will put up a similar amount. I have never
suggested that we needed to quarantine people with this disease. If you
can produce anything that I have ever written or anything that I have ever
said that suggests quarantine, you can have my hundred dollars."

Assemblyman Filante became flustered. Fearing that he was losing
control of the meeting, he quickly rose and said something to the effect
that "The mutual betting window is closed. We don't allow wagers in
this committee." He then went on to confirm his own opposition to the
LaRouche Initiative. He was preparing to call for a vote when I put up
my hand and was recognized.

"Before we vote on the LaRouche Initiative, could you please read the
initiative to the members of this committee?"

Assemblyman Filante looked even more flustered. He searched
through his papers and acknowledged that he did not have a copy of the
initiative. When I pressed him further, he acknowledged he did not even
know what the initiative said but he was firmly against it.

I queried whether anyone in the room could quote the LaRouche
Initiative. No one could. I then quoted from the initiative and asked the
question, "What's wrong with declaring HIV disease as an infectious,
contagious and communicable disease and carriers of the ...virus as
infectious, contagious and communicable?"

The vote of the HHS Committee members was taken. The vote was
18 to 0, against the initiative.

As I stood there in the back of the room, the homosexual man who had
attacked me walked over and stood by my side. Looking up at me he said

— almost hesitantly,

"Perhaps I'm wrong. Haven't you ever advocated quarantine?"

I looked down at him and smiled.

"Of course not. I think you have me confused with someone else."

"Could I have one of your cards?" he asked. "If I'm wrong I'll be glad to apologize."

We exchanged cards. His name was Frank Ricchiazze. He had been appointed to a key administrative position in the California Department of Motor Vehicles. He was a gay activist who had come out of the closet and was now working within the Republican Party to convince party leaders to support homosexual goals. In the months that followed, Frank called several times and tried to convince me that the Republican Party should embrace the homosexual agenda and by so doing, it could have homosexual votes to elect Republican candidates. I am certain that he made similar calls to other Republican leaders. Tragically, some of them were willing to sacrifice principles and moral positions for homosexual support.

As the afternoon wore on, we discussed Propositions 102 and 96. In each instance, Dr. Gladden Elliott from the CMA rose to oppose the initiatives.

Congressman Dannemeyer, Larry McNamee and I each spoke to the initiatives. In each instance, the committee voted them down.

As we left the room I could see the various members of the HHS committee hugging one another in the hallway. There were obvious lesbians hugging homosexual men and homosexuals hugging one another. It soon became obvious that the majority of the committee members were gay or lesbian. Later I was told that highly placed Republican officials had violated the rules and regulations of the California Republican Central Committee and added 12 names to the membership list of the HHS committee just the day before the meeting. All of those added were either homosexuals or lesbians, thus assuring that the committee vote would favor the gay position.

It was the following day when Larry McNamee and Congressman Dannemeyer hoped that they would have an opportunity to address the convention. Larry told me that he had requested permission to address the convention but had been informed by the chairman that a representative from the CMA had insisted that he not be allowed to speak.

Preventing Congress Dannemeyer from speaking was an entirely different matter. After all the Congressman had flown all the way from Washington, D. C. to address the convention. He was one of the best known and admired Republicans in the state. It was vitally important to Bill Dannemeyer that he have that opportunity to address Republican leaders for he needed their support for the Gann Initiative. How would the leaders prevent him from speaking? Very simple. They delayed the afternoon meeting until many of those in attendance had left. At that point there was a quorum call and because of the lack of a quorum, the meeting was adjourned. Bill Dannemeyer's trip to California was for naught. In the spring of 1988 there were already powerful forces within the party intent upon blocking efforts to begin addressing the HIV disease as an infectious, contagious and communicable disease.

✳✳✳

March 1988.

The CMA Convention was held at the Convention Hall in Reno, Nevada. In preparation for that meeting, I sent out three separate mailings to every member of the House of Delegates. In those letters I pointed out how CMA leadership had failed to carry out the position taken by the House in 1986. I pointed out how CMA leadership had not only failed to carry out the directives of the House in 1987 but how they had actively lobbied against those positions before the state legislature.

Just before the meeting Dr. Laurens White, then President-elect of the CMA, had given an interview to the San Francisco Chronicle in which he had talked about how many bad doctors there were practicing in California and how many "sleaze-ball doctors" there were in our state. The article was not only in extremely poor taste but deprecated and demeaned the medical profession. I felt it was entirely inappropriate that the President-elect of the CMA should come out and publicly criticize physicians. Not that there can't occasionally be bad doctors, but I can tell you quite honestly that doctors work very hard to make sure that all physicians on hospital staffs and in medical organizations adhere to the highest caliber of medical practice. Through the years in communities all across California doctors have put in hundreds of thousands of hours in peer review and education, attempting to uphold the standards of our profession. Yet here was the President-elect of the CMA referring to doctors in our state as "sleaze-balls." I therefore reproduced copies of the half-page article and sent one to every delegate to the House.

When I arrived at the convention almost half the members were wearing large lapel buttons asking, "What's a sleaze-ball?" As a result of those buttons and the articles, the President-elect of the CMA was required by the Council to go to every delegation and offer an apology for his injudicious remarks.

✳✳✳

In the weeks before the convention, the CMA mailed to all the delegates information on Propositions 102 and 96. Their criticisms were frank distortions of the truth. It was an obvious attempt to convince the delegates that they should oppose both propositions.

✳✳✳

Larry McNamee attended this convention as well. In an effort to present the truth about Proposition 102, he set up a card table in that area of the Convention Hall where information ordinarily could be publicly disseminated. The leadership of the CMA sent guards to close down his table.

Larry then contacted CMA leadership and asked for permission to hand out copies of his material. Permission was denied.

I was in contact with Congressman Dannemeyer's office and they suggested that I call Dr. Frank Judson of the Denver Department of Public Health to get information on the Colorado program. In Colorado, routine HIV testing was being performed without the use of anonymous test sites and with mandatory reporting to public health departments. Dr. Judson told me that Colorado was doing almost twice as much HIV testing per hundred thousand citizens as California was. He faxed me information on the Colorado experience which showed just how effective tracing had been in identifying unsuspected infected people and beginning to break the chain of transmission of the disease. Thirteen percent of those who were contacted by public health officers were found to have unsuspected HIV infection.

Since the hierarchy of the CMA had refused to give Larry permission to pass out fliers, it seemed that there would be no way to reach the doctors. Yet I had new information that showed conclusively that the use of standard public health techniques worked effectively in Colorado. Somehow we had to get that information disseminated. I made up 600 fliers on a copy machine and with the help of three physicians from the Santa Cruz delegation, we went to the convention hall shortly before the meeting was to convene. We placed copies of the material on contact tracing on every seat in the convention hall. When someone in the CMA hierarchy realized what we were doing, monitors were immediately dispatched to pick up those fliers so that the delegates would have no opportunity to understand the truth about Proposition 102.

※※※

I suspected that the hierarchy would move, once again, to limit debate to two minutes to prevent me from effectively addressing the convention but I had no idea just how far they had already gone in making sure that there would be no support for my position.

During my first afternoon in Reno, I was stopped in the hall by one of the delegates.

"Stan," he said, "I want you to know that I am a public health officer. Several of us agree with you and what you're trying to do but we are not going to be able to come out and support you publicly. We've been threatened and told not to support you. I want you to know that you are right and we believe in what you're doing."

I looked at him in disbelief. Here was a public health officer who knew what needed to be done. He knew that people were dying needlessly but he was afraid to speak out publicly. He was afraid for his job; he was afraid for his future and for his family.

※※※

It was Saturday afternoon, the first day of the convention, when I went to "Reference Committee G." Mervyn Silverman was there as were several of the other public health officers and a number of gay activists who I had come to recognize from preceding years. But this year there was a new speaker who opposed my resolution. He was perhaps 6 feet tall with hair that hung down vertically over his ears and forehead and low over his collar. He was dressed in an old brown sports coat. Every time I spoke he was at the microphone to counter my remarks. He spoke clearly and well but his arguments were pure sophistry.

When I presented my resolution suggesting that HIV disease should be considered as an infectious, contagious, sexually transmitted disease and treated like all other diseases, the young man with shaggy hair was at the microphone claiming that HIV disease was different from other diseases. In essence he said this:

"After all, we know that people with HIV disease are discriminated against. What other disease is there where you can have your house burned just because your children are infected?"

When I pointed out the importance of doing contact tracing, the young man was back at the microphone to discredit my position.

There are no minutes taken of the Reference Committee meetings so I have only my memory to rely upon as to what transpired. I do remember that Mervyn Silverman was at the microphone in front of me and was proclaiming that all we needed to stop the epidemic was education and behavioral modification. He pointed out how effective education had been in stopping the epidemic in the homosexuals in San Francisco and how effective the educational program had been in cutting back on the incidence of rectal gonorrhea and new cases of HIV disease.

I try never to become angry during a public debate or discussion. I have found that when one loses his composure he sometimes may say things that he will later regret. But I had heard Mervyn Silverman refer to the success of education in San Francisco too many times in the past and I knew that in the large Cohort Study of 6700 homosexuals, three quarters of them already carried the virus and were going to die. Yet here was the man who had been the public health officer during the height of the epidemic — trying to convince the reference committee that standard public health techniques were unnecessary to try to stem the course of the epidemic as it spread silently across our nation.

I was at the microphone immediately behind Merv Silverman when I was recognized. I said something to the effect,

"Yes, you did a great job in San Francisco, Dr. Silverman. Because you didn't close the bathhouses, because you wouldn't use standard public health techniques, thousands of homosexuals are going to die. That is a tribute to the success of your program of education and behavioral modification. Perhaps we can do as well in the heterosexual community using your same techniques."

As soon as I had finished speaking, I regretted my words. Attacking Silverman served little purpose. After all, he was internationally known as the President of AMFAR. He was a prominent public health leader and the man who was credited with closing the bathhouses in San Francisco.

What surprised me most was the fact that Silverman turned, smiled at me, then turned back to his microphone and spoke again, reinforcing his position that all we needed to stop the epidemic was education and behavioral modification.

***

As we left the Reference Committee and crowded into the elevator on the way to our rooms at the MGM Hotel, I noticed the young man with the brown sports coat and shaggy hair standing almost next to me. I peered down at the name card on his chest to see who my antagonist was. I could hardly believe what I read, for standing next to me, his long hair draped vertically down over his ears and brushing against his coat collar, was the world's foremost clinical epidemiologist, a man who in some ways was almost a living legend. Here was the man who had saved the world from Ebola Fever when the epidemic had broken out in the 1970's in Africa. Here was the man who the WHO had sent to Bangladesh and India to help eradicate smallpox. Much of the credit for the eradication of smallpox worldwide could be credited to his efforts. Yet here was a man who was opposing my efforts to use standard public health techniques to try to stop the spread of HIV disease.

The elevator was crowded. We were pressed against one another and no one was saying anything until I blurted out:

"You are Don Francis?"

The young man looked at me, obviously startled. I pointed a finger at him and shook it in front of his face.

"Why are you arguing against me when you know what needs to be done to stop this epidemic? You know as well as I do that we have to start addressing HIV disease as a disease if we're ever going to be able to bring it under control."

Even in the crowded elevator, Dr. Francis drew back from my unexpected onslaught. I was angry and frustrated. Here was a man who had gone into the Ebola Valley and taken everyone who had come in contact with the infection and put them into concentration camps, allowing them to die so that the disease would not continue to spread. Here was the man who had insisted that the bodies of those infected were burned so that the disease could be arrested. Here was the man who had done what was necessary to stop an epidemic caused by a retrovirus that was so virulent that almost everyone who had come in contact with it had died. Over one hundred and fifty people had died within a matter of just a few short weeks there in the Ebola valley on the southern border of the Sudan. Yet this same man was publicly arguing that we should not

address HIV as an infectious, contagious, sexually transmitted disease.
"I'll talk to you about it later," he stammered.
Everyone in the elevator was looking at the two of us.
"No. I want to talk about it now. I want to know why you're arguing against what you know is right."
The door to the elevator opened and Don Francis passed through the doorway. I followed him into an empty hallway.
"Why are you arguing against me?" I repeated.
"You know that what I am saying is standard public health policy."
Don Francis glanced at his watch.
"I've got to get to a meeting, but I promise you that I'll get in touch with you as soon as we get back to California."
And then he was gone.
I really thought that I would never see Dr. Don Francis again, however, he was a man of his word and though I may disagree with him, he is another one of those men who has played a key part in managing this epidemic. When the ultimate history of the epidemic is written, his name will be recorded as one of the key players in the unfolding drama...although this disease may well be his "Waterloo." In the months that followed, I was to meet him again and gain some insight into why he had identified with the Gay and AIDS Lobbies rather than with those of us who were trying to use a logical approach to try to save human lives.

❄❄❄

In some ways, it seemed almost too good to be true. Coincidental with the convention in Reno, the publishers of Doctors Masters, Johnson and Kolodny's new book, *Crisis*, had started a nationwide campaign to create interest in their publication. What Doctors Masters, Johnson and Kolodny were saying in their book was that the disease was spreading into the heterosexual population and that in their survey of promiscuous heterosexual men and women across America — those with five or more sexual partners a year — 5% of the men and 7% of the women already carried the virus. In very promiscuous women in New York City — with 12 or more sexual partners a year — 14% carried the virus. The results of their study had been obtained from testing equal numbers of heterosexual men and women in New York, Chicago and Los Angeles.
On Sunday evening there had been a television interview with Doctors Masters and Johnson. Since all the delegates were away from

home the majority of the doctors at the convention did not have the opportunity to see that program. On Monday morning the review of their book was published in Reno newspapers and in newspapers all across the nation. When our Seventh District Delegation met Monday morning to discuss the coming House debate on AIDS, our chairman mentioned the television broadcast of the previous evening.

The delegation chairman regularly attends an earlier morning meeting with the CMA Executive Committee before he comes to our delegation meeting. He usually tells us what the hierarchy wants us to know about what is going to transpire each day. Obviously, someone in the leadership of the CMA was upset by the revelations on television the previous evening and feared that it might influence the vote of the House. I can only assume that was the case because the chairman of our delegation got up and told us about the interview and that Masters and Johnson's new work was really of no significance since their entire study had been done in **Baltimore, Maryland** where everyone knew the epidemic was out of control. At the end of the briefing, I went to the chairman and asked him if he had actually seen the television program. He assured me that he had. I was somewhat taken aback because I did not anticipate our chairman would tell me something that was blatantly untrue.

My wife had seen the interview and had given me an entirely different interpretation. Fortunately, she video-taped the program and later I had an opportunity to view it. There was not one mention in that interview about **Baltimore**. But, you see, a lie told convincingly enough will usually be accepted by good people — and the physicians in our delegation had no reason to disbelieve our chairman. Whether he was told what to say at the early morning briefing I do not know but, intentionally or unintentionally, he told our delegation a "fact" which was untrue. I have never gotten used to the pattern of deceit and treachery that has been used by CMA leadership in dealing with the House. I have tried to assume that people were honest and might make mistakes but with the unfolding of the epidemic it became increasingly obvious that most of what was happening was not a mistake but intentional distortions of the truth in an effort to mislead the House and prevent any effective steps from being taken to stop the dying and the death.

It was on the afternoon of March 8, 1988 when the House of Delegates convened to consider the report of Reference Committee G. Dr. Marilyn Koehn, the Chairman of that committee, addressed the House.

"For the second year, AIDS has been the dominant issue before this House of Delegates. Your reference committee again heard the anger and frustration of physicians who increasingly must confront this frightening disease which is epidemic and which has no cure. AIDS will be a growing part of medical practice for the immediate future and we all must come to terms with it. It is imperative that medicine present a united front on AIDS policy in the future. Last year, despite passage of considerable AIDS policy by this House, dissension within our ranks continued with various physicians' groups approaching legislators with their own proposals. As a direct consequence of the internal conflict, the CMA was ineffective as a major force for change in public policy on AIDS. Physicians must work together on these issues or all our efforts will be in vain."

As I listened to the introductory remarks, it was quite obvious that they were aimed at the Santa Cruz County Medical Society and those of us who had tried to enact the policies laid out by the House of Delegates in 1987. Instead of addressing the fact that CMA leadership had steadfastly refused to support House policy, we were to be the subjects of ridicule and deridement. We were the reason that adequate AIDS policy was not being carried out, not those in positions of power who had betrayed the trust of the House.

The first resolution of the afternoon was introduced by Dr. Richard Snyder, a delegate from Marin. It dealt with changing consent and confidentiality restrictions on testing. Richard was one of the handful of concerned doctors who had been willing to take a stand and support me in years past. His resolution was recommended for a "No" vote by the Reference Committee and ended up being referred to the Council for consideration which in effect killed his resolution.

The second resolution was a compilation of three resolutions — 702-88, 703-88 and 719-88.

Resolution 702-88 had been submitted by the CMA Council and stated:

"The CMA urges all physicians to consider HIV screening as an important adjunct to counseling for the purpose of AIDS prevention."

The real intent of the CMA's resolution was to convince doctors that they must spend 10 to 30 minutes on counseling before testing (screening). This requirement for counseling would discourage any doctor with a busy practice from doing routine HIV testing.

The next resolution dealt with mandatory HIV testing for all hospital admissions and allowing the information to be disseminated to HCW's. The third resolution also dealt with the subject of HIV testing. In an effort to neutralize these resolutions, the reference committee came forward with the following:

Be it RESOLVED:

"That physicians be urged to consider the need for HIV evaluation and counseling of all patients, including those in the office setting as well as those seen in pre-operative consultations and hospital admissions."

It was obvious that the last thing that the leadership wanted was routine HIV testing of hospital admissions. It was certainly well known that routine testing for syphilis had been effective and that physicians had brought syphilis under control long before penicillin was available. The amended resolution was simply a clever means of avoiding taking a position which recommended that doctors carry out routine testing.

Dr. Carl Levinson from the Specialty Delegation rose to amend the resolution and presented the following resolution:

"Be it resolved that the CMA encourage legislation for routine prenatal counseling and testing of all pregnant women with the patient having the option of refusal."

Dr. Levinson then said:

> The AIDS issue is in a state of flux...at stake is a fundamental issue of rights, those of the individual and of society. It is our opinion that the laws to date are not properly directed, that currently they are directed at intimidating medical evaluation and management...The CMA is a medical group which should be emphasizing medical care. Many non-medical groups have brought pressure to bear on what should be a medical and public health issue like syphilis and hepatitis. It is time to make a statement to bring a disease process under appropriate medical care. We propose this resolve which would affect two important citizens in our land, the mother and the baby (emphasis added).

Dr. Levinson's resolution was immediately attacked by a series of gay activists and several public health officers.

Then it was my turn to speak. I simply pointed out that the House had supported this concept in 1987 and the hierarchy had actively opposed prenatal testing in Sacramento in 1987. (My remarks are recorded in Appendix III).

The resolution passed shortly thereafter with the full support of the House. Once again, the House of Delegates came out in favor of prenatal testing. That resolution was referred to the Commission on Legislation and, in the year that followed, Senator Doolittle's prenatal testing bill moved through legislative committees in Sacramento. Again CMA lobbyists steadfastly refused to support prenatal testing. However, on January 1, 1989, Senator Doolittle's bill did become law...without CMA support.

The next resolution was mine (705-88). It stated:

"Be it resolved that the California Medical Association seek legislation that will include HIV infection as a communicable, contagious, reportable disease."

The hierarchy attached their comment to my resolution to this effect:

"In November, the Council adopted a position statement on the adverse effects of reporting HIV-infected individuals and discussed how reporting of HIV-positive individuals without any identifiable positive incentive or action serves to undermine the trust and relationship between those at risk, health authorities and physicians."

Dr. Ronald Van Roy from District 10 rose to speak for his entire delegation to support my resolution.

The Speaker of the House, Dr. Corlin, is supposed to be entirely impartial; however, having observed how the Speaker has used his position for years, it was quite obvious that Doctor Corlin actively opposed testing. In order to introduce his personal views, the Speaker called on Dr. Koehn, the Chairman of the Reference Committee and asked for her thoughts on the resolution. This was a clever ploy by which the Speaker was able to have someone else bring out information that he wanted presented.

"The committee was unanimous against mandatory reporting," Dr. Koehn said, "We think that the CMA, the CDC, the Surgeon General, the National Academy of Science continue to oppose this and we oppose it also."

In fairness to the speaker, at this point he did call upon me to respond.

"Ladies and gentlemen, millions of Americans are going to die from this disease. The only question is not whether millions are going to die but how many millions. We have to start treating this as a communicable disease and...break the chain of transmission. Every other major disease is reportable...We are getting better statistics out of Africa than we are getting out of America. This is insanity. We have all sorts of statistics on AIDS but nothing on the HIV epidemic...We are doing the population of this country a grave disservice not to declare that HIV is an infectious disease...(The full text of my remarks are included in Appendix III).

There were several more speakers, for and against the resolution. Then Dr. Mervyn Silverman moved to the microphone.

Silverman, District 8, Chairman of the CMA Task Force on AIDS. I am also President of the American Foundation for AIDS Research and Director of the Robert Wood Johnson Foundation AIDS Health Services Program. First of all, I want to praise the Reference Committee. I think they've done a superb job and District 8 (San Francisco County) totally supports the recommendations of the Reference Committee. We need statistics; we don't need names. What we need is demography. We can get that without names. Case monitoring to stop the chain can only be done if we go around behind each person who is infected and follow them to make sure they don't do anything bad. What we have to do is to encourage people to come in to be tested, and not discourage them, so that they will change their behavior that leads to the spread of this disease. In San Francisco, at the anonymous testing site, they asked 400 people who had come there voluntarily, would they have come if testing were just confidential...in other words reported? 60% of the gay men said absolutely not. 34% of the heterosexual males and females said absolutely not. 22% more of the gay men said they might not. 34% more of the heterosexuals said they might not. At least 50% of the people who, on their own volition, came in because they thought they had a problem, would stay away. We encourage people to be tested prenatally, premaritally in sexually transmitted disease clinics. We've got to get them in there. We've got to get them in where they feel they are safe. If they think it is going to be reported, then they will stay away and we wouldn't want that. We can do all the epidemiology and we can do much more education if we don't have mandatory testing. It sounds like it makes sense. Let me say this. If we make this a communicable disease, that means that if any of you are infected, you will not be able to practice medicine in the hospital, children won't be allowed in schools, teachers will not be allowed in schools and people will be kept out of food handling. All of this is totally unnecessary.

Of course, what Dr. Silverman said was totally preposterous. Listing HIV disease as a communicable disease did not mean that doctors couldn't practice medicine, children wouldn't be allowed in schools or food handlers couldn't handle food. No restrictions had been imposed by health officers on food handlers, teachers or physicians with AIDS and AIDS was already considered a "disease" by state law. But when the Director of the Robert Wood Johnson Foundation made such a statement, it bore an air of authority. You could almost feel the doctors in the audience cringe under Silverman's rhetoric, each physician wondering what would happen to him if he accidently came down with the disease and could no longer work in his profession.

Furthermore, the poll at the clinics in San Francisco had been specifically taken to justify the position of the AIDS Lobby to demonstrate that people wouldn't come for testing if the test results were reported to public health authorities. Homosexuals have been consistently told by gay publications and their leaders that public health reporting would surely lead to the loss of their jobs, housing, insurance and personal relationships. Pre-test counseling warned patients of the danger of breaches in confidentiality. When the question of testing was asked in that context it is understandable that so many responded that they would not have the blood test if it were reportable. Yet, AIDS was a reportable disease and over 50,000 cases had been reported by 1988 without violation of confidentiality and Silverman knew that. But his statements turned the tide against considering HIV disease as a disease.

Several more speakers opposed the resolution. Then Gladden Elliott, former President of the CMA, spoke. This was the same physician who had been at the conference of the Republican Central Committee the previous month and had come out against Propositions 69, 102 and 96. To justify his opposition to my resolution, he stated:

> ...the few alternative testing sites now are overrun by people wanting anonymous testing but they would certainly disappear if reporting were mandated. All the experience in California indicates that the incidence of testing would decrease. The experience in Colorado is frequently cited where mandatory reporting is present. I rise to cite one thing that maybe you're not aware of...Colorado

testing does not require validation of the name of the patient. The most commonly used names are those of the governor and Walt Disney characters. 70% used false names in one clinic. I submit that mandated reporting is not the way to break the cycle. The way to break the cycle is to get the trust of those high risk practicing individuals so they will...report for testing and then use all of the educational efforts at our disposal.

You see here the thrust of his argument. Physicians should only be concerned with the high risk sector of the epidemic, homosexuals and IV drug users. Physicians were not to be concerned with the spread of the disease into our youth and the heterosexual population.

The next significant speaker was Jack Bridgeman, a general practitioner from Orange County and immediate past-president of the Orange County Medical Society. He spoke in support of my resolution, saying:

> The only data that we have is from Colorado which shows that they are testing almost twice as many people per hundred thousand population as they are in California. The gays are coming in. The Mickey Mouse statistics that Dr. Elliott told us, I have no data on how true that is. Let us just do what is right. If people are going to give a false name, that's their privilege. You cannot treat a communicable disease until you know who has it and how fast it's spreading...The benefits of passing this resolution will be that the governor can declare HIV positivity an infectious disease...If (you) think permissive (reporting) will work, think again. Permissive reporting for AIDS means that my patient, if he is positive, can threaten me or intimidate me against reporting the disease...If child abuse (reporting) were permissive rather than mandatory, how many of us would have the courage to go out and say I'm going to report you. If it's a law, the patient conforms. Society must conform. Society must conform to fight this disease. We can no longer go on with this permissive approach (to the epidemic)...

The final speaker was Fred Armstrong, the President of the CMA, who had come to our Medical Society the previous December to plead with our Board of Governors to give him a letter of support. Doctor Armstrong left the podium and descended to a microphone on the floor. Fred was determined to defeat my resolution for he opposed using public health measures to stop the epidemic.

> I support the Reference Committee. During the past year...we have

gone through an awful lot of talking and agonizing over the whole AIDS issue...We came up with what we think is a very sensible policy on AIDS and on AIDS legislation. We have introduced three AIDS bills which are an attempt by the CMA to get rid of some of the onerous provisions of the law...Now, if we change our basic policy at this time, I feel that this would risk some of the excellent legislation that we have already introduced. Now, perhaps we should change in the future, but I would ask that you not change at this time and I support the Reference Committee.

The powerful President of the California Medical Association had come from the podium to plead with the House to oppose my resolution. The delegates had only two choices. It was a choice between supporting my resolution or supporting the CMA hierarchy. The President of the CMA stated that if we declared HIV an infectious disease, we would "risk some of the excellent legislation already introduced."

Tragically, members of the House did not understand that the legislation introduced by the CMA was not intended to stop the epidemic in the heterosexual population. CMA legislation supported anti-discrimination laws and permissive reporting and opposed the legislation introduced by Senator Doolittle.

Unfortunately, the average member of the House and the average doctor in California did not know what was happening in Sacramento. They had only the words of their leaders to go by. Most doctors could not believe, not for one instant, that the leaders of organized medicine would betray them and would betray the public. And so it was that my resolution, a resolution which simply said that HIV disease should be included in the list of communicable, contagious, reportable diseases in the State of California, was voted down by a narrow margin.

The policy that the CMA's Executive Committee endorsed was for permissive reporting of HIV disease. This legislation became law in January 1989. Permissive reporting of HIV disease by doctors is like permissive paying of income taxes or a permissive speed limit on the highways. How many people do you honestly believe would pay their income taxes if there were no legal requirements? How many people would abide by the speed limit if there were no traffic policemen by the wayside?

Since legislation for permissive reporting became law in 1989, there have been very few cases reported to public health officers and there are still no valid statistics on the prevalence of the disease in our state. But that was the intention; that was the objective. Physicians were not to address the epidemic nor try to stop its spread into the heterosexual community.

✳✳✳

The next resolution, 706-88, was also by resolution which simply stated:

"Be it Resolved that the CMA support legislation that will extend the current AIDS/HIV confidentiality requirements for medical personnel to those persons who are notified and contacted during the process of contact tracing, thus extending fines and penalties to those outside the medical profession should they intentionally divulge the identity of an HIV carrier."

I did not believe that those within the AIDS and Gay Lobbies were really concerned about confidentiality. I felt that they were using the issue of confidentiality and the threat of exposure of the identity of those infected as a clever smoke screen to draw attention away from the fact that we were not addressing HIV as an infectious disease. I really wanted to see what the response of the leadership and of the Reference Committee would be to this resolution. As expected, they opposed it. It was quite clear that they did not want to extend legal restrictions to those who might learn of a patient's infection through contact tracing. Confidentiality obviously was not the issue. Confidentiality was simply the smoke screen behind which the epidemic was being allowed to spread.

✳✳✳

Shortly thereafter we came to the resolution presented by Doctor Seymour Albin, Resolution 729-88, which dealt with Proposition 96, the Block Initiative, sponsored by Sheriff Block of Los Angeles.

Doctor Albin outlined the basic tenets of Proposition 96 which allowed a court to order HIV testing if there was a transfer of body fluid during criminal activity such as rape or an attack on a police officer. Doctor Albin asked the CMA to support similar legislation.

The printed comment on this resolution stated that CMA "disapproved of AB117-87, a bill which required an arrested person to submit to testing if they posed the threat of spreading a communicable disease to a public safety officer." In other words, the CMA opposed efforts to protect our police force. They had already come out publicly against the

Block Initiative — Proposition 96 — and it was obvious that the CMA hierarchy was intent upon blocking this proposition for it called for a form of "routine testing."

The discussion on the floor of the House was pro and con. The Reference Committee, as expected, came out firmly against the resolution.

Speaking in favor of the resolution, Doctor Bryan Johnston of Los Angeles said:

"As an emergency physician, I see a lot of rape victims. I think there is great value in being able to give a rape victim at lease some preliminary information and perhaps some definitive information regarding the HIV status of her assailant..."

Efforts were made to refer the resolution to council, a move that would assure its defeat.

I rose to comment:

> First of all...this (resolution) deals with the initiative which came out of the Los Angeles Sheriff's Department so that they could begin to test people who are guilty of criminal and sexual attacks. The CMA has already come out firmly against the Block Initiative which is going to the voters and I think probably the voters will accept it... I speak against referral. I think we should pass this resolution and give the council the information that we support... police officers and we support, in effect, the Block Initiative... That is what the entire issue is, basically, to get the CMA in line with the Block Initiative so that the CMA council will be forced — even though they don't want to — to support that initiative and protect our police officers and the victims of sexual and violent crimes.

Immediately thereafter the House voted on the resolution. It passed overwhelmingly.

Subsequently, in the book published by the CMA entitled, *Actions Of The House Of Delegates,* Resolution 729-88G was referred to as the "Los Angeles County Sheriff's Department Initiative, Proposition 96" and it was noted that it had been adopted by the House. However, that did not keep the hierarchy of the CMA from coming out, speaking for all the physicians of the State of California, stating that the CMA opposed Proposition 96. I am sure that few of the delegates who attended that meeting remembered the discussion or remembered or realized that, once again, the hierarchy of organized medicine had ignored the will of the doctors and utilized their position to perpetuate the epidemic.

✳✳✳

I was surprised that some of the resolutions were voted down that afternoon, especially the resolution asking for support for Proposition 102. However, CMA leadership made preposterous charges against the Gann Initiative and the House voted against it. That ended the AIDS debate in Reno in 1988.

✳✳✳

Early in 1988, in an article in Cosmopolitan magazine, Doctor Robert Gould advised millions of American women that if they had ordinary sexual intercourse, they would run almost no risk of contracting "Acquired Immune Deficiency Syndrome." This article was simply one of a number of articles that began appearing in magazines all across the nation assuring the public that there was little danger from the heterosexual spread of the epidemic. It seemed more than coincidental that so many articles suddenly appeared, assuring citizens that they had little to fear from the disease.

At that time, the Centers for Disease Control readily admitted that at least 4% of AIDS cases resulted from heterosexual contact — and those figures reflected the epidemic in the heterosexual population ten years earlier. In Africa, 80-90% of cases were from heterosexual spread.

A few months later, a report was released by a University of California statistician which assured young people that their chance of getting HIV disease from a casual sexual encounter would be only one in five million and if they used a condom, their chances would be only one in fifty million. Such statistics were not only medically unsound, they were examples of criminal negligence, and insured the eventual spread of the epidemic into the youth of our nation. Indeed, by mid-1989, the CDC determined that there were already several colleges in America where almost 1% of the students carried the virus. By 1990, analysis of anonymous test results from **sentinel** hospitals in New York and Minnesota showed that 1% of 15-16 year olds were infected. We can thank the program of misinformation waged in the 1980's for that tragedy.

✳✳✳

In early 1988, the **World Health Organization** (WHO) recommended that sterile needles and syringes should be distributed to IV drug users in America. The recommendation was based upon very limited experience in the Netherlands. A poll of IV drug users there suggested that the rate of needle sharing had dropped from 75% to 25% with needle distribution programs. To justify needle distribution in America, it was stated: "Just because you gave addicts needles, you weren't necessarily increasing drug usage." Of course, the issue was not whether you were increasing drug usage. The issue at stake was the fact that distribution of needles and syringes to drug users gave them the wrong message. It was the message that society approved of the use of drugs. How can a nation fight a drug epidemic when it is the official policy of that nation to distribute drug paraphenalia?

The WHO seemed oblivious to that contradiction and in 1988 was actively involved in trying to convince Americans that free needle and syringe exchange programs would be an effective means of fighting the HIV epidemic. Of course the WHO was also insisting on extensive counseling **before** HIV testing, on confidentiality and the use of informed consent for testing. Representatives of WHO reiterated that if we tried to do contact tracing in America we would simply "drive the disease underground."

✻✻✻

In Maryland, the Associate Dean of Academic Affairs at the Johns Hopkins School of Hygiene and Vice-chairman of the Governor's AIDS Council came out publicly against contact tracing, stating:
"There are some complicating factors. First, we don't have a cure for AIDS. So one questions whether it is defensible to do contact tracing for a disease for which there is no known treatment. Another issue is maintaining confidentiality..."

✻✻✻

It was early in April 1988 when my secretary told me that Don Francis was coming to Santa Cruz and wanted to go to dinner. I was really quite amazed. I felt that Don Francis' sudden departure in the hall at the MGM Hotel in Reno had simply been a convenient way of avoiding any further discussion. People so often say, "We will get together," but nothing ever comes of it. However, Don Francis was obviously a different type of person. How different he was would become obvious as we met and talked.

Dinner was at the Miramar Restaurant on the Wharf in Santa Cruz overlooking Monterey Bay and the rugged cliffs that grace the shoreline along the northern coast of our seaside community. Dr. Francis is young, energetic and has a typical Type A personality. He has a ready smile, a warm handshake and a way of talking with enthusiasm and sincerity, designed to win one to his position. Although in many respects a living legend by his mid-40's, he was certainly unassuming and tried to convince me with his arguments rather than trying to impress me with his credentials.

My general impression from our conversation was that Don Francis liked homosexuals. He was heterosexual and happily married, but he had dealt with homosexual leaders for years, starting with his hepatitis study in 1978 which had led to the "Cohort Study." He looked upon homosexuals as kind, intelligent, gentle people who have a different perspective of the world than the rest of us. He told of walking down the street with several homosexuals and seeing an attractive man and woman walking towards them. The woman was wearing a mini-skirt and a tight sweater and was quite striking in appearance.

"What do you think of that?" one of the homosexuals queried.

"I think she is really beautiful," Don replied.

"Not the girl, the fellow. Don't you think he's cute?" his homosexual friend proclaimed.

Don had used that example to demonstrate the difference in perspective between homosexuals and heterosexuals.

It was obvious he had come to know and respect homosexuals and did not want to hurt or offend them, feeling that their gentleness and feminine qualities were necessary in a complex world to counterbalance the macho, masculine tendencies of male heterosexuals. It was largely for this reason that he would not take a stand that would offend them or inflame their fears. On the other hand, he recognized the problems inherent in this disease. Realizing that the AZT studies would soon be available which would demonstrate that drugs could alter the course of HIV disease and prevent unnecessary death, he felt that once treatments were available we could justify trying to identify those who were infected.

I queried him on why he was opposed to prenatal testing when it was so important that we identify mothers who were infected. Don said that by 1989 we would perform HIV tests routinely on mothers all across the state. On that issue he was correct.

However, looking back on my conversation with him that evening, I realize how truly naive he really was. With good intentions and certainly with far more knowledge on epidemiology than I will ever have, he was trying to look at the epidemic from a social point of view rather than a medical point of view, hoping to maintain the support of homosexual leaders without realizing that there were other powerful forces intent upon blocking our nation from ever addressing this epidemic as such.

Now, as I write this book several years later, physicians still do not use routine HIV testing. They still have no knowledge as to the prevalence of HIV disease in our land. Despite all the amazing scientific advances in treatment of HIV disease during the intervening years, there is little contact tracing being carried out in California to identify those who carry the disease and get them into treatment. Even today, all the emphasis is centered on education and protecting the identity of infected homosexuals...and the disease continues its silent spread among our children and the young people and HCW's.

Don Francis felt very strongly that an antidiscrimination law was needed and that we needed to continue confidentiality laws. Although I felt that antidiscrimination laws were aimed specifically at justifying the homosexual lifestyle more than stopping discrimination, I was willing to support any legislation that would allow physicians to begin addressing HIV disease as a disease.

Francis alluded to the fact that medical records could be stolen — indeed, apparently some records had been stolen from a public health office in northern California. He felt that because health records could be stolen we could not have public health reporting until antidiscrimination laws were in place. However, he never questioned who had stolen the records and could not show that the stolen information had resulted in discrimination.

Francis was different from most public health officers I have met. Many public health officers go along with the positions taken by their leaders or politicians. After all, these are men who had chosen the security of government jobs rather than venturing into competitive clinical medicine. Many of them are doctors who are afraid to go into private practice. They are willing to settle for the security of government jobs rather than the challenge that exists in the private practice of medicine. Their motto is, "Go along and get along."

Then there are a few public health officers who know what needs to be done and have had the courage to encourage legislators in their states to enact laws to deal with the epidemic. Certainly that was true in Colorado and Idaho and, by late 1988, there were 12 states where some form of contact tracing was being used—although in many of the states, all reporting was done anonymously so there were no records kept as to who was infected.

Then there was another group of public health officers who knew what needed to be done but were fearful for their jobs. They had been frightened into silence and knew that if they took a stand for what they knew was right their jobs and their economic future would be in jeopardy. After all, when you have house payments to make and children in college, sometimes it is too costly to be courageous.

None of these factors influenced Don Francis. Here was a young man who was quite willing to stand alone for what he believed. He could justify the fears of the homosexual community and rationalize the restrictions placed on the use of standard public health techniques to fight the epidemic, based upon the homosexual fear of discrimination, the stealing of medical records from a public health office and the potential for breach of confidentiality by public health officers. More than that, I personally believe that Don Francis was trying to fight the HIV epidemic as he had fought the smallpox epidemic a decade previously. It is important to understand how smallpox was curtailed to understand the thought process that influenced the actions of some public health officials.

Smallpox was ostensibly eradicated from the world, not by universal vaccination, but by going where the disease was and vaccinating the people in the areas immediately adjacent to where the last outbreaks of smallpox occurred. Any time a case of smallpox was reported anywhere in the world, public health officials rushed to that area and vaccinated the surrounding population so they would not become infected.

Time and again, public health officials felt that smallpox had been eradicated only to have a new outbreak somewhere else in the world, but eventually, by preventing the disease from spreading from each outbreak, they were able to accomplish one of the greatest medical feats of all time...the apparent eradication of smallpox from the face of the earth. Don Francis played an important part in that effort. Thus it was that a similar technique was being used with HIV disease.

Public health officials were going to go where the disease was. They were going to try to prevent the spread of disease in the homosexual population and the IV drug population. That is where the entire emphasis of their efforts lay. They were establishing anonymous testing centers and alternative test centers where people could go and be tested. By making it easy for homosexuals and IV drug users to be tested voluntarily, they hoped that they would be able to limit HIV disease as they had eradicated smallpox.

There was only one tragic flaw in their plan. Smallpox had a latency period of 3 weeks while HIV disease has a latency period of up to a decade. In 1988 we had already lost almost a decade in our efforts to try to stop the spread of the disease in the heterosexual population. I suspect public health officers really felt that they could slow the spread of the disease with the voluntary cooperation of the homosexual community, not realizing that there were forces within that community which were doing everything they could to discourage homosexuals from being tested.

Admittedly, by mid-1989, some homosexual leaders had come out in favor of testing for homosexuals, but they still actively opposed contact tracing and the use of the force of law against those who were intentionally spreading the disease. Also, they opposed general testing of the heterosexual community. Thus, more years will be lost as we delay and delay and delay facing the epidemic from a medical point of view, as the hands of the biological clock move ever closer to that point of no return.

❉❉❉

It was in the latter part of April when my secretary informed me that a representative from the U. S. Civil Rights Commission in Washington, D. C. had called. When I returned the call, I was surprised to hear a cheery voice on the other end of the line:

"Hello, this is Mike."

"Mike who?"

"Mike Fumento."

"Mike Fumento? Have we met?"

"Don't you remember — you didn't like my article in *Commentary* magazine."

Suddenly, I remembered the article in the November issue of *Commentary* suggesting that there was little risk from heterosexual transmission of HIV disease. Mike Fumento was now working as the counsel for the U. S. Civil Rights Commission. His reply, along with my letter, were published shortly thereafter in Commentary.

The subject of his call was to invite me to testify before the Commission addressing the danger of casual transmission of HIV disease. Now, I do not really believe that this disease is readily spread outside of people living in close contact in homes (and then only rarely), with deep, passionate kissing and among health care workers...or by the traditional means of sexual contact, transfer of blood or blood products or from a woman to her child. But I agreed to go to Washington to testify.

It was May 1989 when I went to Washington—this time at taxpayers' expense. I arrived during the morning session of the commission meeting. As I entered the hall, I couldn't help noticing a number of young men wearing pink and black arm bands and strange looking T-shirts which bore a face emblazoned on their chests, a face which bore a strong resemblance to Ronald Reagan but that face was painted green, had fangs and looked very much like Dracula. These young men kept wandering in and out of the meeting hall as the testimony was under way.

When I arrived, there were several physicians sitting at a table facing members of the Civil Rights Commission. The Chairman of the Commission was Clarence Pendleton, a conservative black man who had been appointed by Ronald Reagan. On the far right was a militant, angry, black woman who seemed to take great delight in berating any physician who expressed concern about the spread of the epidemic. She would ask each of those who testified if they had been harassed, threatened or intimidated to keep them from speaking freely. Each one of the participants, in turn, dutifully assured her that no pressure had been brought to bear. The majority of those testifying reiterated the liberal lie that nothing needed to be done to stop the epidemic other than to use education and behavioral modification.

As I sat there I was given a copy of the testimony presented to the Commission by representatives from the Department of Public Health in San Francisco. The handout summarized the results of the "Cohort Study" of 6700 homosexuals which I mentioned earlier. Amazingly, the material presented dealt only with the 350 men who had not been exposed to hepatitis in 1978 and were obviously the least promiscuous of the 6700 homosexuals studied. The testimony stated that the incidence of HIV seropositivity in these gay men in San Francisco was only

50%.

Although true, it was an obvious half-truth since the incidence of disease in the 6700 homosexuals was over 76% by that date. Yet the material presented to the Commission referred to test results in only 350 of the 6700 cases. Several other small studies from San Francisco were also mentioned reaffirming the fact that only 50% of San Francisco homosexuals were infected. It was obvious that there were those in the San Francisco Public Health Department who were intentionally deceiving members of the U. S. Civil Rights Commission as to the incidence of HIV disease among the homosexual population of San Francisco.

The Commission adjourned for lunch. I was in the group which was to speak in the afternoon. There were four seats at the table facing the Commission where those of us who were to testify would be seated. I had been assigned the third seat from the right. The first seat was reserved for a doctor from the Centers for Disease Control, the second was for a public health officer from the New York State Health Department, the third seat was mine and the fourth seat was assigned to a former official from the CDC who was convinced that there was really no serious threat from the epidemic.

As fate would have it, there happened to be a table leg immediately in front of the third microphone where I was to sit. To avoid that table leg I moved slightly to my left whereupon the retired CDC official (who was supposed to have been in the fourth seat) moved into the third position. I was a little surprised but it really did not matter. I simply exchanged the name cards which faced the front of the auditorium and the members of the Commission; however, the names were not visible to the audience.

The members of the Civil Rights Commission filed into the room. Clarence Pendleton opened the meeting and the testimony began.

The doctor from the CDC spoke on the rare cases of infection among health care workers which are reported in the literature. The angry black woman on the far right prodded him with questions and asked if he had been threatened and if any pressure had been brought to bear to force him to alter his testimony. He assured her that that was not the case.

The second doctor gave his testimony, downplaying the importance of using public health techniques to try to control the epidemic. He was also questioned as to whether or not efforts had been made to intimidate him.

Next it was my turn, but the retired CDC official had taken my seat so he began his testimony out of turn. He had no sooner begun his presentation when I heard a chorus singing:

"O' beautiful for spacious skies, for amber fields of grain."

I swung around. There in the center of the auditorium sat 40 young men, all dressed in their white T-shirts with the Dracula-like caricature of Ronald Reagan emblazoned in green on their chests. Most of them wore artificial bulbous noses and Mickey Mouse ears perched on the tops of their heads. They sang loudly through several stanzas of "America," as the former CDC official attempted to complete his testimony. Once the singing had finished, the chanting, yelling and screaming began in an obvious effort to disrupt his testimony.

Clarence Pendleton, the Chairman of the Commission, tried to restore order. He patiently asked the demonstrators to refrain from interrupting — but the young men continued their boisterous actions and managed to totally disrupt the presentation of the third speaker.

Then it was my turn to speak. I began my statement quoting from Randy Shilts' book:

"The bitter truth is that AIDS did not have to happen…it was allowed to happen by an array of public institutions all of which failed to carry out their appropriate task, to guard the public health…There was no reason in this time, in this nation, for a new epidemic."

My remarks were met with cheers and applause from the audience but when I went on to point out that there really was no AIDS epidemic, that the epidemic was really HIV disease, my remarks were met with hoots, cheers and condemnation from the demonstrators. As I proceeded to outline the fact that the major problem in America was that we were not addressing the epidemic as an epidemic, the screams, chants and cries grew ever louder.

Clarence Pendleton finally gaveled the meeting to an end and called for a temporary adjournment. He warned the young men that they would either have to leave or he would call the police. I couldn't help but notice that during the break, the angry black woman was standing in front of the leader of the demonstrators, shaking her finger at him, quite obviously telling him that he should leave so that no one could suggest that threats were used to intimidate speakers.

During the intermission several of the members of the staff of the

Commission walked over to assure me that the demonstrators had been waiting until I spoke — because no one was to be allowed to mention the possibility of casual spread of disease. Fortunately, I had gotten into the wrong seat. When the meeting reconvened, the demonstrators filed out singing. I proceeded with my testimony. I then stated that I wanted to talk about all the physicians who I personally knew who had been threatened. As I tried to go on and list them, I was interrupted by the angry black woman. She attacked me for "talking too much" and did everything she could to disrupt my testimony and keep me from getting further information onto the record of the U. S. Civil Rights Commission.

As I left the Commission that day, I gave an audio cassette of my talk on the epidemic to Clarence Pendleton's secretary. My talk outlined the devious techniques that had been used by the CMA hierarchy to circumvent the will of the doctors. I do not know whether Clarence Pendleton ever listened to that tape. Within three weeks he was dead...apparently of a heart attack.

❋❋❋

It was mid-1988 when I was invited to San Francisco to be on a two hour interview on KABL AM-FM with Dr. Lorraine Day and one other researcher in the field of HIV disease. This was my first opportunity to meet Lorraine. I couldn't help being impressed with her knowledge and forceful presentation. As Chief of the Department of Orthopedic Surgery at one of the busiest hospitals in the nation, she had learned to be quick and authoritative in her responses. Certainly she was businesslike as we bantered back and forth with the moderator about the horrifying prospects of the epidemic.

It wasn't until we left the studio and she and I walked up the street towards our cars that she ceased to be the Chief of Orthopedics and suddenly became very human. She told me that she was seriously considering giving up her position at the San Francisco General Hospital. In the months that followed, I would repeatedly hear her accused of being afraid of becoming infected and it was said that it was her personal fears of infection which motivated her desire to test patients. But you see, that was not really the case. She had no personal fear — although she never expressed publicly what she said to me that afternoon. Her remarks gave me insight into the true motives of this courageous woman. As we walked, she said quietly:

"I could never forgive myself if I gave this disease to my husband or to my children."

It was really her concern for those whom she loved which motivated her far more than any thought of her own personal safety.

I was later told that KABL AM-FM radio received more requests for copies of that taped interview than for any other program ever broadcast. The producer called me in the fall of 1989 and asked if I still had my copy of the recording of that radio program. It seemed that the studio's only copy had disappeared and they were no longer able to offer tapes to those who kept writing or calling.

※※※

It was mid-1988 when Channel 42, a Christian television station in Concord, called and asked if I would be willing to give them my opinion on a series of video programs. Doctor Robert Strecker had recorded three, 30-minute interviews with Maureen Salaman, President of the National Health Federation. In the interviews, Doctor Strecker had presented his belief that the HIV virus had been produced in laboratories under the auspices of the World Health Organization; supposedly the retrovirus had then been introduced into the smallpox vaccine sent to Africa and the hepatitis vaccine used extensively on the homosexual population of San Francisco. Because of some of the inflammatory material contained in the taped interviews there had been a great deal of opposition from gay and AIDS activists who threatened the studio with reprisal if they dared to air the programs. The studio management was willing to face their wrath but wanted to be certain that the interviews were accurate. Thus, I was asked to review the films.

By this time I was deeply involved in my political campaign and the last thing I wanted was additional responsibility. On the other hand, I felt that I should support Christian television so I reluctantly agreed. The studio sent copies of the three interviews plus a tape that Doctor Strecker had prepared which was to be commercially distributed across the country.

Within a few days, I received a call from Doctor Strecker's business agent. It seems that they were waiting for the release of the three taped interviews on Christian television to begin their national campaign to sell Doctor Strecker's videotape. The business agent conveyed to me the urgency with which they looked upon the release of the interviews by Channel 42—and, hopefully, on Christian stations all across the nation.

After I received a second call from Channel 42 asking when I would complete my analysis, I decided to spend the following weekend reviewing the tapes.

The crux of Doctor Strecker's argument was based upon his personal research. Apparently he had gone through World Health Organization publications as part of a research project. He had found a notation in a WHO publication in 1972 suggesting that it would be advantageous to produce a retrovirus that could destroy the immune system so that researchers would be able to utilize infected animals for cancer research. Since the immune system tends to fight off and destroy cancer cells, destruction of the immune system would facilitate growing cancer in animals and thus facilitate cancer research.

Based upon this article, there seemed to be a huge leap in logic to the fact that the retrovirus had actually been produced and was then, somehow, introduced into the smallpox vaccine in Africa and the hepatitis vaccine in America. After all, it was in Africa and in the homosexuals in America where the disease seemed to have made its first major inroads. The spread of the disease in these two groups could be readily explained by Doctor Strecker's hypothesis.

The interviews with Maureen Salaman were expertly filmed and Doctor Strecker's revelations would have created a major stir across this country just as circulation of that information throughout the rest of the world had created a furor in other countries. The only difficulty, as I saw it, was that the theory was entirely untenable. According to Robert Gallo, the father of retrovirology, testing of stored, frozen serum specimens from Africa had revealed the presence of the virus in the late 1950's. There was one documented case of the disease in the United States in the late 1960's.

Furthermore, the San Francisco Cohort Study showed that in 1978, before hepatitis vaccination began, there were already 4% of the homosexual population who carried the virus. The hepatitis vaccine had not been administered to the young men until **after** the blood specimens were drawn and stored. Therefore, as far as I was concerned, Doctor Strecker's theories were entirely untenable.

I called both Channel 42 and Dr. Strecker's business agent and told them that the decision would have to be left up to the management at Channel 42, but in my estimation, the best course of action would be to discard the video films. I am sure that Doctor Strecker, who I believe is a sincere individual, was extremely upset at my decision. But faced with an epidemic of this magnitude, it served little purpose to circulate rumors and conjecture. It is vitally important to stick to known facts.

※※※

A few months later, Paul Gann, Lorraine Day, several other participants and I were invited to Channel 42 to discuss the issues surrounding the epidemic. The station was warned ahead of time by gay and AIDS activists that they should not air that program. After the program was broadcast, the station received calls and threats for days. The manager was threatened and told that he would be reported to the FCC and his TV station license would be revoked. This pattern of harassment was consistently used against any television or radio station that dared to air programs which had not been cleared by the gay censors.

※※※

In June, the second LaRouche AIDS Initiative (Proposition 69) was presented to the voters. Once again, LaRouche's supporters called for quarantine of those who were infected and stressed the possibility of mosquito and casual transmission of the illness. Those allegations were medically unsound and, by making absurd statements, LaRouche and his supporters effectively discredited their position. The LaRouche Initiative of 1988 read basically the same as it had in 1986, stating that HIV disease was an infectious, contagious, communicable disease and those who were infected should be reported to local public health officers.

Once again, the CMA, the CNA, the CHA, the CDA, the ACLU, the CPUSA and every other left-wing group in California joined together to condemn the initiative. Once again, LaRouche spent very little money in the closing days of the campaign to educate the public. As anticipated, Proposition 69 went down to defeat and, once again, the citizens of the State of California voted that they did not want to try stopping the dying and the death.

※※※

June was also the month for the Congressional primary election. Until the last week before the vote, I had taken my victory in the congressional primary for granted; however, I suddenly realized that the majority of the voters in the 16th Congressional District had no idea who I was. Neither Lou Darrigo (my opponent) nor I had received **any** significant coverage in the media. Of the hundreds of press releases sent to the major newspapers, only two had been published. In the closing days of the campaign, I invested the meager funds available from public donations in order to place advertisements in newspapers across the 16th Congressional District. Much to my surprise, two days before the election, almost 1,000 political signs appeared on telephone poles and fence posts across the district declaring Lou Darrigo's candidacy.

On election day, when the votes were counted, I led by 195 votes out of the 45,000 votes cast. But there were still the absentee ballots to be counted. It took three weeks before all four counties completed their tallies. When the votes were finally in...I had won by 250 votes. In the weeks that followed, despite the fact that I have lived in Santa Cruz for 35 years, our local newspapers steadfastly refused to publish the fact that I had won the primary election.

That pattern of censorship was used effectively all across my congressional district until the closing days of the campaign in November. Then, suddenly, I received a great deal of publicity, but the publicity I received then was not the type that I desired.

---

1. "AIDS, Policy and the Law" (Buraff Publications, Inc.) Washington, D. C.; December 2, 1987; p. 4.
2. San Francisco Chronicle; Tuesday, December 15, 1987; p. A10.
3. AMA News; December 4, 1987.
4. People's Daily World; Thursday, December 10, 1987; p. 5A.

CHAPTER SEVEN

May, June, July, August 1988

There were several other important events that occurred in mid-year. First, the report of the Presidential AIDS Commission was to be publicly released. The Gay and AIDS Lobbies knew the content of that report and feared that the public would learn of the commission's conclusion. Why? The report suggested that extensive pretest counseling in the general population was unnecessary and all that was necessary was for doctors to provide a pamphlet to those in low risk groups rather than requiring the prolonged, tedious counseling which had been recommended by the AMA, the CMA and by AIDS activists.

Furthermore, the commission recommended testing of the heterosexual population and restrictions being placed on those who were intentionally spreading the disease. The AIDS and Gay Lobbies had decided that general testing of the population must be prevented at all cost. Why? Because widespread testing might show the rapid spread of HIV disease within our nation and the public would demand that public health measures be used to stop the epidemic.

How could the Gay and AIDS Lobbies prevent that information in the report from being released? By May of 1988, the AIDS Commission report had been completed and was ready for distribution. Two weeks before the scheduled release of the report, Admiral Watkins, the Chairman of the Commission, called an **independent** press conference **to discuss his personal views.** Admiral Watkins pointed out the danger of discrimination and the necessity of antidiscrimination laws. Although the Commission had been pressured into accepting a position supporting antidiscrimination legislation, that legislation **was not** the major thrust of the report. The commission wanted to treat HIV disease as a disease. They wanted to address the epidemic from a medical point of view; however, all that Admiral Watkins apparently talked about at his press conference was the importance of antidiscrimination laws because that was the only information the American public ever received concerning the Presidential AIDS Commission report.

As a result, the public and physicians across the nation were never allowed to realize that the AIDS Commission wanted to limit pretest counseling in low risk groups, begin testing the general population and begin trying to stop this epidemic before it destroyed the nation.

❋❋❋

It was during this time period, in mid-1988, that I tried to get accurate figures on the results of the San Francisco Cohort Study. I had read the testimony given before the Civil Rights Commission from the San Francisco Department of Public Health which stated that their analysis of the 6700 homosexuals studied showed that "in the group they had analyzed most carefully," only 50% of the homosexual population carried the virus. They quoted several other smaller studies in San Francisco where only 50% of homosexuals carried the virus. They stated that all studies confirmed a 50% incidence of the disease. They carefully avoided any mention of the overall figures which the Department of Public Health in San Francisco had documented which showed that by 1988, 76% of the 6700 homosexuals in the cohort were infected.

At that point, I did not have ready access to the documentation of the Cohort Study. I had read Randy Shilts' book where he had noted that by 1984, 64% of the homosexuals in the cohort were infected. To get the correct figures, I wrote directly to the Department of Public Health in San Francisco and asked for their data on the incidence of HIV infection in the Cohort Study. To my surprise, I received a reply stating that only 50% of homosexuals in the group "studied most carefully" were infected.

I began to question my memory and my very sanity. Certainly the San Francisco Department of Public Health would not intentionally deceive the Civil Rights Commission; they would not intentionally deceive a physician asking for information! To confirm the figures, I contacted Don Francis' office in San Mateo and was able to get references to the Cohort Study in public health journals. These articles confirmed that 75% of the 6700 homosexuals in the cohort were already infected by 1985. Yet that information had been intentionally misrepresented to the U. S. Civil Rights Commission and to me by those in the San Francisco Department of Public Health who did not want the public to realize the extent of infection in the homosexual population of San Francisco.

❋❋❋

It was in the latter part of June 1988 when the 2nd International Conference on HIV disease was held by Shepherd Smith in Washington under the auspices of ASAP. It was here that I had the privilege of meeting that small cadre of zealots involved in the battle, trying to stop the epidemic.

This was my first opportunity to meet Councilman Lisa from New York City. The councilman was a liberal Democrat who would probably not agree with most of those on our side of the battle on most social issues but he was sincerely concerned about his city — for he realized that it would soon be bankrupted and destroyed. As the Chairman of New York City's Health Commission, he had consistently battled Dr. Stephen Joseph and Dr. Axelrod in an effort to try to get them to recognize HIV as a communicable disease and start closing the houses of prostitution, the gay bathhouses and remove the barriers which effectively prevented doctors from doing testing and contact tracing.

Doctor Kolodny was there. He had authored the book, *Crisis* along with Doctors Masters and Johnson. His book had conclusively documented the spread of HIV disease into the heterosexual community. He was still smarting from the vicious attacks by the Centers for Disease Control, the Surgeon General and the media, all of whom had ignored his startling revelations and only reported on one or two minor points in his book in an effort to discredit his carefully documented research.

Penny Pullen, the courageous legislator from Illinois was there. She was the person who had battled to get the fundamental AIDS legislation through the Illinois State Legislature. In mid-1988 every effort was being made by the AIDS Lobby to put an end to mandatory premarital testing in Illinois. In the months that followed, massive political pressure was brought to bear and her premarital testing bill was repealed.

Lt. Col. Robert Redfield and Col. Burke of Walter Reed Hospital were both there — they were two of the most outstanding researchers in the field of AIDS.

Doctor Braathen from the University Medical School in Oslo, Norway was there. He was the scientist who had done scientific studies to demonstrate that the Langerhans cell (which lies in the subcutaneous tissue of the skin and the mucosal membranes of the rectum, vagina and nasopharynx) was the primary cell responsible for carrying the HIV retrovirus into the body and infecting the lymphocytes.

Shepherd Smith had done an outstanding job of gathering together this handful of people from across the nation who recognized the implications of the epidemic, an epidemic which would soon threaten the very survival of our society.

✳✳✳

The last event which occurred during mid-year was the attempt by Senator Doolittle to negotiate a deal with the CMA. The antidiscrimination legislation pushed by the CMA, the AIDS activists and the Gay Lobby had passed through the state legislature and was on the governor's desk. Senator Doolittle offered to convince the governor to sign the legislation if the CMA and the AIDS Lobby would withdraw their opposition to Proposition 102. Obviously, discrimination was not the issue.

The CMA and the AIDS Lobby steadfastly refused to withdraw their opposition to the Gann Initiative in return for antidiscrimination legislation. Discrimination, like confidentiality, was simply a smoke screen behind which the epidemic has been allowed to continue spreading across our nation, like the ripples on the surface of a glassy pond — with ever increasing circles of death and devastation.

✳✳✳

Up until three weeks before the November election, I had had almost no news coverage of my campaign. Suddenly there were calls from newspapers all across the state. There were calls from television stations and radio stations. They all wanted to know about **that letter** I had written where I was quoted as stating that AIDS was…"God's gift." You will recall that in November of 1987 I had written a letter to a long-time friend asking him to help get out information on the epidemic. The letter had been stolen either from my office, from the mail or from the recipient and held for eleven months. Of course I did not say that AIDS was God's gift — but that statement was misquoted in every newspaper in my congressional district (in an effort to discredit me) and in every major newspaper in the State of California in an effort to discredit Proposition 102.

I sent copies of the letter to anyone who requested it, since my private letter was now part of the public record. I asked each newspaper to simply quote what I really had said in its proper context, not to take my remarks totally out of context as the AIDS activist had done.

In those weeks before the election, not one newspaper published the full text of the letter. Rather, they kept reiterating that I had said that AIDS was…"God's gift." With the AIDS Lobby firmly in control of the media, there was no opportunity to refute the often repeated lie. (The full text of that letter is reproduced in Appendix V).

Paul Gann was questioned by reporters to find out if he knew me and if he also believed that AIDS was..."God's gift." Dr. Larry McNamee, President of California Physicians For A Logical AIDS Response was challenged by reporters because I was listed on their letterhead as a supporter. Congressman Dannemeyer was besieged by reporters who demanded to know if he knew me and if he supported my statement that AIDS was..."God's gift." My letter was gleefully misquoted in every major newspaper in the state over and over to demonstrate the radical, extremist position of those who supported Proposition 102.

The AIDS Lobby used that letter very effectively. Since every major newspaper in the State of California opposed Proposition 102, it was not surprising that they all repeated the lie.

After the election, I polled 100 newspapers in the state. I could find only three small newspapers which supported Proposition 102 and one newspaper which took a neutral position. The People's Daily World quoted the opponents of Proposition 102 as saying, "Every major newspaper will oppose Proposition 102."

All the major newspapers and almost every minor newspaper reiterated that: 1) Proposition 102 required mandatory testing; 2) Proposition 102 would allow employers to test their employees without consent; 3) Proposition 102 would cost the taxpayers hundreds of millions of dollars and it was far too expensive to use standard public health techniques to try to stop the epidemic; 4) Proposition 102 did away with confidentiality; 5) Proposition 102 would drive the disease underground and prevent doctors from stopping the epidemic.

None of these statements were true but, repeated over and over by the media, the lies came to be accepted as truth.

Our opponents kept stating that trying to stop the spread of the disease "would cripple the efforts of physicians, researchers and public health officials to halt the spread of AIDS...it would only make the epidemic worse."

How could trying to identify those who were infected and spreading the virus unknowingly make the epidemic worse? The thrust of their argument was that homosexuals would not be tested if they knew that they would be reported to public health authorities. But the vast majority of homosexuals in San Francisco and Los Angeles (where the majority of homosexuals live) were already infected and every homosexual in California should have considered himself potentially infectious.

In 1988, the major public health effort should have been to try to stop the second and third epidemics, the spread of the disease into IV drug users and the heterosexual population. Our opponents were determined that we would not be allowed to stop the last two epidemics and prevent further spread of disease into the youth of our nation. In 1988, the STD Clinics of America were filled to overflowing and the incidence of new cases of syphilis was steadily rising.

✳✳✳

Initial statewide voter polls showed that over 70% of voters supported the Gann Initiative. In the final weeks before the election, support was down to 53% with 35% opposing Proposition 102 and 12% undecided.

During the ten day period immediately before the November election, the radical left and the Gay Lobby launched a massive attack to defeat Proposition 102. The CMA came out strongly against Proposition 102 (which had been opposed by members of the House) and against Proposition 96 which had been supported by the House. It was obvious that it really didn't matter how the members of the House voted. The hierarchy had its own policies and those policies were intent on preventing any form of routine HIV antibody testing.

The People's Daily World published their voting recommendations. The CPUSA suggested that their supporters vote "YES" on all the state propositions which involved spending large sums of money, except those propositions funding the prison system. Why? Their goal was the bankruptcy of the state economy and a breakdown in the criminal justice system.

However, they specifically opposed Proposition 96 and 102 stating: "Proposition 96 and 102 are new right-wing punitive attacks on people with the AIDS virus. Both measures would inhibit efforts to combat AIDS..."

Shortly before the election, I received a letter from the Non-Partisan Candidate Evaluation Council, Inc. of Los Angeles, California. Basically, what they proposed was that their organization would send out a slate card to every Republican voter in my congressional district suggesting how they should vote. In my district the slate card would recommend George Bush for President, Dan Quayle for Vice-President, Pete Wilson for Senator and Stanley Monteith for Congress. Then they

308 AIDS: THE UNNECESSARY EPIDEMIC

would list the various state propositions. For only $1,000.00 they would do a mailing to every registered Republican voter in my congressional district, putting me on the slate with George Bush and other popular Republican leaders. I called the council to find their position on Proposition 102. They were opposing it.

Although the slate would have been a very economical means of getting my name to Republican voters and I might very well have picked up a good deal of support, I reluctantly refused to compromise my position. To associate my name with that of George Bush, Dan Quayle and Pete Wilson and then use my name to oppose Proposition 102 would be unprincipled. After several telephone calls to the council, I withdrew my name from the slate.

On October 27, the People's Daily World revealed that their reporter had obtained an interview with Dana Van Gorda, coordinator of the Northern California No on 102 Committee. Ms. Van Gorda told representatives of the People's Daily World:

"Opponents of (Proposition 102) have the endorsements of most major politicians and newspapers and **will appear on a slate card to be mailed to millions of Californians.**" She went on to say, "Voters would prefer to have the AIDS epidemic managed by health officials rather than politicians. Our strategy...is working."

In the Soviet Union, according to the People's Daily World of December 2, 1988, Communist authorities were carrying out mandatory testing of those in "risk groups" and screening the population. In America, the People's Daily World objected to routine testing because of the danger to "constitutional rights." In Russia, as of December 1988, there were less than 100 people known to be infected with the virus and only 3 or 4 deaths. In America, probably close to 2 million were already infected. By 1990, 50 million had been tested in Russia and 3/4 of the population had been tested in Cuba. In the Soviet Union and Cuba, they treated HIV infection as a disease, not as a civil rights issue.

❋❋❋

On October 20, 1988 a number of religious leaders in northern California joined together in condemning Proposition 102. At a press conference at St. Mary's Cathedral in San Francisco, the leader of the Episcopalian diocese, Rev. James Emerson of the Presbyterian Church, Archbishop John Quinn of the Catholic Church, Rabbi Robert Kirschner of San Francisco's Temple Emanu-el and Bishop Lyle Miller of the

Evangelical Lutheran Church of America, all joined together in denouncing the Gann Initiative.[1]

***

The Los Angeles Times, in its editorial of October 20, 1988, proclaimed that Proposition 102 would "squander millions of dollars on mandated programs of limited value...From the face of it, the initiative offers a beguiling, simplistic solution to fight AIDS, doing to this disease what has been done to other communicable diseases by insisting on complete reporting and case by case contact tracing."

The article went on to say how foolish this was because there was no cure for AIDS and so it really was rather preposterous that we should try to identify those who had the disease. The initiative was also ridiculed because it mandated that "a doctor is required to report anybody he reasonably thinks might have the disease."

Of course, the editorial did not mention that current public health law in California required that a doctor must report anyone "suspected of being infected" with any reportable disease such as TBC, syphilis, gonorrhea or 55 other reportable diseases. The editorial went on to suggest that the cost of the initiative might be as much as 765 million dollars in the first year and that all the evidence suggested that treating HIV like other diseases would be of no benefit.

They added that Proposition 102 was opposed by the CMA, the CHA, the CNA, the State Health Officers Association, the regional representatives of the CDC (Don Francis), the California AIDS leadership which included top state, county and local public health representatives, in addition to the California Catholic Conference, the League of California Cities, the State Chamber of Commerce and the League of Women Voters of California. They all agreed that Proposition 102 should be defeated. (See Appendix VI for the full text of the article).

***

It was suggested in an article published in the San Jose Mercury on October 28, that 1 of 4 current blood donors would stop giving blood if Proposition 102 passed. The article said that if Proposition 102 became law, the current blood shortage would become far worse and precipitate a crisis that could cripple health care delivery.

The California State Chamber of Commerce came out against Proposition 102 as did the California State Farm Bureau.

✳✳✳

On October 28, Governor George Deukmejian announced his support for Proposition 102. In one of his more heroic acts, the governor publicly stated that he would vote for Proposition 102. Gay activists were furious. The Watsonville Register-Pajaronian newspaper reported, "George Deukmejian, outraging his own AIDS advisors, Friday announced his support for a November ballot measure that would relax confidentiality protection for AIDS virus carriers and require that their sexual and drug use contacts be traced by health officials."

The governor was attacked and vilified by every major newspaper in California. Then why did he support Proposition 102? A few weeks before the governor's announcement, Congressman William Dannemeyer visited his old friend, George Deukmejian. The two men had served together in the State Legislature years before and had maintained their friendship. When Dannemeyer asked the governor to support Proposition 102, the governor protested that his advisors, the CMA and public health groups all opposed the initiative. At that point, Dannemeyer pointed out that the Medical Society of New York State held a position 180 degrees opposed to that of the CMA and New York doctors were actively supporting reporting and contact tracing to control the epidemic.

The Congressman asked why it was that New York doctors supported his initiative while California doctors opposed it. Furthermore, there were several thousand doctors in California supporting Larry McNamee's California Physicians for a Logical AIDS Response in open defiance of the CMA. I can only assume that this visit from Bill Dannemeyer, along with other information relayed to the governor earlier, convinced him to support Proposition 102.

Senator Pete Wilson came out firmly against Proposition 102, saying that it could cost 750 million dollars or more a year to use contact tracing and public health measures. Senator Wilson's advisor on the AIDS issue was an avowed homosexual activist, Bruce Decker, who also headed the Stop Proposition 102 Committee. When Paul Gann tried to dissuade Senator Wilson, the Senator was adamant. He was firmly convinced that it was far too expensive to try to stop the epidemic. He felt that it was our obligation to take care of the dead and dying but the senator insisted that it would be far too expensive to try to prevent further spread of the disease.

✳✳✳

On the same day that Governor Deukmejian announced his support for Proposition 102, I was scheduled to go to Monterey to a Catholic Church and discuss the AIDS epidemic. The AIDS is...."God's gift" letter had been widely circulated in the region and I had been repeatedly attacked in local newspapers. Monsignor McLaughlin, a Catholic priest from Monterey had invited me to speak before the publication of the stolen letter and had sent out notices to his parishioners. He was not about to withdraw his invitation, although he may well have felt somewhat uncertain as to the response we would receive.

As the Monsignor and I crossed the street to the meeting hall, we could hear the chants of the demonstrators. The Bishop from the Monterey diocese had sent the editor of the diocese newspaper (The Observer) to the meeting to hear what was said and make sure that I was not an embarrassment to local church authorities. When we arrived, the Bishop's representative was outside the meeting hall picketing with the demonstrators. There were perhaps 25 angry gays, lesbians and activists with their signs and posters. Television cameras from two local stations were busy photographing the demonstrators for the 11:00 News. The cameras took pictures of the priest admonishing the demonstrators when they came into the small auditorium and tried to disrupt the meeting. The cameramen were only interested in recording the priest shouting, "Sit down and be quiet or get out!" They didn't bother to record one word I said that evening.

There were perhaps half a dozen women from the local diocese and 25 angry demonstrators in the audience. There was one young man, obviously horribly debilitated, walking with a cane, in the terminal stages of AIDS. He sat in the front row, his prominent, sad eyes fixed on me with an intense, angry stare. He carried a sign proclaiming: "MY GOD IS A COMPASSIONATE GOD." At the beginning, he tried several times to disrupt the meeting but was silenced by the Monsignor with the admonition that he would either have to behave or leave. During the entire talk, he fixed me with his sad, intense stare. I responded by looking at him directly during the entire talk. The anger and hostility in his eyes gradually faded as he listened to my discussion of the tragedy of this unnecessary epidemic.

There was another Catholic priest in the audience, a man who worked with AIDS victims. He had been with over thirty-five AIDS patients when they died and he was obviously consumed with the tragedy. He was also consumed with anger and hostility towards me because I wanted to use testing and tracing to try to stop further spread of the disease.

The audience was well-behaved as I talked quietly and unemotionally about the fact that President Reagan and physicians had been prevented from doing what was necessary to stop the epidemic.

When it came time for questions, everyone in the audience wanted to speak. To avoid chaos, the demonstrators decided to allow the activist priest to be their spokesman. As the priest rose to his feet, it was clear from his tone of voice that he was hostile to everything I had said. He hated President Reagan because the President didn't want to address the epidemic. He disliked me because I wanted to use testing to stop the epidemic rather than education and behavioral modification.

"Do you think that patients should be tested before they go into surgery?" he demanded.

"Yes."

"Do you think that doctors should be tested?"

"Yes."

"Have you been tested?"

"Certainly."

"How often should surgeons be tested?"

"About every 6 months."

"Well, if you think patients should be tested every time they go into surgery then why shouldn't doctors be tested every time they go into surgery?" he demanded.

"That is ridiculous."

"No it isn't," the priest said, seizing on what he felt was a weakness in my argument. "A doctor could be infected in any case then he could cut his finger and bleed into the wound during the next case and infect the next patient. That's why if testing is really important then doctors should be tested before every operation."

I looked at the priest intently. He must have been a very kind and dedicated human being to have spent years caring for people who were dying of this horrible illness, yet he was using a totally illogical line of argument in an effort to discredit my pleas for a logical, medical approach to the epidemic. I could see the frustration and anger in his eyes.

"Why are you arguing with me in this way?" I asked quietly. "Why are you using this line of sophistry? Haven't you seen enough dying? Don't you really want to stop the unnecessary death? Don't you want to stop the unnecessary killing?"

I spoke without emotion, staring at him intensely.

The priest started to answer—then hesitated—then looked away and sat down. That ended the meeting. All of their hopes for a confrontation vanished.

✳✳✳

By mid-October 1988, three national public health organizations had recommended that states adopt programs for partner notification and contact tracing. The Association of State and Territorial Health Officers, the National Association of County Health Officials and the U. S. Conference of Local Public Health Officials...all urged state and local governments to aggressively educate citizens about how contact tracing works. Dr. Thomas Vernon, President of the Association of State and Territorial Public Health Officers, stated:

"Public health officials have, for years, successfully used partner notification programs to slow the spread of sexually transmitted diseases...The use of partner notification for HIV can help protect the public health while simultaneously protecting the rights of the individuals."

Yet on Monday, November 7, 1988 a news release appeared in newspapers all across the state. Surgeon General C. Everett Koop had come out against Proposition 102 and was quoted as saying, "There is no one in public health who supports this measure. (Proposition 102). It is contrary to every principle of public health I know."

✳✳✳

In the week immediately before the election, I made contact with the ABC radio station (KGO) in San Francisco to try to get Larimore onto their evening program. Since three national public health organizations had come out favoring contact tracing and contact tracing was the basic thrust of the Gann Initiative, it was vitally important that people understand Proposition 102 and what it covered.

Lee Rogers was the talk show host on the evening program. Despite several letters and personal telephone calls between Larimore and Mr. Rogers, no invitation was forthcoming. Obviously there were those at

KGO who firmly opposed Proposition 102 and would not allow the facts
about the initiative to be presented to the public.

✳✳✳

In Santa Cruz County, 120 doctors signed an advertisement supporting Proposition 102. The local newspaper carried a headline stating:
"Three doctors say NO to ad for the AIDS plan."
The newspaper quoted the names of those three doctors and their
statement as to why Proposition 102 was bad. There was almost no
mention in the article of what was said by the 120 doctors who supported
Proposition 102. The article went on to say, "Proposition 102 has been
opposed by the California Medical Association, the Red Cross, the Los
Angeles and Orange County Medical Societies, the California Nurses
Association, President Gerald Ford, Bank of America, AT&T" etc., etc.

✳✳✳

All across California none of the major newspapers, radio or television stations allowed information to be presented to the public as to the
true facts concerning Proposition 102 and why it would save money and
human lives. The gay censorship was frighteningly effective.[2]

✳✳✳

When the statewide vote was finally counted on November 8,
Proposition 102 went down to defeat almost 2 to 1.
When the congressional race votes were counted across the nation,
98.6% of all incumbent congressmen were re-elected. It became pat-
ently obvious that congressional elections were simply a facade —
carefully staged to allow the American public to continue to believe that
somehow they could influence elections. Tragically, they could not.
With the bias of the media and censorship of the news, the public
could not get the truth. With congressional franking, the gerrymander-
ing of political districts, with the expenditure of massive sums of money
by special interest groups and with powerful forces working behind the
scenes intent upon bringing ever more governmental control over the
lives of our citizens, there was no way in 1988 that the American public
could regain control of the federal government.
Only a spiritual revival and an awakening of the desire for freedom
on the part of every American could change the political balance in our
nation's capital. However, few of our citizens realized in 1988 that their

freedom was endangered or that powerful political forces at the state and national level were perpetuating the epidemic.

1. San Francisco Chronicle; October 20, 1988, p. 8.
2. Santa Cruz Sentinel; Tuesday, November 1, 1988.

CHAPTER EIGHT

In mid-November, I returned to my medical practice. In some ways it was good to get back to medicine. It had cost me well over a hundred thousand dollars to run for political office in expenses and lost income. Few people understand the discouragement that occurs when so few people help to finance political candidates. I know of many professional people in our town who made $500,000 or more a year but they would not contribute as much as $100 towards my campaign. There were others to whom $5 was a sacrifice but they gave that and much more to help support a candidate in whom they believed.

By the time the election was over, only one Republican candidate replaced one Democratic incumbent in Congress. I came to realize that the entire electoral process was simply a facade, an exercise carried out every 2 years to convince the American public that our government ruled with the consent and support of the governed.

✳✳✳

December 1988

It was in December that a group of gay activists attacked the KRON television station in San Francisco. Two-hundred fifty gay activists held a noisy and violent demonstration in front of the television studio because the station dared to air a program that had not been approved by the gay censors who previewed the script. That was the program I alluded to in the introduction — "Midnight Caller."

This program depicted a bisexual man who was intentionally spreading the infection to women. The program was handled very sensitively to the point where the viewer had a feeling of sympathy for the bisexual man. But that was not the message that the gay censors wanted the American people to see.

Representatives from ACT UP (the AIDS Committee To Unleash Power) coordinated the demonstration. Terry Bostwick, spokesman for ACT UP, stated: "It's time to let people know the truth. That show is full of lies and misconceptions. We are not purposely spreading the virus." Tragically, however, there were people within the gay and bisexual community who were intentionally spreading the disease. There were also people within the heterosexual community who were intentionally spreading the disease. Since most of them have been tested anonymously, there is nothing that can be done to stop further spread. But the American public was not allowed to hear that message. It was not acceptable to the gay censors.[1]

✳✳✳

Dr. Lorraine Day presented a paper on HIV disease at the San Francisco meeting of the American Back Society. She reported that Dr. G. Johnson of the Department of Orthopedic Surgery at Stanford had carried out an experiment to determine whether or not there was danger to physicians and operating room personnel from aerosolization of the virus during surgery.

In the experiment, bone was drilled inside an air-tight compartment as HIV-infected blood was dripped onto the field. Air from the enclosed environment was then funnelled onto a petrie dish covered with human lymphocytes. The lymphocytes became infected with the retrovirus. According to a report in the "Family Research Newsletter," Dr. Johnson then went to the physician in charge of the AIDS Unit at San Francisco General Hospital and asked if he would write a letter to the Army Research Unit at Fort Detrick, Maryland asking them to carry out a similar test on chimpanzees. The doctor is reported to have said that he "would not write such a letter because if infection of a chimpanzee occurred, then where would we be?"

From this response, it was obvious that the San Francisco AIDS expert feared such a study might conclusively demonstrate spread of the disease by the respiratory route. If respiratory spread of the disease were confirmed, it would alarm the public.

✳✳✳

Bruce Decker was an avowed homosexual. He had been Chairman of the "No On 102" campaign committee and personal advisor to Senator Pete Wilson. During the month following the defeat of Proposition 102, he expressed concern that another AIDS initiative would be submitted at some future date. The Bay Area Reporter, a gay San Francisco newspaper, reported that,

"Decker stunned other opponents of the Dannemeyer initiative by saying that a legislative compromise should be reached with physician groups that would include some form of HIV reporting."

Decker was reported as saying: "We have to do whatever we can to avoid future initiatives. It is too draining on us...The other side is going to get better and better at writing these initiatives...and eventually will wear us down and beat us." Gay and AIDS activists throughout the state attacked Decker as a renegade, irresponsible homosexual because he was willing to compromise the gay position on HIV testing and contact tracing. Gay and AIDS activists remained firm in their opposition to the use of standard public health techniques.

***

January 1989

In January, the new laws on HIV testing went into effect in California. These laws included **permissive HIV** reporting and **permissive** contact tracing, followed by **the destruction of all records containing names of infected patients.** Also, **informed consent** replaced **written consent** for HIV testing. Yet, doctors were told in 1989 that because of the complexities of testing, they should use an extensive **informed consent** and should still have the patient sign a **written consent**...because it might be construed that physicians were doing something harmful to their patients by testing for HIV disease. This approach worked very effectively to continue to discourage physicians from testing.

There was another new law that went into effect in January of 1989. The CMA supported legislation which allowed doctors to inform their surgical nurses and other physicians when a patient was infected but the threat of a $10,000 fine and a year imprisonment for disclosure outside the medical profession remained as an effective barrier to testing.

***

In January 1989, it was time once again to write my resolutions to be presented to the House of Delegates in March of 1989. I felt it was important that the members of the House of Delegates realized how they had been betrayed by their leaders; therefore I presented the following resolution to the Constitution and Bylaws Committee of the CMA.

> WHEREAS in 1986 the members of the House of Delegates voted to seek legislation to change consent and confidentiality requirements for HIV testing; and
> WHEREAS the Council of the CMA refused to carry out the House mandate; and
>
> WHEREAS in 1987 the House of Delegates voted to support voluntary premarital and prenatal testing to change consent and confidentiality requirements, to allow reporting to public health officers and an antidiscrimination law; and

WHEREAS the CMA actively lobbied against legislation written to correspond to CMA policy and only backed an antidiscrimination law; and

WHEREAS in 1988, the House of Delegates voted to encourage legislation for prenatal counseling and testing and to support the Block Initiative; and

WHEREAS the Council failed to support prenatal testing and came out publicly (speaking for all the doctors of this state) against the Block Initiative; and

WHEREAS it makes little sense for the House of Delegates to vote on issues while the Council refuses to abide by the position taken by the House; now therefore, be it

RESOLVED: That the Council be instructed in the future to abide by and support positions taken by the House.

I presented a second resolution which would have encouraged routine testing and reporting but allowed anonymous testing sites to continue to operate. I do not approve of anonymous testing, but if conceding to anonymous test sites would have allowed physicians to stop the epidemic within the IV drug users and heterosexual population then I was willing to make that concession. To that end the following resolution was presented:

WHEREAS the Centers for Disease Control announced that by 1993 there will be 450,000 people dead and dying of AIDS, yet for every person dying of AIDS, there may be 10 to 20 (or 30) people who are infected with the virus, thus within five years between 5 and 10 million people may be infected with the virus and will ultimately die; and

WHEREAS the social, human and financial implications of this catastrophe are beyond the ability of our society to handle; and

WHEREAS to date California law fails to consider HIV disease as a communicable, infectious, sexually transmitted disease; and

WHEREAS declaring HIV as a communicable, infectious, sexually transmitted disease would not prevent utilization of anonymous testing sites by the homosexual component of our society but would allow the reporting of heterosexual cases to the public health officer for contact tracing as has been supported by the President's Commission; now, therefore be it

RESOLVED: That the CMA seek legislation that will declare HIV infection as a communicable infectious, sexually transmitted disease; and, be it further

RESOLVED: That the CMA support contact tracing for HIV (disease) in heterosexual AIDS cases which are picked up in routine screening in doctors' offices and hospitals; and be it further
RESOLVED: That homosexuals and drug users who will voluntarily cooperate with public health officers be encouraged to identify their sexual partners so in those instances where it is reasonable to do contact tracing that it be carried out; and be it further
RESOLVED: That the CMA demand that the legislature provide sufficient funds to carry out the public health techniques that are necessary to begin to try to limit this epidemic before it destroys the fabric of our society.

This resolution should have met all the objections of the AIDS and Gay Lobbies.

The CMA replied to this resolution by stating: "Resolution 704A-87 defined AIDS as a communicable disease which is not casually transmitted and which should be subject to the proven methods of communicable disease control appropriate for it...Support for contact tracing is outlined in the Policy on AIDS as established in Resolution 735A-87. The CMA affirms the need to protect confidentiality and prevent discrimination against seropositive individuals..."

Resolution 704A-87 was the resolution I presented in 1987 but the CMA had added the phrase "subject of the proven methods of communicable disease control appropriate for it." The result of their addition was to insure that no standard public health techniques would be used to stop this disease. Furthermore, Resolution 735A-87 was the Santa Cruz County Medical Society's resolution which I had also presented in 1987.

Although the CMA stated that they supported contact tracing, by adding "where appropriate" they had changed the entire meaning of the resolution, for only those within the CMA hierarchy knew where tracing "was appropriate." The CMA AIDS Committee had specifically opposed any efforts to do general contact tracing in California.

Looking back on what occurred in March of 1989, I once again marvel at the ingenuity, dedication and subtlety of the opposition. Under no circumstances would they allow my resolution to be adopted. The ends they went to to prevent effective steps from being taken to control the epidemic bordered on the unbelievable. Even more unbelievable was the fact that CMA leadership was, once again, able to deceive the House of Delegates. They would lie to the members of the Reference Committee; my resolution would be singled out for attack in the parting speech by the CMA President and, once again, the hierarchy would be successful — and the dying and the death would continue.

By early 1989, homosexual groups in San Francisco had begun training with weapons so they would be able to defend themselves from acts of discrimination and violence which homosexual leaders said were becoming increasingly commonplace. And so it was, in 1989, we saw the preliminary preparation for that period of conflict and crisis which I anticipate will occur in the latter part of the 1990's as various groups within our society resort to demonstrations and violence to obtain their "civil rights."

By early 1989, states throughout the nation were spending increasing amounts of money to control the epidemic. California was spending 76 million dollars a year, New York was spending 52 million dollars a year while Florida, Massachusetts and New Jersey were spending 17 million, 14 million and 13 million respectively. A great deal of money was being spent on caring for AIDS patients and funding gay organizations but very little money was being spent on efforts to try to stop the spread of the HIV epidemic.

---

1. San Francisco Chronicle; December 14, 1988, p. A4.

CHAPTER NINE

MARCH 1989

It was in March that the CMA once again held its annual meeting at the Disneyland Hotel in Anaheim. It was obvious that the hierarchy would go to any length to try to block my resolution, a resolution that simply said that "HIV disease should be considered as an infectious, communicable disease for legal purposes and should be reportable to public health officers."

My second resolution which pointed out how the CMA hierarchy had refused, year after year, to carry out the dictates of the House, put the CMA hierarchy on the defensive. That second resolution carried readily in the Constitution and Bylaw Committee with minor amendments and, when presented to the House, it was voted in by a resounding majority.

The meeting of Reference Committee G was held on Saturday and was a replay of the three previous years. The gay and AIDS activists were there along with Doctor Silverman. The Chairman of the Reference Committee was John L. Bourne, M. D. of Torrance. He seemed like a kindly, older, gray-haired gentleman and I hoped that his Reference Committee would be more objective in dealing with my resolution than the Reference Committee had been in Reno in 1988. I did not find out until after the convention (when I talked to Dr. Bourne) that experts were brought in to address the Reference Committee during their deliberations. The so-called experts told the members of the Reference Committee that the epidemic had peaked out and that the incidence of new AIDS cases was dropping off. The experts assured the committee members that there was no need to change current CMA policies because they had been successful in controlling the epidemic.

✳✳✳

On Sunday morning, the departing President of the CMA ordinarily gives his final address, covering his accomplishments during his tenure in office. I had little desire to hear Laurens White discuss his accomplishments so I went to Disneyland, feeling that I might well discover far more reality in Fantasyland than I would in the speeches being delivered at the convention.

Unfortunately, I missed Dr. White's parting remarks because he took this occasion to attack me personally and my AIDS resolution. He stated that he disagreed with everything that I had said in my resolution on HIV disease other than the fact that public health officers needed more money for contact tracing. Never before or since that Sunday morning, to my knowledge, has a speech by a departing CMA President been used to attack a resolution and a physician. But Dr. White obviously felt that the defeat of my resolution was vital. He concluded his attack stating:

"There is no one in the California Medical Association with whom I disagree more than Stan Monteith; however, he is a good doctor and I would trust him with my life. For in our diversity is our strength."

Those were flattering words but I was being damned with faint praise. For the issue was not whether or not I was a good doctor or whether Dr. White would trust me with his life. The issue was whether or not we were going to address HIV disease as an infectious, communicable, sexually transmitted disease in the State of California.

✳✳✳

Monday morning came and we read over the recommendations of Reference Committee G. In all the years that I have attended meetings of the CMA, I have never seen any resolution that received two pages of comments. Usually the commentary was simply a line or a paragraph recording the opinions of the Reference Committee. But with **my** resolution in 1989 those who wrote the Reference Committee report wanted to make sure that the members of the House would believe that disastrous events would occur if HIV disease were considered an infectious disease. What the Reference Committee did was to outline current public health laws in the State of California as they apply to **every one of the 58 reportable diseases in the state.** Most of these laws have never been implemented by a public health officer and have not been used with AIDS, the terminal stage of HIV disease. In part, this is what their report said:

"Legislating HIV disease as a communicable disease would have far reaching, legal ramifications which are onerous and undesirable. In California, designating a disease as reportable triggers a wide array of reporting duties:

1. Every physician...or any other person knowing of, or in attendance on, a case or suspected case of such disease must notify the local public health officer immediately.

2. Any and every individual who lives with or visits any person afflicted with such a disease, no matter where located, must reveal

that fact to the local public health officer.

3. If there is no physician in attendance, any individual having knowledge of a case or suspected case must report the case to a local public health officer.

4. Anyone in charge of a public or private school, kindergarten, boarding school or day nursery must report all cases to the local public health officer.

5. The local health officer must report all cases or suspected cases of such a disease to the Department.

Designating a disease as a reportable, communicable disease also permits or requires the implementation of a variety of other measures.

1. The Department **may** (emphasis added) adopt or enforce regulations requiring isolation or quarantine of infected or exposed persons.

2. The local health officer **may** also require isolation or quarantine **when necessary.**

3. **Under certain circumstances,** the health officer **must** require isolation or quarantine.

4. Upon being notified of a case or suspected case of such a disease, the public health officer must take any measures that are necessary to prevent the spread of the disease or occurrence of additional cases.

5. Persons afflicted with a reportable disease **must** be excluded from certain occupations and services (schools and food handling).

B. The CMA supported public health policy for voluntary testing and contact tracing is proving effective in reducing HIV infection.

C. If resolution 709-89 were adopted, patients would be dissuaded from seeking testing and treatment.

Of course, what the Reference Committee had listed were the standard public health laws **for all diseases in the State of California.** These laws applied to AIDS, syphilis, gonorrhea, aseptic meningitis and every one of the 54 other diseases which are presently reportable. The members of the Reference Committee presenting this list knew that there was no reason to quarantine HIV-infected carriers any more than those with AIDS, syphilis or gonorrhea. Presenting this material to the House was clearly a deceptive effort to frighten the House into opposing my resolution.

During the debate, CMA leaders assured the House that their policies were working to reduce the spread of HIV infection. How did they know? Since there was no reporting of HIV disease in California, there was no way of knowing the prevalence of the disease or how far it had spread.

The discussions on Monday were very much as they had been in 1987 and 1988. The same speakers were at the microphone. My remarks are included in Appendix III. Doctor Kennedy of Santa Clara remarked:

"Doctor Monteith and I have debated this Proposition for so long and on so many occasions that I would like to suggest that we each number our arguments. Stan could get up and say number 23 and then I could stand up and say number 11 and we could both sit down."

His remarks were greeted with laughter but it was not a laughing matter. The epidemic was continuing to spread and people were dying unnecessarily in an epidemic which never had to happen.

Dr. Carl Treiling of Los Angeles tried to point out the inconsistency of the arguments that were being used and the fact that AIDS, the terminal stage of HIV disease, was reportable, yet no one ever suggested that reporting AIDS discouraged anyone from treatment or testing. But the members of the AIDS and Gay Lobbies and some others who were ill-informed were there to speak against the resolution.

Actually, I had more support in 1989 than ever before. When the vote was taken, it was very close and had I been a better parliamentarian, I would have been on my feet demanding a standing vote rather than simply a voice vote.

As the vote was being called one of the six members of the Executive Committee hurried from the podium and sat down next to me. I will not mention his name because I cannot verify what he said and I have no desire to incur a charge of libel. However, this member of the CMA hierarchy has been one of my most persistent opponents.

"Stan," he said, "we have got to get together and come up with a resolution for next year that we can both live with."

"You know this epidemic will destroy this country if we don't get it under control," I replied.

"I know. I will call you next week after the convention."

We shook hands but, once again, I had been deceived. I am still awaiting his call **despite the fact that he acknowledges that the epidemic "will destroy this country."**

***

It was April of 1989 when the results of scientific studies on prevention of Pneumocystis pneumonia were released to the public. The multi-center studies demonstrated conclusively that the use of AZT and Pentamidine would prevent Pneumocystis pneumonia in the vast majority (80%-90%) of those infected with the HIV virus. In April of 1989, HIV disease was definitely treatable. It was at this point that many of the gay leaders began recommending that homosexuals should be tested. However, those same leaders still objected to routine HIV testing of the heterosexual population. Strangely, it was permissible for homosexuals to be tested anonymously but the AIDS Lobby was still intent upon blocking efforts to test the general population.

***

There were two other important events that occurred in April. The first was my trip to Washington to a special program put on by Americans For A Sound AIDS Policy. The second was my visit to the CDC in Atlanta.

An organization affiliated with ASAP had received a small grant from the CDC to develop a program to encourage the churches of our nation to mobilize and prepare for the care of the overwhelming numbers of victims of the epidemic in the next few years. It was here I had a chance to meet James Johnson, a former homosexual who had accepted the Christian faith and had dedicated his life to organizing hospices in Southern California to care for AIDS victims.

Homosexual groups in Los Angeles had mobilized to destroy his ministry. Anyone who left the "homosexual brotherhood" had to be destroyed. James had received numerous death threats and his ministry "Beyond Rejection" was under constant pressure and attack from the AIDS and Gay Lobbies intent upon undermining his efforts to minister to the bodies and souls of those who were dying in the terminal stages of HIV disease.

This meeting was my first opportunity to personally meet Lt. Col. Redfield who also told me of the death threat that he had received because of his support for Proposition 102. It was the same story that I had heard all across our nation. Anyone who dared to speak out in support of a sound public health program could expect to be threatened and possibly destroyed.

✳✳✳

A few days later, I went to Atlanta to the CDC where I had appointments with several key individuals. It was here that I learned what few Americans understand. What I came to realize was that there are people in the CDC who know what needs to be done but they are either afraid or unable to speak out because the reins of power in Washington are in the hands of the AIDS activists and those who are beholden to the Gay Lobby. Anyone in governmental service who dares to speak out in support of a sound public health policy will be attacked and if they cannot be silenced they will be destroyed.

Furthermore, there are people working within the CDC who are dedicated to the policies of the far left and are determined to prevent the use of testing and contact tracing to stop the epidemic. I found that there are some people at the CDC who will intentionally lie to visitors in an effort to deceive them.

Before I went to Atlanta, a friend had written to the CDC under the Freedom of Information Act and requested information on horizontal transmission of HIV disease (i.e., transmission within families). In response to his request he received an unmarked package containing a large, IBM computer tape about the size of a 16 mm movie film reel. By running this through a computer we were able to come up with over 20,000 entries consisting of long series of numbers on several hundred pages of computer paper — a compilation of CDC information from 1987. Unfortunately, my computer consultant was unable to interpret the data. Therefore, one of the first things I did on arriving at the CDC was to ask for the codes. There was a tremendous amount of suspicion and curiosity on the part of everyone I contacted as to how I had gotten the coded information.

I readily told them that I had gotten the information under the Freedom of Information Act but needed the codes to decipher the figures. A number of barriers were put in my way to prevent me from obtaining the codes. It was suggested that I surely would want much more up-to-date information than that contained on a 1987 IBM tape. However, I persisted and eventually I did get the code. What was so fascinating was that someone from the CDC called my office in Santa Cruz, pretending to be calling at my request, asking for the identification numbers from the IBM tape.

It was obvious that certain people from the CDC were frightened that

I might have gotten significant information under the Freedom of Information Act. It appeared that there was some sort of underground organization within the CDC, intent upon protecting information from inquisitive outsiders.

My first interview was with a very pleasant gentleman who was involved in compiling statistics. He told me about the CDC "family of studies," about 40 **anonymous** testing programs being carried out across the nation sponsored by the U. S. Public Health Service. The purpose of the programs was to determine the prevalence of the disease by measuring the incidence of the disease nationwide in certain small groups.

There was to be no general testing of the population — only a few isolated anonymous studies so that there would be **no** possibility of identifying those who were infected. I have serious doubts as to the accuracy of the information presented because when I mentioned the fact that the CDC had reported that over 50% of the prostitutes tested in Newark, N.J. had HIV disease, this representative of the CDC adamantly denied that any such study existed.

Now when you are talking to the man who is in charge of compiling CDC statistics you would expect that he would know those statistics. Despite the fact that the CDC had reported their study in the MMWR in March of 1987, the CDC employee responsible for compiling statistics adamantly denied that any such report existed. Thus it was readily apparent from my first interview that there were those at the CDC who were intent upon deceiving me as to the prevalence of the disease.

My second interview was with a man who I will refer to as Dr. Mark. This physician was obviously one of the more prominent bureaucrats in the venereal disease division of the CDC. His replies to my questions gave me tremendous insight into why our nation is losing the battle against the epidemic.

One of the questions that had always intrigued me was, "Why didn't the CDC try to stop Gaetan Dugas from continuing to spread the disease after they identified him as a primary vector in April of 1982? Why did they let him continue spreading the disease in San Francisco for six months and then let him return to Canada to continue spreading the disease for another year and a half before he died?" I posed that very question to Dr. Mark.

Long ago, I learned that in any sort of debate the best way of avoiding answering a question is to ask a question. That is exactly what Dr. Mark did.

"What would you have done with Gaetan?" he inquired.

"He was a foreigner," I replied, "I would have deported him from America. He was intentionally spreading a contagious disease. There are laws in this country — especially in California — which makes it illegal for a person to intentionally spread an infectious disease. Why weren't those laws enforced?"

"Do you think that foreigners who are infected with the virus should be kept out of America?"

"Of course," I answered, since we were talking about Gaetan Dugas, a foreign national who had been intentionally spreading a lethal illness.

"How about a 70-year-old professor from the University of Leipzig who acquired the disease from a transfusion. Now he wants to come to an AIDS conference in America to present information that will help save American lives?"

I looked at Dr. Mark incredulously. On one hand, I was talking about Gaetan Dugas, a man who was known to have spread the disease directly or indirectly to at least 40 people and probably indirectly to hundreds or thousands of others and, as a foreigner, should have been deported from America. To counter my remarks, Dr. Mark brought up an entirely different subject, describing a 70-year-old, probably impotent man with AIDS who had gotten it from a transfusion and certainly would not be spreading the disease. It was obvious that Dr. Mark was playing word games to justify the fact that in 1982 and 1983 no effort had been made to stop the spread of the disease.

I went on to ask him why the CDC objected to mandatory premarital HIV testing. In reply to my query, Dr. Mark reiterated the official CDC-AIDS Lobby line...that it was far too costly to try to stop the spread of the disease by premarital HIV testing because there were a finite number of government health dollars and the government needed that money for other, more important, public health projects.

When I pointed out that premarital testing was ordinarily paid for by those who were applying for marriage licenses, Dr. Mark's response gave me a penetrating insight into the thought processes of those who are directing our battle against HIV disease.

"But if the young people have to spend their own money for premarital testing, they won't have those same health dollars to spend for other medical expenses such as Well Baby Clinics or for having proctoscopic examinations."

Here I was talking about marriage applicants spending their money to have a blood test to try to prevent one marital partner from infecting his/her partner and Dr. Mark was talking about people needing those same health care dollars for "Well Baby Clinics" and he was concerned that young couples would not have funds to pay for proctoscopic examinations. For the reader who does not know what proctoscopy is, it is the insertion of a small metal tube into a patient's rectum so that a physician can visualize the rectal mucosa. Of all the medical examinations that I can think of that would be **unnecessary** for most young couples, a proctoscopic examination would be at the top of the list. I could not help but wonder why Dr. Mark was so concerned about the availability of proctoscopic examinations. Most physicians might have mentioned the need for PAP smears, mammograms or blood tests. Dr. Mark, however, seemed to be deeply concerned that young couples would not have money for **proctoscopic examinations.**

When a high official in the CDC makes such a ridiculous statement to justify his opposition to mandatory premarital blood testing, it is little wonder that our nation faces destruction today.

It was the following day that I had an opportunity to visit with Dr. James Curran who heads the Venereal Disease Section of the CDC. In that position, he leads the CDC program to combat HIV disease. When I walked into his office I found it to be of moderate size. On the far wall there was a white blackboard (a white background on which you write with a black ink pen). At the bottom of the board there was a drawing of a large, lopsided heart containing the inscription, "I love my doctor daddy Curran," written in a childish scrawl. Here was the office of the single most important man in the CDC as far as the AIDS epidemic was concerned. Distinguished visitors from across the nation and around the world came to that office. Yet Jim Curran had left a lopsided heart on the bottom of his blackboard — obviously written by one of his children. That may not have impressed most politicians or AIDS researchers — but it did impress me. I knew that I was going to like Jim Curran.

Doctor Curran is small in size — probably not more than 5' 2 or 3" tall. He is athletic in build with sharp, handsome features. He speaks clearly although he is occasionally guarded in his answers. I felt he was trying to tell me as much as he could within the limitations that were placed on him by being in government service.

I started out asking him the same question that I had asked Dr. Mark — "Why did the CDC allow Gaetan Dugas to continue spreading HIV disease when the CDC had identified him as a primary vector of transmission?" What was Jim Curran's response?

"We have made a lot of mistakes."

That was an honest answer from an honest man. There was no attempt to cover up; there was no attempt to answer a question with a question; there was no attempt to mislead me. Who among us has not made serious mistakes, but how many of us are willing to admit to them? I am sure that the mistake of releasing Gaetan Dugas and allowing him to continue spreading HIV disease was not the fault of Jim Curran. I am sure it primarily reflected the position of Doctor James O. Mason and others in positions of authority at the CDC in 1982.

I then asked Jim Curran if he knew of any specific instances of discrimination which had resulted from patients with AIDS or HIV disease having their names reported to public health officers. Jim Curran stated that he knew of no such cases.

I then asked him why the CDC opposed routine testing. He said that he personally supported the use of testing to try to bring the disease under control. He went on to say that every time he testified before governmental committees in support of testing, he kept "getting beaten up by politicians." He repeated that statement several times during our interview. It was obvious that he had been repeatedly attacked by left-wing politicians for supporting HIV testing. At one point he said:

"I'm caught in the middle...between Congressman Waxman on one side and Bill Dannemeyer and Lorraine Day on the other."

Then he added: "A lot of what Lorraine Day says is exaggeration and she has misquoted us, but if there weren't a lot of truth to what she says, she would not have the following that she does."

He then mentioned the fact that the CDC has been accused of down-playing the risk of HIV infection to health care workers and he in no way denied that this was the case. One point he made very clearly:

"What are we going to do when the first patient gets infected from an HIV-infected surgeon? Because it is going to happen sooner or later. This disease is spread just like infectious hepatitis and we don't allow doctors with hepatitis who are contagious to practice surgery."

AIDS: The Unnecessary Epidemic

I shall never forget one of the last things that Curran said to me that morning. He asked a simple question:

"Why do you think that we are not trying to identify the people in New York City who carry the virus? Let me tell you why. There are so many people there who are infected, what can we possibly do with all of them? We don't have enough money to do blood testing on them, much less give them Pentamidine. And if we had to give them AZT? There just isn't enough money to treat all the people who are infected in New York City today."

He stressed that America was going to have to nationalize this epidemic. Our nation was going to have to make treatment for this disease free and there must be a massive infusion of government funds to begin caring for those who are infected. He felt there was no other way to deal with the disease. I personally agreed with him — but I also believe that money must be spent to try to stop the disease from spreading, since prevention is always far more economical than therapy.

As I was about to leave, Doctor Curran insisted that I must read the book by Ronald Bayer on the AIDS epidemic. Indeed, he took over five minutes to track down the title and publisher of that book, a book I have alluded to earlier which describes, in great detail, how gay activists have been able to control the course of this epidemic since its inception. (*Public Acts, Social Consequences* by Ronald Bayer).

I left the headquarters of the CDC with mixed emotions. It was obvious that there were those within the CDC who represented the interests of the Gay and AIDS Lobbies. There were other people there who were simply going along with the government program to keep their job. Then there were good people, like Jim Curran, who knew what needed to be done but were unable to effectively influence government policy.

※※※

It was in June of 1989 when I journeyed to Montreal to the 5th International Conference on AIDS, a trip which I described in Chapter One. One story which I did not tell bears repeating. It involved the conversation I had with Councilman Lisa. As the Chairman of the City Health Commission in New York, the councilman wanted to have a prominent brothel closed. He had gone to the public health department and requested the closure of the house. Public health officials refused, insisting that there was no reason for closing houses of ill-repute because brothels in New York City were used to disseminate information on safe sex and educate customers as to safe means of avoiding HIV infection. Councilman Lisa was not convinced. He knew that this was simply the rhetoric of the AIDS Lobby, intent upon blocking the implementation of logical steps to stop the spread of HIV disease. So the councilman went to the leader of the garbagemen's union and pointed out that garbage was being left on the street in front of the brothel, enclosed in green plastic bags. He asked union leaders if they felt it was safe for garbagemen to pick up the green bags since they contained infected refuse and condoms which would be covered with vaginal and seminal secretions. Did the union leaders really want their members collecting those green bags and take a chance on becoming infected?

The leaders of the union agreed and informed the brothel operator that the refuse from the brothel must be placed in red bags and collected by the special division of the Sanitation Department which dealt with contaminated materials. The brothel then started putting red bags onto the street on collection days but the Contaminated Material Division of the Sanitation Department refused to pick them up. Week by week, the pile of red and green bags grew higher in front of the brothel until eventually the proprietor closed the brothel and moved elsewhere.

What is so incredible about that story is that in New York City in 1989 public health authorities refused to close down a brothel where HIV disease was being spread. The Chairman of the Health Commission of the Council of the City of New York could not close down that brothel. It could only be closed down by garbagemen who refused to pick up infected refuse. That is certainly a sad commentary on the status of public health in America today.

***

It was in August of 1989 when exciting new studies on the use of AZT were released. These studies demonstrated conclusively that AZT could slow the progression of HIV disease to AIDS in the majority of cases. By August of 1989, it was definitely established that HIV disease was a treatable disease. At that point, every effort should have been made to identify those who were infected. But that was not to happen. America was not to be allowed to try to stop the spread of this disease; America was not to be allowed to stop the dying and the death. Subsequent to the release of scientific data confirming that HIV is a treatable disease, every imaginable type of barrier continued to be used to thwart doctors who wanted to try to stop the epidemic.

✳✳✳

In the fall of 1989, Paul Gann died following a hip fracture. Larimore Cummins gave up the battle and returned to full-time medical practice. His personal efforts to pass Proposition 102 had been costly and his income had been severely curtailed. Yet no one seemed to care or be concerned with the fact that no significant efforts were being made to control the epidemic. No one seemed concerned with the personal sacrifices of those of us who remained in the battle. In the fall of 1989 in California, there were only Congressman Dannemeyer, Dr. Larry McNamee, Dr. Lorraine Day and myself who were still engaged in the struggle.

✳✳✳

In the fall of 1989, Americans were increasingly optimistic over events in the Soviet Union. President Gorbachev was talking about Glasnost and Perestroika and imminent changes in the Eastern Bloc. In the August issue of Soviet Life, a magazine directed to Communist sympathizers in America, an article was published written by Georgi Shakhnazarov, President of the Soviet Association of Political Sciences. At the beginning of the article there were two cartoon pictures side by side. The first picture showed a large black statue standing on a plateau of land, pointing across a canyon to a plateau of land on the opposite side. Behind the statue stood a mass of little people carrying signs, obviously representing the World Socialist Movement. In the second cartoon the statue had fallen forward and its head was resting on the far plateau, its feet on the near plateau. The socialist masses with their signs were walking across the back of the statue to the opposite side. The message was clear. With the fall of the old order, the Socialist Movement would move towards its ultimate goal, "A New World Order" and the establishment of Socialist governments. The title of the article was "East-West — Maybe the Twain Can Meet." The theme presented was that one day soon Russian Socialism and the Socialism of America (Social Democracy) would merge. Strangely, no one in America has ever publicly commented on this article, but every revolutionary in America understood that the purpose of Perestroika was to facilitate Socialism in America.

It was in September of 1989 when the Convention of the Republican State Central Committee convened in Anaheim at the Hilton Hotel. Congressman Dannemeyer, Larry McNamee and I were there. The major issues at the convention were centered around the Health and Human Services Committee (of which I was now a member). On this occasion, the Republican hierarchy had appointed 90 people to membership on that committee — knowing full well that they would never be able to get a quorum of voting members. Thus the Republican hierarchy could maintain that the committee was not officially constituted and therefore the issues that were addressed before the committee could not be brought to the convention floor without a two-thirds vote.

Bill Dannemeyer presented a resolution to the HHS Committee stating that the Republican Party should decertify the Log Cabin (homosexual) Club. The Congressman did not object to homosexuals belonging to the Republican party. He did object to those who openly advocated the homosexual lifestyle (of fisting, rimming, golden showers, oral sex and sodomy) organizing a club within the Republican Party.[1] By accepting a homosexual club in the party, the Republicans were legitimizing the homosexual lifestyle. Members of the governing board of the State Republican Committee objected to his resolution stating that

"The subject material in Congressman Dannemeyer's resolution should **not** be presented to the general conference because the content is obscene."

Dannemeyer jumped to his feet when that statement was read and pointed out that the leaders of the Republican Party had confirmed his point of view. Certainly these activities **were** obscene and the Republican Party should not be certifying a club that openly advocated obscene practices.

Tragically, the leaders of the State Republican organization had come to fear the power of the homosexuals. George Deukmejian had taken a courageous stand in October of 1988 in support of Proposition 102. When the AIDS and Gay Lobbies had been able to convert a statewide support of 70% for Proposition 102 to a position of 70% opposed in just three weeks, the governor recognized the **apparent** awesome power of the Gay Lobby. Henceforth he would not oppose their efforts to dominate the Republican Party. Apparently Governor Deukmejian and Senator Pete Wilson both sent directives to the Chairman of the State

Republican Central Committee in September of 1989 requesting that the issues of AIDS and homosexuality **not** be discussed.

The vast majority of the delegates at that convention supported Bill Dannemeyer and wanted to discuss those issues and decertify the homosexual club. The Republican leadership used parliamentary techniques and delays until late in the afternoon and then, with a quorum call, they adjourned the meeting.

By September of 1989, the AIDS and Gay Lobbies were effectively in control of both the Democrat and Republican Parties in the State of California.

***

It was in October of 1989 when the Hudson Institute of Indianapolis, Indiana released its report on the epidemic. The Hudson Institute analyzed the same figures that the CDC had used to determine the incidence of HIV disease in America and concluded that in all probability there were close to two and a half million Americans already infected. Furthermore, they felt that if our nation continued the same programs that we had in the past, in the worst case scenario we could expect to have over fourteen million people infected by the year 2002. In their worst case scenario, it was anticipated that we could lose as many as 41% of the black youth of America as well as a significant portion of Hispanic youth. Their press release was circulated on the wire services but few of the major newspapers and television networks felt that the report was newsworthy.

***

By the fall of 1989, the medical society of the State of New York had appealed its lawsuit against Doctor Axelrod. The New York State Medical Society had initially sued Doctor Axelrod demanding that HIV disease be designated as a disease in their state. The suit had been rejected by a "liberal" judge. In the fall of 1989, their case was being appealed to a higher court. In New York State, medical leaders wanted to address the epidemic as a disease, unlike their counterparts in California.

***

It was in October of 1989 when Dr. Lorraine Day was on "60 Minutes" with Dr. Curran. It was here that Dr. Curran admitted that the incidence of infection of HCW's after a needle stick is 1 in 200 cases and that rate of infection is considered "low risk." On the other hand, the incidence of infection with unprotected rectal intercourse is 1 in 200 contacts and that type of activity is considered "high risk." As a result of Lorraine Day's appearance on national television, she was invited to testify before at least three state legislatures and to attend OSHA hearings to bring out the background of her assertions that there was an intentional downplaying of the danger of infection to health care workers.

✳✳✳

It was early in November 1989 that Lorraine and I were on KABL AM-FM in San Francisco. She and I were on one side of the table, the Director of the AIDS Hotline and the San Francisco public health officer in charge of research were on the other. This public health officer announced that he was responsible for monitoring the 6700 members of the Cohort Study. It was during our interview that I asked the incidence of infection among the 6700 homosexuals in the Cohort Study.

"About 1/5 of them have AIDS," he said, somewhat hesitantly.

"But how many of that 6700 are infected with the HIV virus?"

"Of the group we have studied most carefully, about 50% of them are infected."

"But of the entire group of 6700, how many of them are infected with the HIV virus?"

"Somewhere between 70% and 75%."

This doctor was responsible for monitoring the epidemic for the Department of Public Health in San Francisco. By the fall of 1989, the incidence of infection among the homosexuals in the cohort was over 76%, yet this public health officer was intentionally concealing the truth from the public, for there has been a continuing effort to cover up the true facts about the epidemic since its inception. Copies of that tape should be available from KABL in San Francisco for anyone who would like to hear what was actually said.

✳✳✳

During November, the Berlin Wall came down. Americans were overjoyed at the prospect of victory. Headlines across America proclaimed,

"The Cold War Is Over" and "Communism has Failed."

Strangely, no one questions why communist authorities had allowed the destruction of the Berlin Wall when there were 340,000 communist troops stationed in East Germany. Immediately, liberal congressmen and senators proclaimed a peace dividend and demanded that America cut back on military expenditures. Soviet officials came to Washington to testify before congressional committees discussing America's military expenditures. Amazingly, newspapers and television broadcasts across America failed to note that during 1989, the Soviet Union was launching a new Red October class submarine every six weeks, increasing tank and artillery production and updating their first-strike SS18 intercontinental ballistic missiles to carry 30 one-megaton missiles instead of 10.[2]

❄❄❄

It was later during the month of November when I finally hit upon the idea of trying to involve the Federal Bureau of Investigation. It seemed like such a natural undertaking. After all, the FBI was assigned the task of preserving law and order across our nation. Agents were involved in sting operations — trapping such men as John De Lorean, the congressmen involved in the ABSCAM incident and state legislators in California. Certainly if the FBI was that concerned about law and order and the proper running of the government, it ought to be concerned about an organized movement across America which had effectively blocked the use of testing and contact tracing and would eventually result in the deaths of countless millions of our citizens.

I called the FBI office in Santa Cruz. I left my number on several occasions but the agent assigned would never return my call. Finally, I did reach him in San Francisco and explained the situation. I brought up the material from the Hudson Institute report stating that if we continued our present suicidal course, we could be dealing with the loss of 14 million Americans shortly after the turn of the century. The agent promised to contact me upon his return to Santa Cruz. I am still awaiting his call.

You see, no one employed by the Federal Government would dare to take a stand against the AIDS and Gay Lobbies, not even those employed by the Federal Bureau of Investigation. For the reins of power are firmly held by those who are intent upon allowing this unnecessary epidemic to continue to spread across our nation.

It was in the early part of December 1989 when the AMA met in the Hawaiian Islands. Doctor Larry McNamee, his brother Brian and Dr. Billy Jones of Arkansas were there. By a clever parliamentary technique, they were able to introduce a resolution stating that: "The American Medical Association strongly recommends the reportability of HIV-seropositive patients to the Departments of Public Health of the 50 states for the purpose of contact tracing and partner notification."

Those leaders of the AMA who were intent upon blocking contact tracing were not prepared for this resolution. The resolution passed by an overwhelming vote of the House of Delegates of the AMA. In December of 1989 contact tracing became official AMA policy. There was nothing that the leaders of the AMA or the AIDS or Gay Lobbies could do about it. I am sure that you did not read about this in your local newspapers and I am equally sure that the AIDS Lobby will continue to work to prevent implementation of the new policy...just as they have done so effectively for years at the CMA.

❋❋❋

It was also in December when 4000 angry demonstrators paraded in front of St. Patrick's Cathedral in New York City to voice their opposition to Cardinal O'Connor's position opposing the gay lifestyle and distribution of condoms. While police tried to control the demonstrators outside, activists planted within the cathedral disrupted the service with their screams and chanting. Some of the demonstrators lay down in the aisles and handcuffed themselves to the pews. The Holy Eucharist was seized and thrown onto the floor. All across the nation, the media actively suppressed the news of the desecration of the Cathedral and the Eucharist.

❋❋❋

It was in January of 1990 when Doctor Jewett, Professor of Orthopedic Surgery at the University of California in San Francisco, testified before a meeting of OSHA. Dr. Jewett announced that investigators at UC had carefully monitored operating rooms and found that blood could be aerosolized by drilling, cutting and the use of the Bovie. They found evidence that aerosolized blood could be transmitted into the lungs of surgeons and operating room personnel.

Doctor Jewett's study independently verified the findings of the Stanford University group which suggested that health care workers were, indeed, in danger when operating on HIV-infected patients. Doctor Jewett stressed, however, that if doctors knew that a patient was infected, proper equipment could be used and physicians could protect themselves. Tragically, the CDC, the AMA, the CMA, the ACLU and other radical groups still objected to doctors routinely testing patients being admitted to hospitals. As a result, the dying and the death will continue.

***

In late January, I attended a meeting at the Washington Sheraton Hotel in Washington, D. C. on "Homosexual Healing." There were only 50 people in attendance. Half the participants were homosexuals and lesbians who had come out of the gay lifestyle and were working to help others who wanted to change their sexual orientation. The meeting room had to be checked repeatedly for bombs. It took 150 riot police to control the 1500 demonstrators who marched on the hotel. Those of us who attended were locked in the meeting room as bands of activists surged through the halls, yelling and screaming. Yet the confrontation received the conspiracy of silence from the media across America.

***

In January 1990, Dr. Stephen Joseph, public health director of New York City, was fired. After his public statement in Montreal in June of 1989 supporting contact tracing, political pressure was brought to bear and Dr. Joseph was discharged. His replacement, Dr. Meyer, a black public health officer from the middle west, also supported contact tracing. Every effort was then made to block Dr. Meyer's appointment.

March 1990
In Sacramento, the meeting of the Coalition for Traditional Values was attacked by gay activists. Thirty angry members of ACT UP stormed into the meeting room knocking down several bystanders including a pregnant woman who had to be taken to the hospital. The demonstrators seized the microphone and proceeded to disrupt the meeting until the police arrived. The organizer of that meeting, Reverend Lou Sheldon, was plagued with bomb threats for months after the incident.

May 1990

On May 8, 1990 Larry Kramer, one of the founders of ACT UP was quoted in the Wall Street Journal as saying:

"It hurts me to say (that) I think the time for violence has now arrived...I'd like to see an AIDS terrorist army like the IRGUN which led to the State of Israel."[3]

Larry Kramer was calling for rebellion in America.

June 1990

The 6th International Conference on AIDS was held in San Francisco from June 20 to 24. Every day, hordes of black-shirted young men and lesbians rioted in one or another area of the city. On Wednesday, June 20, the demonstrators gathered in front of the Moscone Convention Center. I watched as professional organizers inflamed the emotions of the young men and women. Using blow horns, leading chants, stripping off their shirts and jumping up and down on them, the level of tension mounted until, finally, the order was given to jump the barricades. As I stood close by filming the demonstrators, several black-shirted youths climbed the barricades and ran towards the police. One police officer fell, writhing at my feet, as several demonstrators ran over him.

The next day, hundreds of demonstrators were at the Federal Immigration building condemning our nation's immigration policy. Although infected foreigners had been allowed to come to the conference, U. S. Immigration policy prevented those infected from coming to live in America. Ninety demonstrators were arrested that day. The following day, hundreds of young men lay down in the middle of Market Street in the center of San Francisco to block traffic.

On Sunday, June 24, the final day of the conference, Dr. Louis Sullivan, the Secretary of Health and Human Services was the final scheduled speaker. As Dr. Sullivan was introduced, members of ACT UP marched to the front of the auditorium and unfurled a pink banner which read,

"He talks, we die."

Other protestors shouted, whistled and used air horns. The noise was so deafening that many of the 6000 people in the audience covered their ears. Dr. Sullivan finally approached the podium and gave his speech. Few in the audience could hear because of the intense noise generated by the 500 protestors.

During the conference, gay and AIDS activists once again dominated the meetings. No one was allowed to speak who supported the use of accepted health techniques to control this sexually transmitted epidemic. No one was allowed to speak from the podium who wanted to identify those who were infected and intentionally or unintentionally spreading the deadly illness.

New figures on the prevalence of the disease were released. Anonymous blood specimens had been taken from men in their mid-twenties who had gone to general practitioners across the nation. The tests revealed that almost 2% of sexually active young men carried the virus. They will continue spreading the disease because the testing was done anonymously. Thus there was no means of identifying them, educating them or trying to stop further spread of the disease.

In children 15 to 16 years of age in the Northeast and in Miami, 1.24% of children tested already carried the virus but the testing was done anonymously so nothing could be done to stop them from continuing to spread the disease.

Talking to those working in New York, it was felt that between 450,000 to 500,000 people were already infected in their city. It was only a matter of time before those infected progressed to AIDS.

It was on Friday, June 22 that I attended a talk on AIDS Activism sponsored by the conference organizers. Representatives from ACT UP were there and spoke openly of their program for continuing to control the epidemic. Reference was made to Larry Kramer's call for a terrorist army but members of ACT UP insisted he was speaking only for himself. It was said that Kramer had called for violence because,

"He felt that we have lost the war against AIDS."

Others spoke openly of "revolutionary acts."

A black activist from the National AIDS Network in Washington, D. C. personally disavowed violence but cautioned,

"We must deal with the reality of our history...As we look at the history of progressive movements, changes have not come about until people have done battle. We are in a revolution...Our cities are about to singe (burn). People are angry...It won't take much...Either AIDS, substance abuse, homelessness, overcrowding of prisons, unemployment...People will take to the streets..."

No one spoke against his remarks. Everyone at that meeting on "activism" had a feeling of inevitability as we approach the coming period of chaos and crisis. For indeed, there are those within the AIDS and gay movements who are dedicated, as was the IRGUN, to the destruction of existing society. Tragically, as the tempo of violence grows, many Americans will mobilize to lash back against homosexuals, never realizing that the majority of gay activists are frightened, immature young men who are plagued with a compulsive, addictive sexual disorder, and have been manipulated since the advent of this epidemic by the radical left which has its own agenda for our nation.

---

1. For the reader who is unfamiliar with the activities involved in the homosexual lifestyle:
   a) "Fisting" is the insertion of a man's fist and/or his forearm into another man's rectum.
   b) "Rimming" involves licking your partner's anus and often involves ingestion of feces.
   c) "Golden Showers" consists of one man lying naked while one or several other men urinate on him. Homosexual leaders insist that safe sex demands that the recipient keep his mouth closed during these "water sports."

2. In 1990, the Soviet Union continued its massive armament build-up, turning out over 3400 advanced heavy tanks and over 2000 artillery pieces. The updating of their first-strike nuclear potential continued with further deployment of their new, mass destruction SS18's, and the launching of nine more typhoon-class first-strike nuclear submarines. However, the Soviet plan for world conquest has always anticipated that America would fall from within without a struggle as a result of moral decay resulting from capitalism and affluence. What few Americans realize is that as long ago as 1968, a British television producer, Bryan Magee, spent a year researching homosexuality throughout the world. In his book, *The Gays Among Us* (page XI) he noted that many homosexuals felt "a radical rejection of society altogether — society (had) persecuted them, humiliated them, derided them: very well, then, they will try to destroy society...(their attitude) tends to ally itself with Marxist revolutionary theories...(and to embrace) Marxism because it provides them with a ready-made social revolutionary theory."

The Gay Liberation Movement in America was founded by Harry Hay, an avowed Marxist and revolutionary who founded the Mattachine Society to mobilize the homosexuals of our nation and the world. (Los Angeles Times Magazine, November 25, 1990) The advent of the AIDS epidemic gave the gay revolutionary movement their opportunity to mould the frightened, alienated homosexuals of our country into an angry militant movement that could be utilized for their goal, i.e., the destruction of the society that had rejected them. Many other revolutionary, radical groups have joined the gay leadership in their effort to disrupt our society. Tragically, if they are successful, today's society will be replaced by a socialist system that will be totally intolerant of the gay lifestyle. However, should this happen, all Americans will lose their freedom and the dream that was America shall become a nightmare.

3. Quoted from an article by Paul Cameron entitled, "Gay Leader Calls for AIDS Terrorist Army" — Family Research Institute, Box 2091, Washington, D.C. 20013

CHAPTER TEN

It is natural for man to indulge in the illusion of hope.
We are apt to shut our eyes against a painful truth...
For my part, whatever anguish of spirit it may cost, I
am willing to know the whole truth: to know the worst
and to provide for it.

— Patrick Henry's Speech to the Virginia Convention,
Richmond, March 23, 1775.

In war, to fight and conquer in all of your battles is not
supreme excellence. Supreme excellence consists of
breaking the enemy's resistance without fighting.

— Sun Tsu (written approximately 400 years BC).

Today our nation is at war. America is under attack from an enemy
that lurks within. Every day, the casualty list mounts. By the end of
1991, the CDC estimates there may be as many as 271,000 Americans
dead or dying in that terminal stage of HIV disease which we refer to as
AIDS. By the end of 1993, they estimate there may be 435,000
Americans dead or dying but for every person dead or dying, there may
be 10, 20 or 30 who are infected and will ultimately die. We do not know
how many people are infected in our land today and no effective effort
is being made to find out who carries the virus, who is spreading the
virus and no effective effort is being made to stop the spread of this
epidemic within our nation.

During the 1960's and 1970's, America was engaged in a different
war — at that time the war was in South Vietnam. Our nation, with all
its vast resources and military power, was unable to defeat a small nation
the size of the State of Mississippi. Do you really believe for one instant
that we lost the war in South Vietnam because we were incapable of
winning? No. We lost the war in Vietnam because we were never
allowed to win. Our congress and senate were under the control of those
who were dedicated to the concept of socialism — and ever increasing
governmental power and control over our lives. Our elected representatives did not have the will to win; they did not have the character or
integrity to win. They sent our young men to fight, bleed, suffer and die

in the rice paddies of Vietnam. But our soldiers were never allowed to win that war.

In the 1980's and 1990's, we are engaged in another war. This time we fight against an enemy which lies within our own borders. The enemy, however, is not the virus. The enemy is the same enemy which prevented us from winning in Vietnam two decades ago. At any time in the 1960's and 1970's we could have won the war in Vietnam if we had attacked North Vietnam and destroyed the enemy's stronghold. At any time during this last decade we could have slowed or stopped the epidemic had we used standard accepted public health measures. But there are those in Washington, D. C. and in high places in state governments who have no desire to win this war.

In the 1960's and 1970's, there were demonstrations across our land. In the 1980's and 1990's, there are demonstrations across our land.

In the 1960's and 1970's, the left-wing media consistently told us we could never win in Vietnam. In the 1980's and 1990's, our left-wing media tells us if we try to stop this epidemic we will drive it underground — yet the epidemic is already underground for we have no idea how far this epidemic has spread within our tragic land.

In the 1960's and 1970's, the liberals and socialists within the congress of the United States put every barrier in the way of our fighting men to keep them from winning the war in Vietnam. In the 1980's and 1990's, those same forces among our elected and nonelected representatives have erected barrier after barrier to keep us from winning this war within our own borders.

In the 1960's and 1970's, we spent billions of dollars fighting a war that we never intended to win, but the American public felt that with the tremendous expenditure of funds and the loss of ever more American lives, we must be doing something to try to be victorious. In the 1980's and 1990's, we are spending billions of dollars to take care of the tragic victims of HIV disease and to desensitize our youth to the subject of sex and to fund gay organizations, but we are spending very little to try to win the war or stop the spread of the epidemic.

In the 1970's, Richard Nixon was put in a defensive position because of his involvement in the Watergate scandal. There was talk of impeachment and the President was unable to effectively govern our nation or to pursue the Vietnam war.

In the 1980's, Ronald Reagan was put in a defensive position by the

Iran-Contragate scandal. There was talk of impeachment and the embattled President was unable to effectively pursue his efforts to try to stop the epidemic.

In the 1960's and the 1970's, we called those young men "cowards" who refused to go to fight in Vietnam. In the 1980's and 1990's, it is the American public who should be involved in the battle — to once again regain control of our legislative halls. What should we call those citizens who are too busy today to be involved in the battle for the very survival of America? In the 1980's and 1990's, the youth of our nation are not going overseas to die. They are dying here — in our own villages, towns and cities.

We lost the war in Vietnam in the 1960's and 1970's. We must not lose this war in the 1980's and the 1990's. If we do lose, then America's promise of freedom will be lost for all time.[1]

The Hudson Institute, Herman Kahn's "think tank" in Indianapolis, Indiana, gives the worst case scenario for America. Their estimate is that over 41% of the black and 25% of the Hispanic youth of America may die in this epidemic. What percentage of the whites? It is unimportant. The blacks, Hispanics and homosexuals are as much America's children as the whites.

Who then are the cowards in the 1990's? They are the citizens of this republic who are not involved daily in the battle to save our nation. Freedom is not maintained by going to the polls every 2 or 4 years to vote for the political candidate picked by someone else to represent your district. Freedom is only maintained by total commitment on the part of every citizen every day of the year.

Paul Gann often started his speeches by saying, "Freedom is never free — it had to be purchased with struggle, sacrifice and suffering by those who came before us. It cannot be maintained without our struggle and our sacrifice."

In this battle for the very survival of America, **you** must be involved not yearly, monthly or weekly. **You** must be involved daily — just as those boys we sent to Vietnam were involved daily.

What then can be done?

Everyone who reads this book must commit himself or herself to working full-time to change the political, moral and spiritual climate of our nation. How? You can work in your local precinct to educate your neighbors so that we can begin electing men of integrity and principle to the legislative halls of our states and the Federal Government. You must work to help instill an understanding of the fact that America is a Christian nation built upon Judeo-Christian concepts and that our freedoms come not from government but from God. (See appendix VII for a detailed assessment of what can be done).

Today, America is moving rapidly towards Socialism. The structure of government grows ever larger and will soon control our citizenry from the cradle to the grave. We move progressively towards a society which is controlled by the KGB (the kinder and gentler bureaucracy). The move to total government must be stopped. We must replace the liberal-socialistic politician who believes in a paternalistic and regulatory government with men of courage, integrity and character. But such men have no hope of being elected unless you become personally involved.

We must mobilize the citizens of our nation against the American Civil Liberties Union and other radical groups which are intent upon corrupting our courts. We must demand that our courts enforce laws against drugs, crime, pornography and prostitution. We must begin impeaching judges all across this nation who refuse to support moral laws. We must boycott any and all television and radio programs which encourage immorality and launch a campaign to boycott all those who advertise on immoral television and radio stations. We must boycott stores which sell pornographic material and support those businesses which embrace our Judeo-Christian heritage.

We must return to moral teaching in our classrooms and replace the modern concepts of sex education and desensitization of our youth with the teaching of religious and spiritual values.

We must each seek to re-evaluate our own religious concepts which are the basis for our morality for if the people of our nation are immoral then how can our nation be moral?

We must begin to address this epidemic as an epidemic rather than as a civil rights issue. We need routine HIV testing in doctors' offices, schools and hospitals and contact tracing. We need to remove the legal barriers to testing. We need to close down the houses of prostitution, get drug users into treatment and make drug dealing an offense with life imprisonment without possibility of parole.

Every American must be willing to stand against the attack, vilification and intimidation of those domestic enemies who have used the homosexuals as the shock troops for their own devious purposes, purposes which have allowed this epidemic to spread unnecessarily.

Is there a better way to destroy this great and noble nation than to allow a major epidemic to continue to spread across our land and lead our nation into that period of chaos and conflict that lies ahead? Today must be the day of **your** commitment. Is there a more noble or worthy cause than to fight for the preservation of a society based upon the concepts of individual liberty under God? Can we hope to survive as a nation when we have forgotten the basic foundations of our society? America's greatest libertarian, the man who wrote the Declaration of Independence, expressed those concepts far better than anyone else. As recorded earlier, the words of Thomas Jefferson have long since been forgotten by our citizens, but are still chiseled in the granite of the Jefferson Monument on the shores of the tidal basin in Washington, D.C.

"God who gave us life gave us liberty. Can the liberties of a nation be secure when we have removed a conviction that these liberties are the gift of God? Indeed, I tremble for my country when I reflect that God is just, that His justice cannot sleep forever."

It has also been said that,

"Some men die in foxholes and some go down in flames.

But most men die just bit by bit playing foolish little games".

The challenge is yours. I would remind you, again, of the words of James Russell Lowell, written over 150 years ago, when America faced a far different crisis — the crisis of slavery. In part, he said this:

"Once to every man and nation comes the moment to decide,
In the strife of truth with falsehood for the good or evil side.
Then it is the brave man chooses while the coward stands aside,
Til the multitudes make virtue of the faith they have denied.
Though the cause of evil prospers yet tis truth alone tis strong.
Though its portion be the scaffold and upon the throne be wrong.
Yet that scaffold sways the future and behind the dim unknown,
Standeth God within the shadows, keeping watch above His own."

---

1. The idea of comparing the war in Vietnam with the war against the epidemic is derived from a speech by Dr. David Pence.

Appendix I

(For the sake of readability this report has been typeset rather than photographically reproduced. — Publisher)

The Surgeon General's Report on
ACQUIRED IMMUNE DEFICIENCY SYNDROME

This is a report from the Surgeon General of the U. S. Public Health Service to the people of the United States on AIDS. Acquired Immune Deficiency Syndrome is an epidemic that has already killed thousands of people, mostly young, productive Americans. In addition to illness, disability, and death, AIDS has brought fear to the hearts of most Americans — fear of disease and fear of the unknown. Initial reporting of AIDS occurred in the United States, but AIDS occurred in the United States, but AIDS and the spread of the AIDS virus is an international problem. This report focuses on prevention that could be applied in all countries.

My report will inform you about AIDS, how it is transmitted, the relative risks of infection and how to prevent it. It will help you understand your fears. Fear can be useful when it helps people avoid behavior that puts them at risk for AIDS. On the other hand, unreasonable fear can be as crippling as the disease itself. If you are participating in activities that could expose you to the AIDS virus, this report could save your life.

In preparing this report, I consulted with the best medical and scientific experts this country can offer. I met with leaders of organizations concerned with health, education, and other aspects of our society to gain their views of the problems associated with AIDS The information in this report is current and timely.

This report was written personally by me to provide the necessary understanding of AIDS.

The vast majority of Americans are against illicit drugs. As a health officer I am opposed to the use of illicit drugs. As a practicing physician for more than forty years, I have seen the devastation that follows the use of illicit drugs — addiction, poor health, family disruption, emotional disturbances and death. I applaud the President's initiative to rid this nation of the curse of illicit drug use and addiction. The success of his initiative is critical to the health of the American people and will also help reduce the number of persons exposed to the AIDS virus.

Some Americans have difficulties in dealing with the subjects of sex, sexual practices, and alternate lifestyles. Many Americans are opposed to homosexuality, promiscuity of any kind, and prostitution. This report must deal with all of these issues, but does so with the intent that information and education can change individual behavior, since this is the primary way to stop the epidemic of AIDS. This report deals with the positive and negative consequences of activities and behaviors from a health and medical point of view.

Adolescents and pre-adolescents are those whose behavior we wish to especially influence because of their vulnerability when they are exploring their own sexuality (heterosexual and homosexual) and perhaps experimenting with drugs. Teenagers often consider themselves immortal, and these young people may be putting themselves at great risk.

Education about AIDS should start in early elementary school and at home so that children can grow up knowing the behavior to avoid to protect themselves from exposure to the AIDS virus. The threat of AIDS can provide an opportunity for parents to instill in their children their own moral and ethical standards.

Those of us who are parents, educators and community leaders, indeed all adults, cannot disregard this responsibility to educate our young. The need is critical and the price of neglect is high. The lives of our young people depend on our fulfilling our responsibility.

AIDS is an infectious disease. It is contagious, but it cannot be spread in the same manner as a common cold or measles or chicken pox. It is contagious in the same way that sexually transmitted diseases, such as syphilis and gonorrhea, are contagious. AIDS can also be spread through the sharing of intravenous drug needles and syringes used for injecting illicit drugs.

AIDS is *not* spread by common everyday contact but by sexual contact (penis-vagina, penis-rectum, mouth-rectum, mouth-vagina, mouth-penis). Yet there is great misunderstanding resulting in unfounded fear that AIDS can be spread by casual, non-sexual contact. The first cases of AIDS were reported in this country in 1981. We would know by now if AIDS were passed by casual, non-sexual contact.

Today those practicing high risk behavior who become infected with the AIDS virus are found mainly among homosexual and bisexual men and male and female intravenous drug users. Heterosexual transmission is expected to account for an increasing proportion of those who become infected with the AIDS virus in the future.

At the beginning of the AIDS epidemic many Americans had little sympathy for people with AIDS. The feeling was that somehow people from certain groups "deserved" their illness. Let us put those feelings behind us. We are fighting a disease, not people. Those who are already afflicted are sick people and need our care as do all sick patients. The country must face this epidemic as a unified society. We must prevent the spread of AIDS while at the same time preserving our humanity and intimacy.

AIDS is a life-threatening disease and a major public health issue. Its impact on our society is and will continue to be devastating. By the end of 1991, an estimated 270,000 cases of AIDS will have occurred with 179,000 deaths within the decade since the disease was first recognized. In the year 1991, an estimated 145,000 patients with AIDS will need health and supportive services at a total cost of between $8 and $16 billion. However, AIDS is preventable. It can be controlled by changes in personal behavior. It is the responsibility of every citizen to be informed about AIDS and to exercise the appropriate preventive measures. This report will tell you how.

The spread of AIDS can and must be stopped.

C. Everett Koop, M.D., Sc.D.,*Surgeon General*

AIDS Caused by Virus

The letters A-I-D-S stand for Acquired Immune Deficiency Syndrome. When a person is sick with AIDS, he/she is in the final stages of a series of health problems caused by a virus (germ) that can be passed from one person to another chiefly during sexual contact or through the sharing of intravenous drug needles and syringes used for "shooting" drugs. Scientists have named the AIDS virus "HIV or HTLV-III"[1] These abbreviations stand for information denoting a virus that attacks white blood cells (T-Lymphocytes) in the human blood. Throughout this publication, we will call the virus the "AIDS virus." The AIDS virus attacks a person's immune system and damages his/her ability to fight other disease. Without a functioning immune system to ward off other germs, he/she now becomes vulnerable to becoming infected by bacteria, protozoa, fungi, and other viruses and malignancies, which may cause life-threatening illness, such as pneumonia, meningitis, and cancer.

No Known Cure

There is presently no cure for AIDS. There is presently no vaccine to prevent AIDS.

Virus Invades Blood Stream

When the AIDS virus enters the blood stream, it begins to attack certain white blood cells (T-Lymphocytes). Substances called antibodies are produced by the body. These antibodies can be detected in the blood by a simple test, usually two weeks to three months after infection. Even before the antibody test is positive, the victim can pass the virus to others by methods that will be explained.

Once an individual is infected, there are several possibilities. Some people may remain well but even so they are able to infect others. Others may develop a disease that is less serious than AIDS referred to as AIDS Related Complex (ARC). In some people the protective immune system may be destroyed by the virus and then other germs (bacteria, protozoa, fungi and other viruses) and cancers that ordinarily would never get a foothold cause "opportunistic diseases" — using the *opportunity* of lowered resistance to infect and destroy. Some of the most common are *pneumocystis carinii* pneumonia and tuberculosis. Individuals infected with the AIDS virus may also develop certain types of cancers such as Kaposi's sarcoma. These infected people have classic AIDS.

Evidence shows that the AIDS virus may also attack the nervous system, causing damage to the brain.

Signs and Symptoms

No Signs

Some people remain apparently well after infection with the AIDS virus. They may have no physically apparent symptoms of illness. However, if proper precautions are not used with sexual contacts and/or intravenous drug use, these infected individuals can spread the virus to others. Anyone who thinks he or she is infected or involved in high risk behaviors should not donate his/her blood, organs, tissues, or sperm because they may now contain the AIDS virus.

ARC

AIDS Related Complex (ARC) is a condition caused by the AIDS virus in which the patient tests positive for AIDS infection and has a specific set of clinical symptoms. However, ARC patients' symptoms are often less severe than those with the disease we call classic AIDS. Signs and symptoms of ARC may include loss of appetite, weight loss, fever, night sweats, skin rashes, diarrhea, tiredness, lack of resistance to infection, or swollen lymph nodes. These are also signs and symptoms of many other diseases and a physician should be consulted.

AIDS

Only a qualified health professional can diagnose AIDS, which is the result of a natural progress of infection by the AIDS virus. AIDS destroys the body's immune (defense) system and allows otherwise controllable infections to invade the body and cause additional diseases. These opportunistic diseases would not otherwise gain a foothold in the body. These opportunistic diseases may eventually cause death.

Some symptoms and signs of AIDS and the "opportunistic infections" may include a persistent cough and fever associated with shortness of breath or difficult breathing and may be the symptoms of *Pneumocystis carinii* pneumonia. Multiple purplish blotches and bumps on the skin may be a sign of Kaposi's sarcoma. The AIDS virus in all infected people is essentially the same; the reactions of individuals may differ.

Long Term

The AIDS virus may also attack the nervous system and cause delayed damage to the brain. This damage may take years to develop and the symptoms may show up as memory loss, indifference, loss of coordination, partial paralysis, or mental disorder. These symptoms may occur alone, or with other symptoms mentioned earlier.

AIDS: the present situation

The number of people estimated to be infected with the AIDS virus in the United States is about 1.5 million. All of these individuals are assumed to be capable of spreading the virus sexually (heterosexually or homosexually) or by sharing needles and syringes or other implements for intravenous drug use. Of these, an estimated 100,000 to 200,000 will come down with AIDS Related Complex (ARC). It is difficult to predict the number who will develop ARC or AIDS because symptoms sometimes take as long as nine years to show up. With our present knowledge, scientists predict that 20 to 30 percent of those infected with the AIDS virus will develop an illness that fits an accepted definition of AIDS within five years. The number of persons known to have AIDS in the United States to date is over 25,000; of these, about half have died of the disease. Since there is no cure, the others are expected to also eventually die from their disease.

The majority of infected antibody positive individuals who carry the AIDS virus show no disease symptoms and may not come down with the disease for many years, if ever.

No Risk from Casual Contact

There is no known risk of non-sexual infection in most of the situations we encounter in our daily lives. We know that family members living with individuals who have the AIDS virus do not become infected except through sexual contact. There is no evidence of transmission (spread) of AIDS virus by everyday contact even though these family members shared food, towels, cups, razors, even toothbrushes, and kissed each other.

Health Workers

We know even more about health care workers exposed to AIDS patients. About 2,500 health workers who were caring for AIDS patients when they were sickest have been carefully studied and tested for infection with the AIDS virus. These doctors, nurses and other health care givers have been exposed to the AIDS patients' blood, stool and other body fluids. Approximately 750 of these health workers reported possible additional exposure by direct contact with a patient's body fluid through spills or being accidentally stuck with a needle. Upon testing these 750, only 3 who had accidentally stuck themselves with a needle had a positive antibody test for exposure to the AIDS virus. Because health workers had much more contact with patients and their body fluids than would be expected from common everyday contact, it is clear that the AIDS virus is not transmitted by casual contact.

Control of Certain Behaviors Can Stop Further Spread of AIDS

Knowing the facts about AIDS can prevent the spread of the disease. Education of those who risk infecting themselves or infecting other people is the only way we can stop the spread of AIDS. People must be responsible about their sexual behavior and must avoid the use of illicit intravenous drugs and needle sharing. We will describe the types of behavior that lead to infection by the AIDS virus and the personal measures that must be taken for effective protection. If we are to stop the AIDS epidemic, we all must understand the disease — its cause; its nature, and its prevention. *Precautions must be taken.* The AIDS virus infects persons who expose themselves to known risk behavior, such as certain types of homosexual and heterosexual activities or sharing intravenous drug equipment.

Risks

Although the initial discovery was in the homosexual community, AIDS is not a disease only of homosexuals. AIDS is found in heterosexual people as well. AIDS is not a black or white disease. AIDS is not just a male disease. AIDS is found in women; it is found in children. In the future AIDS will probably increase and spread among people who are not homosexual or intravenous drug abusers in the same manner as other sexually transmitted diseases like syphilis and gonorrhea.,

Sex Between Men

Men who have sexual relations with other men are especially at risk. About 70% of AIDS victims throughout the country are male homosexuals and bisexuals. This percentage probably will decline as heterosexual transmission increases. *Infection results from a sexual relationship with an infected person.*

Multiple Partners

The risk of infection increases according to the number of sexual partners one has, *male or female.* The more partners you have, the greater the risk of becoming infected with the AIDS virus.

How Exposed

Although the AIDS virus is found in several body fluids, a person acquires the virus during sexual contact with an infected person's blood or semen and possibly vaginal secretions. The virus then enters a person's blood stream through their rectum, vagina or penis.

Small (unseen by the naked eye) tears in the surface lining of the vagina or rectum may occur during insertion of the penis, fingers, or other objects, thus opening an avenue for entrance of the virus directly into the blood stream; therefore, the AIDS virus can be passed from penis to rectum and vagina and vice versa without a visible tear in the tissue or the presence of blood.

Prevention of Sexual Transmission — Know Your Partner

Couples who maintain mutually faithful monogamous relationships (only one continuing sexual partner) are protected from AIDS through sexual transmission. If you have been faithful for at least five years and your partner has been faithful too, neither of you is at risk. If you have not been faithful, then you and your partner are at risk. If your partner has not been faithful, then your partner is at risk which also puts you at risk. This is true for both heterosexual and homosexual couples. Unless it is possible to know with *absolute certainty* that neither you nor your sexual partner is carrying the virus of AIDS, you must use protective behavior. *Absolute certainty* means not only that you and your partner have maintained a mutually faithful monogamous sexual relationship, but it means that neither you nor your partner has used illegal intravenous drugs.

AIDS: you can protect yourself from infection

Some personal measures are adequate to safely protect yourself and others from infection by the AIDS virus and its complications. Among these are:

• If you have been involved in any of the high risk sexual activities described above or have injected illicit intravenous drugs into your body, you should have a blood test to see if you have been infected with the AIDS virus.

• If your test is positive or if you engage in high risk activities and choose not to have a test, you should tell your sexual partner. If you jointly decide to have sex, you must protect your partner by always using a rubber (condom) during (start to finish) sexual intercourse (vagina or rectum).

• If your partner has a positive blood test showing that he/she has been infected with the AIDS virus or you suspect that he/she has been exposed by previous heterosexual or homosexual behavior or use of intravenous drugs with shared needles and syringes, a rubber (condom) should always be used during (start to finish) sexual intercourse (vagina or rectum).

• If you or your partner is at high risk, avoid mouth contact with the penis, vagina, or rectum.

• Avoid all sexual activities which could cause cuts or tears in the linings of the rectum, vagina, or penis.

• Single teen-age girls have been warned that pregnancy and contracting sexually transmitted diseases can be the result of only one act of sexual intercourse. They have been taught to say NO to sex! They have been taught to say NO to drugs! By saying NO to sex and drugs, they can avoid AIDS which can *kill* them! The same is true for teenage boys who should also not have rectal intercourse with other males. It may result in AIDS.

• Do not have sex with prostitutes. Infected male and female prostitutes are frequently also intravenous drug abusers; therefore, they may infect clients by sexual intercourse and other intravenous drug abusers by sharing their intravenous drug equipment. Female prostitutes also can infect their unborn babies.

Intravenous Drug Users

Drug abusers who inject drugs into their veins are another population group at high risk and with high rates of infection by the AIDS virus. Users of intravenous drugs make up 25 percent of the cases of AIDS throughout the country. The AIDS virus is carried in contaminated blood left in the needle, syringe, or other drug related implements and the virus is injected into the new victim by reusing dirty syringes and needles. Even the smallest amount of infected blood left in a used needle or syringe can contain live AIDS virus to be passed on to the next user of those dirty implements.

No one should shoot up drugs because addiction, poor health, family disruption, emotional disturbances and death could follow. However, many drug users are addicted to drugs and for one reason or another have not changed their behavior. For these people, the only way not to get AIDS is *to use a clean, previously unused* needle, syringe or any other implement necessary for the injection of the drug solution.

Hemophilia

Some persons with hemophilia (a blood clotting disorder that makes them subject to bleeding) have been infected with the AIDS virus either through blood transfusion or the use of blood products that help their blood clot. Now that we know how to prepare safe blood products to aid clotting, this is unlikely to happen. This group represents a very small percentage of the cases of AIDS throughout the country.

Blood Transfusion

Currently all blood donors are initially screened and blood is *not* accepted from high risk individuals. Blood that has been collected for use is tested for the presence of antibody to the AIDS virus. However, some people may have had a blood transfusion prior to March 1985 before we knew how to screen blood for safe transfusion and may have become infected with the AIDS virus. Fortunately there are not now a large number of these cases. With routine testing of blood products, the blood supply for transfusion is now safer than it has ever been with regard to AIDS.

Persons who have engaged in homosexual activities or have shot street drugs within the last 10 years should *never* donate blood.

Mother Can Infect Newborn

If a woman is infected with the AIDS virus and becomes pregnant, she is more likely to develop ARC or classic AIDS, and she can pass the AIDS virus to her unborn child. Approximately one third of the babies born to AIDS-infected mothers will also be infected with the AIDS virus. Most of the infected babies will eventually develop the disease and die. Several of these babies have been born to wives of hemophiliac men infected with the AIDS virus by way of contaminated blood products. Some babies have also been born to women who became infected with the AIDS virus by bisexual partners who had the virus. Almost all babies with AIDS have been born to women who were intravenous drug users or the sexual partners of intravenous drug users who were infected with the AIDS virus. More such babies can be expected.

Think carefully if you plan on becoming pregnant. If there is any chance that you may be in any high risk group or that you have had sex with someone in a high risk group, such as homosexual and bisexual males, drug abusers and their sexual partners, see your doctor.

Summary

AIDS affects certain groups of the population. Homosexual and bisexual males who have had sexual contact with other homosexual or bisexual males as well as those who "shoot" street drugs are at greatest risk of exposure, infection and eventual death. Sexual partners of these high risk individuals are at risk, as well as any children born to women who carry the virus. Heterosexual persons are increasingly at risk.

AIDS: what is safe

Most Behavior is Safe

Everyday living does not present any risk of infection. You *cannot* get AIDS from casual social contact. Casual social contact should not be confused with casual *sexual* contact which is a major cause of the spread of the AIDS virus. Casual *social* contact such as shaking hands, hugging, social kissing, crying, coughing or sneezing, will not transmit the AIDS virus. Nor has AIDS been contracted from swimming in pools or bathing in hot tubs or from eating in restaurants (even if a restaurant worker has AIDS or carries the AIDS virus.) AIDS is not contracted from sharing bed linens, towels, cups, straws, dishes, or any other eating utensils. You cannot get AIDS from toilets, doorknobs, telephones, office machinery, or household furniture. You cannot get AIDS from body massages, masturbation or any non-sexual contact.

Donating Blood

Donating blood is *not* risky at all. *You cannot get AIDS by donating blood.*

Receiving Blood

In the U. S. every blood donor is screened to exclude high risk persons and every blood donation is now tested for the presence of antibodies to the AIDS virus. Blood that shows exposure to the AIDS virus by the presence of antibodies is not used either for transfusion or for the manufacture of blood products. Blood banks are as safe as current technology can make them. Because antibodies do not form immediately after exposure to the virus, a newly infected person may unknowingly donate blood after becoming infected but before his/her antibody test becomes positive. It is estimated that this might occur less than once in 100,000 donations.

There is no danger of AIDS virus infection from visiting a doctor, dentist, hospital, hairdresser or beautician. AIDS cannot be transmitted non-sexually from an infected person through a health or service provider to another person. Ordinary methods of disinfection for urine, stool and vomitus which are used for non-infected people are adequate for people who have AIDS or are carrying the AIDS virus. You may have wondered why your dentist wears gloves and perhaps a mask when treating you. This does not mean that he has AIDS or that he thinks you do. He is protecting you and himself from hepatitis, common colds or flu.

There is no danger in visiting a patient with AIDS or caring for him or her. Normal hygienic practices, like wiping of body fluid spills with a solution of water and household bleach (1 part household bleach to 10 parts water), will provide full protection.

Children in School

None of the identified cases of AIDS in the United States are known or are suspected to have been transmitted from one child to another in school, day care, or foster care settings. Transmission would necessitate exposure of open cuts to the blood or other body fluids of the infected child, a highly unlikely occurrence. Even then routine safety procedures for handling blood or other body fluids (which should be standard for all children in the school or day care setting) would be effective in preventing transmission from children with AIDS to other children in school.

Children with AIDS are highly susceptible to infections, such as chicken pox, from other children. Each child with AIDS should be examined by a doctor before attending school or before returning to school, day care or foster care settings after an illness. No blanket rules can be made for all school boards to cover all possible cases of children with AIDS and each case should be considered separately and individualized to the child and the setting, as would be done with any child with a special problem, such as cerebral palsy or asthma. A good team to make such decisions with the school board would be the child's parents, physician and a public health official.

Casual social contact between children and persons infected with the AIDS virus is not dangerous.

Insects

There are no known cases of AIDS transmission by insects, such as mosquitoes.

Pets

Dogs, cats and domestic animals are not a source of infection from AIDS virus.

Tears and Saliva

Although the AIDS virus has been found in tears and saliva, no instance of transmission from these body fluids has been reported.

AIDS comes from sexual contacts with infected persons and from the sharing of syringes and needles. There is no danger of infection with AIDS virus by casual social contact.

Testing of Military Personnel

You may wonder why the Department of Defense is currently testing its uniformed services personnel for presence of the AIDS virus antibody. The military feel this procedure is necessary because the uniformed services act as their own blood bank in a time of national emergency. They also need to protect new recruits (who unknowingly may be AIDS virus carriers) from receiving live virus vaccines. These vaccines could activate disease and be potentially life-threatening to the recruits.

AIDS: what is currently understood

Although AIDS is still a mysterious disease in many ways, our scientists have learned a great deal about it. In five years we know more about AIDS than many diseases that we have studied for even longer periods. While there is no vaccine or cure, the results from the health and behavioral research community can only add to our knowledge and increase our understanding of the disease and ways to prevent and treat it.

In spite of all that is known about transmission of the AIDS virus, scientists will learn more. One possibility is the potential discovery of factors that may better explain the mechanism of AIDS infection.

Why are the antibodies produced by the body to fight the AIDS virus not able to destroy that virus?

The antibodies detected in the blood of carriers of the AIDS virus are ineffective, at least when classic AIDS is actually triggered. They cannot check the damage caused by the virus, which is by then present in large numbers in the body. Researchers cannot explain this important observation. We still do not know why the AIDS virus is not destroyed by man's immune system.

Summary

AIDS no longer is the concern of any one segment of society; it is the concern of us all. No American's life is in danger if he/she or their sexual partners do not engage in high risk sexual behavior or use shared needles or syringes to inject illicit drugs into the body.

People who engage in high risk sexual behavior or who shoot drugs are risking infection with AIDS virus and are risking their lives and the lives of others, including their unborn children.

We cannot yet know the full impact of AIDS on our society. From a clinical point of view, there may be new manifestations of AIDS — for example, mental disturbances due to the infection of the brain by the AIDS virus in carriers of the virus. From a social point of view, it may bring to an end the free-wheeling sexual lifestyle which has been called the sexual revolution. Economically, the care of AIDS patients will put a tremendous strain on our already overburdened and costly health care delivery system.

The most certain way to avoid getting the AIDS virus and to control the AIDS epidemic in the United States is for individuals to avoid promiscuous sexual practices, to maintain mutually faithful monogamous sexual relationships and to avoid injecting illicit drugs.

Look to the Future

The Challenge of the Future

An enormous challenge to public health lies ahead of us and we would do well to take a look at the future. We must be prepared to manage those things we can predict, as well as those we cannot.

At the present time there is no vaccine to prevent AIDS. There is no cure. AIDS, which can be transmitted sexually and by sharing needles and syringes among illicit intravenous drug users, is bound to produce profound changes in our society, changes that will affect us all.

Information and Education
Only Weapons Against AIDS

It is estimated that in 1991 54,000 people will die from AIDS. At this moment, many of them are not infected with the AIDS virus. With proper information and education, as many as 12,000 to 14,000 people could be saved in 1991 from death by AIDS.

AIDS will Impact All

The changes in our society will be economic and political and will affect our social institutions, our educational practices, and our health care. Although AIDS may never touch you personally, the societal impact certainly will.

Be Educated — Be Prepared

Be prepared. Learn as much about AIDS as you can. Learn to separate scientific information from rumor and myth. The Public Health Service, your local public health officials and your family physician will be able to help you.

Concern About Spread of AIDS

While the concentration of AIDS cases is in the larger urban areas today, it has been found in every state and with the mobility of our society, it is likely that cases of AIDS will appear far and wide.

Special Educational Concerns

There are a number of people, primarily adolescents, that do not yet know they will be homosexual or become drug abusers and will not heed this message; there are others who are illiterate and cannot heed this message. They must be reached and taught the risk behaviors that expose them to infection with the AIDS virus.

High Risk Get Blood Test

The greatest public health problem lies in the large number of individuals with a history of high risk behavior who have been infected with and may be spreading the AIDS virus. Those with high risk behavior must be encouraged to protect others by adopting safe sexual practices and by the use of clean equipment for intravenous drug use. If a blood test for antibodies to the AIDS virus is necessary to get these individuals to use safe sexual practices, they should get a blood test. Call your local health department for information on where to get the test.

Anger and Guilt

Some people afflicted with AIDS will feel a sense of anger and others a sense of guilt. In spite of these understandable reactions, everyone must join the effort to control the epidemic, to provide for the care of those with AIDS, and to do all we can to inform and educate others about AIDS, and how to prevent it.

Confidentiality
Because of the stigma that has been associated with AIDS, many afflicted with the disease or who are infected with the AIDS virus are reluctant to be identified with AIDS. Because there is no vaccine to prevent AIDS and no cure, many feel there is nothing to be gained by revealing sexual contacts that might also be infected with the AIDS virus. When a community or a state requires reporting of those infected with the AIDS virus to public health authorities in order to trace sexual and intravenous drug contacts — as is the practice with other sexually transmitted diseases — those infected with the AIDS virus go underground out of the mainstream of health care and education. For this reason current public health practice is to protect the privacy of the individual infected with the AIDS virus and to maintain the strictest confidentiality concerning his/her health records.

State and Local AIDS Task Forces
Many state and local jurisdictions where AIDS has been seen in the greatest numbers have AIDS task forces with heavy representation from the field of public health joined by others who can speak broadly to issues of access to care, provision of care and the availability of community and psychiatric support services. Such a task force is needed in every community with the power to develop plans and policies, to speak, and to act for the good of the public health at every level.

State and local task forces should plan ahead and work collaboratively with other jurisdictions to reduce transmission of AIDS by far-reaching informational and educational programs. As AIDS impacts more strongly on society, they should be charged with making recommendations to provide for the needs of those afflicted with AIDS. They also will be in the best position to answer the concerns and direct the activities of those who are not infected with the AIDS virus.

The responsibility of State and local task forces should be far reaching and might include the following areas:
• Insure enforcement of public health regulation of such practices as ear piercing and tattooing to prevent transmission of the AIDS virus.
• Conduct AIDS eduction programs for police, firemen, correctional institution workers and emergency medical personnel for dealing with AIDS victims and the public.
• Insure that institutions catering to children or adults who soil themselves or their surroundings with urine, stool, and vomitus have adequate equipment for cleanup and disposal, and have policies to insure the practice of good hygiene.

School
Schools will have special problems in the future. In addition to the

guidelines already mentioned in this pamphlet, there are other things that should be considered such as sex education and education of the handicapped.

Sex Education

Education concerning AIDS must start at the lowest grade possible as part of any health and hygiene program. The appearance of AIDS could bring together diverse groups of parents and educators with opposing views on inclusion of sex education in the curricula. There is now no doubt that we need sex education in schools and that it must include information on heterosexual and homosexual relationships. The threat of AIDS should be sufficient to permit a sex education curriculum with a heavy emphasis on prevention of AIDS and other sexually transmitted diseases.

Handicapped and Special Education

Children with AIDS or ARC will be attending school along with others who carry the AIDS virus. Some children will develop brain disease which will produce changes in mental behavior. Because of the right to special education of the handicapped and the mentally retarded, school boards and higher authorities will have to provide guidelines for the management of such children on a case-by-case basis.

Labor and Management

Labor and management can do much to prepare for AIDS so that misinformation is kept to a minimum. Unions should issue preventive health messages because many employees will listen more carefully to a union message than they will to one from public health authorities.

AIDS Education at the Work Site

Offices, factories, and other work sites should have a plan in operation for education of the work force and accommodation of AIDS or ARC patients *before* the first such case appears at the work site. Employees with AIDS or ARC should be dealt with as are any workers with a chronic illness. In-house video programs provide an excellent source of education and can be individualized to the needs of a specific work group.

Strain on the Health Care Delivery System

The health care system in many places will be overburdened as it is now in urban areas with large numbers of AIDS patients. It is predicted that during 1991 there will be 145,000 patients requiring hospitalization at least once and 54,000 patients who will die of AIDS. Mental disease (dementia) will occur in some patients who have the AIDS virus before they have any other manifestation such as ARC or classic AIDS.

State and local task forces will have to plan for these patients by utilizing conventional and time honored systems but will also have to investigate alternate methods of treatment and alternate sites for care including homecare.

The strain on the health system can be lessened by family, social, and psychological support mechanisms in the community. Programs are needed to train chaplains, clergy, social workers, and volunteers to deal with AIDS. Such support is particularly critical to the minority communities.

Mental Health

Our society will also face an additional burden as we better understand the mental health implications of infection by the AIDS virus. Upon being informed of infection with the AIDS virus, a young, active, vigorous person faces anxiety and depression brought on by fears associated with social isolation, illness, and dying. Dealing wit these individual and family concerns will require the best efforts of mental health professionals.

Controversial Issues

A number of controversial AIDS issues have arisen and will continue to be debated largely because of lack of knowledge about AIDS, how it is spread, and how it can be prevented. Among these are the issues of compulsory blood testing, quarantine, and identification of AIDS carriers by some visible sign.

Compulsory Blood Testing

Compulsory blood testing of individuals is not necessary. The procedure could be unmanageable and cost prohibitive. It can be expected that many who *test* negatively might actually be positive due to *recent* exposure to the AIDS virus and give a false sense of security to the individual and his/her sexual partners concerning necessary protective behavior. The prevention behavior described in this report, if adopted, will protect the American public and contain the AIDS epidemic. Voluntary testing will be available to those who have been involved in high risk behavior.

Additional Information

Telephone Hotlines (Toll Free)

PHS AIDS Hotline 800 342-AIDS, 800 342-2437

National Sexually Transmitted Diseases Hotline, American Social Health Association, 800 227-8922

National Gay Task Force, AIDS Information Hotline 800 221-7044, (212) 807-6016 (NY State)

Information Sources

US Public Health Service Public Affairs Office, Hubert H. Humphrey Building, Room 725-H, 200 Independence Avenue, SW, Washington, D.C. 20201, Phone (202) 245-6867

Local Red Cross or American Red Cross, AIDS Education Office, 1730 D Street, NW, Washington, D.C. 20006, Phone (202) 737-8300

American Association of Physicians for Human Rights, P. O. Box 14366, San Francisco, CA 94114 Phone (415) 558-9353

AIDS Action Council, 729 Eighth Street, SE, Suite 200, Washington, D.C. 20003 Phone (202) 547-3101

Gay Men's Health Crisis, P. O. Box 274, 132 West 24th Street, New York, NY 10011 Phone (212) 807-6655

Hispanic AIDS Forum, c/o APRED, 853 Broadway, Suite 2007, New York, NY 10003 Phone (212) 870-1902 or 870-1864

Los Angeles AIDS Project, 7362 Santa Monica Boulevard, Los Angeles, CA 90046 Phone (213) 876-AIDS

Minority Task Force on AIDS, c/o New York City Council of Churches, 475 Riverside Drive, Room 456, New York, NY 10115 Phone (212) 749-1214

Mothers of AIDS Patients (MAP), c/o Barbara Peabody, 3403 E Street, San Diego, CA 92102 Phone (619) 234-3432

National AIDS Network, 729 Eighth Street, SE, Suite 300, Washington, D.C. 20003 Phone (202) 546-2424

National Association of People with AIDS, P. O. Box 65472, Washington, D.C. 20035 Phone (202) 483-7979

National Coalition of Gay Sexually Transmitted Disease Services, c/o Mark Behar, P. O. Box 239, Milwaukee, WI 53201 Phone (414) 277-7671

National Council of Churches AIDS Task Force, 475 Riverside Drive, Room 572, New York, NY 10115 Phone (212) 870-2421

San Francisco AIDS Foundation, 333 Valencia Street, 4th Floor, San Francisco, CA 94103 Phone (415) 863-2437

APPENDIX II

Publisher's note: This document has been typeset rather than photographically reproduced in the interest of readability.

U. S. Department of Health & Human Services
Public Health Service
Centers for Disease Control
P. O. Box 6003
Rockville, MD 20850
HHS Publication NO. (CDC) HHS-88-8404

Understanding AIDS

A Message From The Surgeon General

This brochure has been sent to you by the Government of the United States. In preparing it, we have consulted with the top health experts in the country.

I feel it is important that you have the best information now available for fighting the AIDS virus, a health problem that the President has called "Public Enemy Number One."

Stopping AIDS is up to you, your family and your loved ones.

Some of the issues involved in this brochure may not be things you are used to discussing openly. I can easily understand that. But now you must discuss them. We all must know about AIDS. Read this brochure and talk about it with those you love. Get involved. Many schools, churches, synagogues, and community groups offer AIDS education activities.

I encourage you to practice responsible behavior based on understanding and strong personal values. This is what you can do to stop AIDS.

C. Everett Koop, M. D., Sc. D.
Surgeon General

What AIDS Means To You

AIDS is one of the most serious health problems that has ever faced the American public. It is important that we all, regardless of who we are, understand this disease.

AIDS stands for *acquired immunodeficiency syndrome*. It is a disease caused by the Human Immunodeficiency Virus, HIV — the AIDS virus.

The AIDS virus may live in the human body for years before actual symptoms appear. It primarily affects you by making you unable to fight other diseases. These other diseases can kill you.

Many people feel that only certain "high risk groups" of people are infected by the AIDS virus. This is untrue. *Who you are has nothing to do with whether you are in danger of being infected with the AIDS virus. What matters is what you do.*

People are worried about getting AIDS. Some should be worried and need to take some serious precautions. But many are not in danger of contracting AIDS.

The purpose of this brochure is to tell you how you can, and just as important, how you can't become infected with the AIDS virus.

Your children need to know about AIDS. Discuss it with them as you would any health concern.

How Do You Get AIDS?

There are two main ways you can get AIDS. First, you can become infected by having sex — oral, anal or vaginal — with someone who is infected with the AIDS virus.

Second, you can be infected by sharing drug needles and syringes with an infected person.

Babies of women who have been infected with the AIDS virus may be born with the infection because it can be transmitted from the mother to the baby before or during birth.

In addition, some persons with hemophilia and others have been infected by receiving blood.

The Difference Between Giving And Receiving Blood

1. Giving blood. You are not now, nor have you ever been in danger of getting AIDS from giving blood at a blood bank. The needles that are used for blood donations are brand-new. Once they are used, they are destroyed. There is no way you can come into contact with the AIDS virus by donating blood.

2. Receiving blood. The risk of getting AIDS from a blood transfusion has been greatly reduced. In the interest of making the blood supply as safe as possible, donors are screened for risk factors and donated blood is tested for the AIDS antibody. Call your local blood bank if you have questions.

Can You Become Infected?

Yes, if you engage in risky behavior.

The male homosexual population was the first in this country to feel the effects of the disease. But in spite of what you may have heard, the number of heterosexual cases is growing.

People who have died of AIDS in the U. S. have been male and female, rich and poor, white, Black, Hispanic, Asian and American Indian.

How Do You Get AIDS From Sex?

The AIDS virus can be spread by sexual intercourse whether you are male or female, heterosexual, bisexual or homosexual.

This happens because a person infected with the AIDS virus may have the virus in semen or vaginal fluids. The virus can enter the body through the vagina, penis, rectum or mouth.

Anal intercourse, with or without a condom, is risky. The rectum is easily injured during anal intercourse.

Remember, AIDS is sexually transmitted, and the AIDS virus is not the only infection that is passed through intimate sexual contact.

Other sexually transmitted diseases, such as gonorrhea, syphilis, herpes and chlamydia, can also be contracted through oral, anal and vaginal intercourse. If you are infected with one of these diseases and engage in risky behavior you are at greater risk of getting AIDS.

What Behavior Puts You At Risk?

You are at risk of being infected with the AIDS virus if you have sex with someone who is infected, or if you share drug needles and syringes with someone who is infected.

Since you can't be sure who is infected, your chances of coming into contact with the virus increase with the number of sex partners you have. Any exchange of infected blood, semen or vaginal fluids can spread the virus and place you at great risk.

The following behaviors are risky when performed with an infected person. You can't tell by looking if a person is infected.

RISKY BEHAVIOR

Sharing drug needles and syringes.

Anal sex, with or without a condom.

Vaginal or oral sex with someone who shoots drugs or engages in anal sex.

Sex with someone you don't know well (a pickup or prostitute) or with someone you know has several sex partners.

Unprotected sex (without a condom) with an infected person.

SAFE BEHAVIOR

Not having sex.

Sex with one mutually faithful, uninfected partner.

Not shooting drugs.

You Won't Get AIDS From Insects — Or A Kiss

No matter what you may have heard, the AIDS virus is hard to get and is easily avoided.

You won't just "catch" AIDS like a cold or flu because the virus is a different type. The AIDS virus is transmitted through sexual intercourse, the sharing of drug needles, or to babies of infected mothers before or during birth.

You won't get the AIDS virus through everyday contact with the people around you in school, in the workplace, at parties, child care centers, or stores. You won't get it by swimming in a pool, even if someone in the pool is infected with the AIDS virus. Students attending school with someone infected with the AIDS virus are not in danger from casual contact.

You won't get AIDS from a mosquito bite.

The AIDS virus is not transmitted through a mosquito's salivary glands like other diseases such as malaria or yellow fever. You won't get it from bed bugs, lice, flies or other insects, either.

You won't get AIDS from saliva, sweat, tears, urine or a bowel movement.

You won't get AIDS from a kiss.

You won't get AIDS from clothes, a telephone, or from a toilet seat. It can't be passed by using a glass or eating utensils that someone else has used. You won't get the virus by being on a bus, train or crowded elevator with a person who is infected with the virus, or who has AIDS.

What About Dating?

Dating and getting to know other people is a normal part of life. Dating doesn't mean the same thing as having sex. Sexual intercourse as a part of dating can be risky. One of the risks is AIDS.

How can you tell if someone you're dating or would like to date has been exposed to the AIDS virus? The bad news is, you can't. But the good news is, as long as sexual activity and sharing drug needles are avoided, it doesn't matter.

You are going to have to be careful about the person you become sexually involved with, making your own decision based on your own best judgment. That can be difficult.

Has this person had any sexually transmitted diseases? How many people have they been to bed with? Have they experimented with drugs? All these are sensitive, but important, questions. But you have a personal responsibility to ask.

Think of it this way. If you know someone well enough to have sex, then you should be able to talk about AIDS. If someone is unwilling to talk, you shouldn't have sex.

Do Married People Get AIDS?

Married people who are uninfected, faithful and don't shoot drugs are not at risk. But if they engage in risky behavior, they can become infected with the AIDS virus and infect their partners. If you feel your spouse may be putting you at risk, talk to him or her. It's your life.

What Is All The Talk About Condoms?

Not so very long ago, condoms (rubbers or prophylactics) were things we didn't talk about very much.

Now, they're discussed on the evening news and on the front page of your newspaper, and displayed out in the open in your local drugstore, grocery, and convenience store.

For those who are sexually active and not limiting their sexual activity to one partner, condoms have been shown to help prevent the spread of sexually transmitted diseases. That is why the use of condoms is recommended to help reduce the spread of AIDS.

Condoms are the best preventive measure against AIDS besides not having sex and practicing safe behavior.

But condoms are far from being foolproof. You have to use them properly. And you have to use them every time you have sex, from start to finish. If you use a condom, you should remember these guidelines:

(1) Use condoms made of latex rubber. Latex serves as a barrier to the virus. "Lambskin" or "natural membrane" condoms are not as good because of the pores in the material. Look for the word "latex" on the package.

(2) A condom with a spermicide may provide additional protection. Spermicides have been shown in laboratory tests to kill the virus. Use the spermicide in the tip and outside the condom.

(3) Condom use is safer with a lubricant. Check the list of ingredients on the back of the lubricant package to make sure the lubricant is water-based. Do not use petroleum-based jelly, cold cream, baby oil or cooking shortening. These can weaken the condom and cause it to break.

What Does Someone With AIDS Look Like?

It is very important that everyone understands that a person can be infected with the AIDS virus without showing any symptoms at all.

It is possible to be infected for years, feel fine, look fine and have no way of knowing you are infected unless you have a test for the AIDS virus.

During this period, however, people infected with the AIDS virus can pass the virus to sexual partners, to people with whom drug needles are shared, and to children before or during birth. That is one of the most disturbing things about AIDS.

Once symptoms do appear, they are similar to the symptoms of some other diseases. As the disease progresses, they become more serious. That is because the AIDS virus keeps your body's natural defenses from operating correctly.

If you are concerned whether you might be infected, consider your own behavior and its effects on others. If you feel you need to be tested for the AIDS virus, talk to a doctor or an AIDS counselor for more information.

Is There A Cure For AIDS?

There is presently no cure for AIDS.

Medicines such as AZT have prolonged the lives of some people with AIDS. There is hope that additional treatments will be found.

There is also no vaccine to prevent uninfected people from getting the infection. Researchers believe it may take years for an effective, safe vaccine to be found.

The most effective way to prevent AIDS is avoiding exposure to the virus, which you can control by your own behavior.

Should You Get An AIDS Test?

You have probably heard about the "AIDS Test." The test doesn't actually tell you if you have AIDS. It shows if you have been infected with the virus. It looks for changes in blood that occur after you have been infected.

The Public Health Service recommends you be confidentially counseled and tested if you have had any sexually transmitted disease or shared needles; if you are a man who has had sex with another man; or if you have had sex with a prostitute, male or female. You should be tested if you have had sex with anyone who has done any of these things.

If you are a woman who has been engaging in risky behavior and you plan to have a baby or are not using birth control, you should be tested.

Your doctor may advise you to be counseled and tested if you are a hemophiliac, or have received a blood transfusion between 1978 and 1985.

If you test positive, and find you have been infected with the AIDS virus, you must take steps to protect your partner.

People who have always practiced safe behavior do not need to be tested.

There's been a great deal in the press about problems with the test. It is very reliable if it is done by a good laboratory and the results are checked by a physician or counselor.

If you have engaged in risky behavior, speak frankly to a doctor who understands the AIDS problem, or to an AIDS counselor.

For more information, call your local public health agency. They're listed in the government section of your phone book. Or, call your local AIDS hotline. If you can't find the number, call 1-800-342-AIDS.

The Problem Of Drugs And AIDS

Today, in some cities, the sharing of drug needles and syringes by those who shoot drugs is the fastest growing way that the virus is being spread.

No one should shoot drugs. It can result in addiction, poor health, family disruption, emotional disturbances and death. Many drug users are addicted and need to enter a drug treatment program as quickly as possible.

In the meantime, these people must avoid AIDS by not sharing any of the equipment used to prepare and inject illegal drugs.

Sharing drug needles, even once, is an extremely easy way to be infected with the AIDS virus. Blood from an infected person can be trapped in the needle or syringe, and then injected directly into the bloodstream of the next person who uses the needle.

Other kinds of drugs, including alcohol, can also cause problems. Under their influence, your judgment becomes impaired. You could be exposed to the AIDS virus while doing things you wouldn't otherwise do.

Teenagers are at an age when trying different things is especially inviting. They must understand how serious the drug problem is and how to avoid it.

Drugs are also one of the main ways in which prostitutes become infected. They may share needles themselves or have sex with people who do. They then can pass the AIDS virus to others.

For information about drug abuse treatment programs, contact your physician, local public health agency or community AIDS or drug assistance group.

AIDS And Babies

An infected woman can give the AIDS virus to her baby before it is born, or during birth. If a woman is infected, her child has about one chance in two of being born with the virus.

If you are considering having a baby, and think you might have been at risk of being infected with the AIDS virus, even if it was years ago, you should receive counseling and be tested before you get pregnant.

You must have a long talk with the person with whom you're planning to have a child. Even if you have known this person for a long time, there's no way to be sure he or she hasn't been infected in the past, possibly without realizing it. That person needs to think hard and decide if an AIDS test might be a good idea. So should you.

Talking With Kids About AIDS

Children hear about AIDS, just as we all do. But they don't understand it, so they become frightened. They are worried they or their friends might get sick and die.

Children need to be told they can't get AIDS from everyday contact in the classroom, cafeteria or bathrooms. They don't have to worry about getting

AIDS even if one of their schoolmates is infected.

Basic health eduction should be started as early as possible, in keeping with parental and community standards. Local schools have the responsibility to see that their students know the facts about AIDS. It is very important that middle school students — those entering their teens — learn to protect themselves from the AIDS virus.

Children must also be taught values and responsibility, as well as skills to help them resist peer pressure that might lead to risky behavior. These skills can be reinforced by religious and community groups. However, final responsibility rests with the parents. As a parent, you should read and discuss this brochure with your children.

Helping A Person With AIDS

If you are one of the growing number of people who know someone who is infected, you need to have a special understanding of the problem.

No one will require more support and more love than your friend with AIDS. Feel free to offer what you can, without fear of becoming infected.

Don't worry about getting AIDS from everyday contact with a person with AIDS. You need to take precautions such as wearing rubber gloves only when blood is present.

If you don't know anyone with AIDS, but you'd still like to offer a helping hand, become a volunteer. You can be sure your help will be appreciated by a person with AIDS.

This might mean dropping by the supermarket to pick up groceries, sitting with the person a while, or just being there to talk. You may even want to enroll in a support group for caregivers. These are available around the country. If you are interested, contact any local AIDS-related organization.

Above all, keep an upbeat attitude. It will help you and everyone face the disease more comfortably.

APPENDIX III

Remarks Delegate Stanley Monteith made to the CMA Convention in March of 1986:

I think we have an obligation to protect the individual. I think we have an obligation to protect those people who work with us. In October of last year... Weis, et al in JAMA, reported four cases of needlesticks that turned from negative to positive. It is not very often. But if it's your nurse and she gets stuck, wouldn't you like to be able to at least draw an HTLV (test)? That information should be kept confidential except to the person who got stuck. But I think we certainly shouldn't have politicized this disease to the point where we can't practice good public health. That is what has happened. The hysteria is on the other side. They are just frightened to death that anybody is going to get a blood test and find out there might or might not be a problem. Let's hope there isn't a problem, but if there is, I think that the person who gets stuck deserves to know it.

The other thing is, you are prevented by law, if you know that a patient has a positive HTLV (test), from telling your operating room staff who might very well take additional precautions. In fact, things are so ridiculous that you may receive a $10,000 fine and a year in jail if you tell your nurse that she ought to double-glove and be extra careful. That is insanity. Let's not be hysterical. Let's be logical and sensible, and let's do what is right from the public health point of view. (applause)

※※※

The following is my letter, which I sent to a number of newspapers in California in the fall of 1986 in support of Proposition 64:

The epidemic of AIDS sweeping across our nation today threatens to destroy the very fabric of our society. In San Francisco, the health department had the opportunity to stem the spread of the infection when only 25% of the homosexual population was infected. Tragically, because of bureaucratic inertia and lack of conviction, public health authorities refused to act until over 50% of the gay population was infected. Today, 75% of San Francisco's homosexual men will carry the HTLV virus through the rest of their lives. 20% - 40% of them will ultimately die needless deaths, because action was not taken early enough. (In 1986, I didn't realize the disease was almost 100% fatal).

Today, the disease is spreading into the heterosexual population in America as it has in Africa and in Europe:

No one questions that the HTLV-III infection is a contagious, venereal disease and spread by sexual contact. The tragedy is that many influential organizations in our society refuse to deal with the HTLV-III infection as they do other contagious, venereal diseases.

The current AIDS Initiative is backed by Lyndon LaRouche — a political radical who I personally detest, but because he advocates a rational approach to the spread of this disease does not mean that the approach is necessarily wrong. There is nothing in Proposition 64 that violates confidentiality within the framework of medical practice. There is nothing in Proposition 64 that requires isolation or quarantine of a venereal disease. This decision is to be left to the public health officers.

We cannot depend upon the politicians to solve our problems. Tragically, we cannot depend on the medical establishment which is taking an unrealistic attitude and has even opposed the institution of premarital blood testing to prevent heterosexual spread of this disease.

Will we wait until there are 1 million cases in California before we become concerned? Will we wait until there are 2 or 5 million people infected? I suggest that you read Proposition 64, as I have, and see what it says, not what people say it says. Then, vote your conscience. I would far rather rely upon the collective intelligence of the people of the State of California...than on leadership which has failed to accept its responsibility.

※※※

Remarks by S. Monteith to the CMA Convention in 1987:

Last year we voted in favor of voluntary — or to encourage voluntary — prenatal testing. Unfortunately, when a bill of that sort went to the legislature, it did not have the firm support of the CMA and so it is now bound up in committee. I think prenatal testing is vitally important for a number of reasons.

The most important one is the protection of that child. If indeed a child is born, there is only a 50% (now known to be 35%) chance that they are going to have AIDS, but mothers may go right ahead and breast feed. There are instances of transmission through breast milk. If we don't start testing, we are condemning a certain number of these children to die of secondary infection. The fact that we have not done this (advocated prenatal testing) to date, I think shows tremendous negligence on the part of organized medicine to protect the children who are born without the virus. We need to know who has the virus and to...limit the mother's access to breast feeding. I speak in favor of this resolution very strongly.

※※※

Remarks of Delegate Stanley Monteith made to the CMA Convention in

Reno, Nevada in March 1988:

Ladies and gentlemen, millions of Americans are going to die of this disease. The only question is not whether millions are going to die but how many millions. We have to start treating this as a communicable disease. We have to begin to break the chain of transmission. Every other major disease is reportable. We have no statistics. Masters & Johnson came up with some statistics based on 800 people, but we do not have nationwide statistics. I can only give you isolated "statistics." We are getting better statistics out of Africa than we are getting out of America. This is insanity. We have all sorts of statistics on AIDS, but nothing on the HIV epidemic.

First of all, we need statistics. Secondly, we need case monitoring and contact tracing to begin to break the chain of transmission. And thirdly, the people who have HIV infection ought to know, because there are many things that can be done to protect their own health. If you are a woman and you have it, you shouldn't get pregnant. We are doing the population of this country a grave disservice not to declare that HIV is an infectious disease.

Do you know why health officers in California can't take the prostitutes, who have HIV and are communicating it, off the streets? Do you know why? Because in California, as in...other states, HIV infection is not a contagious disease and not reportable. Ladies and gentlemen, this is the first politically protected disease in all history. Please join me in making the first major step towards bringing this disastrous epidemic under control. Declare this as an infectious, communicable — not necessarily contagious — but infectious, communicable disease which should be reported....

※※※

Additional remarks by S. Monteith to the CMA Convention in Reno, Nevada, March, 1988:

I saw a bumper sticker not too long ago. It asked if there was intelligent life on other planets, but when I hear these discussions, I sometimes wonder if there is intelligent life on earth. (Laughter)

Ladies and gentlemen, we are dealing with a disease where millions of Americans are going to die and we have made it as difficult as possible for doctors to do testing. There are three types of consent. There is a written consent, there is an informed consent and there is a consent we get when we do tests for any other disease except this disease which we are somehow told is different from other diseases and is terrible. And it is terrible when you put barriers in the way of doctors doing what doctors need to do...and that is simply to do routine testing of all patients who come into our hospitals; not mandatory (testing), but certainly on a routine basis.

Let doctors test when they want to. Don't make them give an informed consent, because if you read what AB87 says about "informed consent" it makes it incredibly difficult. When I have three or four people I am going to put in the hospital two or three days hence, and I have to do an informed consent on every one of those... one of the things you are supposed to tell in informed consent is that if they have the blood test and a third party finds out about it, it can impact on their insurability. Things of this sort.

Don't make it difficult for doctors. Let's treat this like any other disease. Let's start getting it under control. Because if we don't, the public is going to lose all confidence in organized medicine as justifiably they should.

Please, let's get around to just a regular straight consent (for HIV blood testing) like we would with any disease. Don't listen to those people who are intent upon blocking doctors from doing what doctors must do to begin to bring this epidemic under control.

Appendix IV

California Medical Association
44 Gough Street
San Francisco, California 94103

March 10, 1987

AIDS WHITE PAPER

The California Medical Association House of Delegates adopted a package of resolutions at its March 9 session which urges significant changes in present law governing confidentiality of persons who have tested positive for HIV.

John McNally, M.D., chairman of the reference committee which presented the recommended resolutions, made this statement to the House:

> (The) Reference Committee heard extensive testimony on the subject of AIDS covering many areas of physician concern and frustration. CMA policy on AIDS to date has been consistent with the policies of the National Institutes of Health, the Centers for Disease Control, the AMA, and California public health authorities. We believe it is important to maintain that consistency because medical knowledge in this field is changing rapidly and there is great need for a clear, consistent public education on AIDS. However, there are issues on which no policy exists; some may be unique to the California medical community. Such issues and problems were well described by many physicians who spoke to the resolutions before us.

> In the following resolutions recommended for adoption, it is our intent to give strong impetus to CMA to emphasize in its policies on AIDS that a sound, scientifically based medical approach to prevention, diagnosis and treatment is essential, even though such an approach may at times be socially unpopular or politically sensitive. It is our further intent to emphasize that CMA can have great impact on the AIDS epidemic by aggressively seeking adequate state and federal funding for education and research.

Testimony before the Reference Committee emphasized the necessity of counseling persons in high-risk groups. Such action could be the most important counseling of all, in the view of testifying physicians.

Resolution no. 704-87 adopted March 9 declares: "that CMA policy recognize that AIDS is a communicable disease which is not casually transmitted and should be subject to the proven methods of communicable disease control which are appropriate for it." The resolution also encourages counseling and voluntary HIV testing.

A single recommended action which combined provisions of a series of resolutions (nos. 702-87, 703-87, 727-87, and 729-87) won approval on a voice vote after a series of proposed amendments was defeated. The combined resolution, adopted by voice vote, contains the following provisions:

> 1. That the CMA seek to delete legal requirements for consent to HIV testing which are "more extensive than requirements generally imposed for informed consent to medical care."

> 2. That in those circumstances where HIV testing is desired, all physicians are urged "to counsel their patients appropriately before and after testing."

> 3. That CMA seek legislative changes to provide that the results of a positive HIV test may be made available on a confidential basis to physicians involved in caring for the patient and to the local health officer.

> 4. That physicians should have the option, after counseling a patient, to report with immunity to "an endangered third party" that the patient has tested HIV positive.

> 5. That CMA take whatever action is necessary to allow blood banks and health departments to share information for the purpose of locating and informing persons who have any transmissible blood-borne disease — including, of course, AIDS.

The above resolution places the Association squarely behind efforts to relax existing law on confidentiality as it relates to those infected with HIV. Under present law, physicians must have written consent to notify a patient's spouse or "significant other" that they may be in danger of contracting HIV infection through sexual contact with the already-infected patient. Under present law, failure to obtain such written consent could subject the notifying physician to fines of up to $10,000 and a year in jail for each unauthorized disclosure.

The effect of the above, if placed into law, would provide legal immunity for physicians who, after counseling the patient, notify an "endangered third party" (such as a sexual partner) that the physician's patient has tested positive. The presumption here is that the physician would urge the patient to notify sexual partners of the positive test result, and, if the patient refuses to do so, the physician would be provided legal protection if he or she chose to notify.

The resolution also urges that physicians be allowed to notify public health officers of AIDS virus carriers. Debate on this section of the resolution revolved around the question of such notification would cause persons in high-risk groups to avoid testing, out of fear that their names would become known, or placed in a central registry of some kind.

An additional resolution (amalgamating nos. 720-87 and 723-87) adopted by the House urged the development of specific educational programs and materials for individuals of various age groups from grade school to college and their parents concerning HIV infection and means of preventing its spread. The resolution declared that CMA will support and assist the California Department of Education in the "immediate development" of these materials.

Greater involvement and "adequate funding" for development and implementation of AIDS/HIV educational programs on both state and national levels will also be encouraged under provisions of the resolution. It declares CMA will "vigorously seek very substantially increased government and private funding" for research in viral illnesses, virology, and HIV infection, including production of a vaccine, and, further, treatment of patients with HIV infection.

Resolution no. 735-87 urged voluntary "premarital, prenatal and perinatal" HIV screening. It also urged that the Association support adequate funding "so that local public health officials may carry out contact tracing for HIV-infected individuals where appropriate, with attention to confidentiality and counseling."

Resolution no. 704-87, also adopted, declares: "That CMA policy recognize that AIDS is a communicable disease which is not casually transmitted and should be subject to the proven methods of communicable disease control which are appropriate for it." The resolution also encourages counseling and voluntary HIV testing.

All of the above actions of the House are to be transmitted to the American Medical Association House of Delegates June meeting for introduction as resolutions by the California delegation. The thought here is that California would assist in development of national health policy on AIDS-related issues.

(Prepared by the Division of Communications March 10, 1987)

Publisher's note: This document has been typeset rather than photographically reproduced in the interest of readability.

Appendix V

Stanley K. Monteith, M.D.
618 Frederick Street
Santa Cruz, California 95062

November 23, 1987

Charles Armour
c/o The John Birch Society
396 Concord Ave.
Belmont, Massachusetts 02178

Dear Chuck:

As you know, I have gotten deeply involved in the battle of AIDS. I think this will be the final battle. Either we win this or we lose altogether. The problem is that there is a specific plan to keep us from doing anything about the epidemic. Part of this is engineered by the homosexuals, but part of this is definitely engineered by the subversive element within our nation.

Most Americans do not understand that we are not in any way monitoring the epidemic. We are monitoring the number of AIDS cases but that simply reflects the end stages of the epidemic. We can tell from the number of AIDS cases that are present today that between 5 and 10 years ago 40,000 people contracted the disease. The tragedy is, we have no idea what is happening in the epidemic today or how many Americans have the virus or even, honestly, how they get the virus.

In California — for the last two years — I have presented resolutions to the House of Delegates of the California Medical Association. Although the members of the House of Delegates are usually extremely liberal in most things, on this issue they solidly backed me. Unfortunately, the small, well organized group within the hierarchy of the CMA has effectively blocked any action from being taken.

I am working very hard with a small group of physicians to try to get the doctors to counter this and work towards getting California to be the first State in the nation that starts doing routine, widespread testing.

What is really needed, however, is an organization, nationwide to begin getting the facts out to the people. It is important that this is done carefully and logically, and sticking with the scientific facts as they are known. We can question the scientific facts, but to date there is no danger from mosquito spread or shaking hands with a patient who has the virus, et cetera. On the other hand, medical personnel, dental personnel, firemen, police officers, et cetera are in real danger of contracting the virus since they come in contact with blood and other body fluids.

I think that if the John Birch Society would set up AIDS committees from every chapter — as I look at it we could establish a national association for AIDS prevention and then have individual chapters in every city that are disseminating information to health care personnel, emergency personnel and to the general public — we could use this as a vehicle to, first of all, educate people on AIDS and get them to bring about legislation so that we could start treating this plague as the species threatening epidemic that it is. Secondly, the entire subject of AIDS gets into sex education, moral breakdown, humanism and all of the sinister forces which work behind the scenes attempting to destroy our society. This will be a tremendous opportunity to educate the general public as to what has gone wrong with America.

The major problem that we face in America is not the AIDS epidemic, it is the moral breakdown that has led to the rapid spread of this epidemic throughout our society and our toleration of promiscuity and perversion on a scale unparalleled since the days of Ancient Rome.

I really believe this may be our one last chance to awaken the American public. Indeed, it may be God's gift to us to give us that one last chance as a nation to change our ways. Otherwise, the outlook for the survival of our society is grim.

I have met with Kirt Kidwell in Washington. He is certainly warm, intelligent and a charming young man. Perhaps we could put our heads together and come up with a program. Whether I will work on the program with you or if you set it up independently is immaterial to me. I would be very glad to help in any way that I can in establishing some separate organization of the John Birch Society into which conservative members could be recruited and yet with the major driving force behind this, the local members of the Birch Society.

At the meeting in San Francisco, you asked if Congressman Dannemeyer's initiative was good. I can assure you it is. It was actually written in Santa Cruz by a very close friend of mine. It deserves the full support of the Chapters in California. We have got to get those signatures in so that we will have an alternative one year down the line to declare this disease a communicable, contagious disease. I hate to have to wait that long to start doing something about the epidemic, but it certainly gives us an alternative if we fail in the political arena.

In many ways, this horrible epidemic gives us a chance to rejuvenate the John Birch Society, to rejuvenate many of the people who have fallen by the wayside. I have talked to a number of the local members of the John Birch Society who long ago dropped out. Almost all of them are willing to get involved again working towards educating people on the AIDS epidemic. Now the threat is very real, it is not something that is going to happen in the distant future or is happening in South Africa or Vietnam. The threat is here. I believe that if we seize this opportunity, we can rekindle that spark of patriotism and dedication in the hearts of people all across America. In my humble opinion, this will be the last great battle, win or lose.

Warm Personal Regards,

Stanley K. Monteith, M.D.

SKM:jh

Publisher's note: This letter has been typeset from the original.

APPENDIX VI

Los Angeles Times
A Times Mirror Newspaper
Part II/Thursday, October 20, 1988

*Publisher's note: This document has been typeset rather than
photographically reproduced in the interest of readability.*

Fighting AIDS: No on 102

There are two reasons why most public-health professionals strongly oppose Proposition 102, the AIDS reporting initiative: It would outlaw the single most effective prevention program now in place, and it would squander millions of dollars on mandated programs of limited value.

On the face of it, the initiative offers a beguilingly simplistic solution to fight AIDS, doing to this disease what has been done to other communicable diseases by insisting on complete reporting and case-by-case contact tracing. This familiar solution has an attractive ring to it. But the proposal ignores the fundamentals of AIDS, above all that it is a disease without known cure.

The initiative goes further, however. It mandates not only reporting of all who test positive to the human immunodeficiency virus (HIV) that causes AIDS, but also requires that a doctor who "has reasonable cause to believe" that a person has been infected to report his suspicions. And anyone who learns that he or she has been infected must report to the local health officer.

The effect of this will be to eliminate the anonymous test centers that have proven the most effective means of reaching persons at risk, particularly intravenous drug users and homosexuals, who fear discrimination, including job and housing loss, if their infection becomes known.

There is another awesomely negative effect: The cost, according to the official estimate by the legislative analyst, "could be as high as tens or hundreds of millions of dollars"—$765 million the first year, according to a UC Berkeley School of Public Health study. The sponsors argue that this is a small price to pay to reduce the number of infected persons. True, if it works. But they offer no evidence to support their contention that this extremely costly approach would be more effective than the existing program. In fact, the evidence points overwhelmingly in the opposite direction.

A recent study in Oregon showed the extraordinary effectiveness of anonymous test sites, which would be eliminated by the initiative.

In the absence of a cure, the AIDS pandemic can be controlled only by programs that encourage testing of high-risk populations. The final report of the Presidential Commission on the Human Immunodeficiency Virus Epidemic, headed by Adm. James D. Watkins, emphasized the crucial importance of "voluntary cooperation" in a testing program, the only avenue to changing behavior that places others at risk. That very strategy, so carefully developed in California over the last five years, would be destroyed by the provisions of the initiative. And the damage would be compounded by diverting scarce resources from urgently needed current programs into a wasteful program mandated to trace every sexual contact over the last seven years of every infected person.

The last session of the Legislature adopted new laws on sharing HIV test information among health-care providers, on reporting and on contacting partners of infected persons. These measured and constructive proposals contrast with the punitive and carelessly drawn provisions of Proposition 102.

The existing AIDS program has the support of the California Medical Assn., the California Dental Assn., the California Nurses Assn., the State Health Officers Assn., the regional representative of the Centers for Disease Control, the California AIDS Leadership Committee, including top state, county and local public-health professionals. They are unanimous in their opposition to Proposition 102. And, in their opposition, they are joined by a long list of responsible civic organizations, among them the California Catholic Conference, the League of California Cities, the State Chamber of Commerce and the League of Women Voters of California. We agree with them. Vote *no*.

The New York Times

(Editorial on AIDS tests. Type reset by publisher)

A Treacherous Paradox: AIDS Tests

Present tests for the AIDS virus antibody are highly accurate. Yet if applied to the population at large, they could falsely brand nine people infected for every true case identified. The President's AIDS commission had better be sure it understands this treacherous paradox if it intends to recommend the widespread testing favored by some Administration officials.

Applied to groups at high risk for AIDS, like gay men and drug abusers, the tests are highly reliable, and the minute number of false positives is dwarfed by the large number of true positives. The testing of prostitutes, as suggested last week by Stephen Joseph, New York City's health commissioner, is worth considering because 20 to 60 percent may be addicts, and the proportion of false positives would probably be minute.

But that's not true of groups at low risk, among whom the very small number of true positives can easily be less than the number of false positives. If a low-risk group — like blood donors in Peoria, for instance — were screened for AIDS by the Elisa test, with its positive results confirmed by the Western blot test, 89 people out of 100,000 would be labeled as carrying the virus. But the real incidence of AIDS infection among this group probably is 10 per 100,000. The tests would miss one of the 10, catch the other nine and falsely describe 80 other people as carriers of the virus, according to new estimates by Lawrence Miike of the Congressional Office of Technology Assessment.

Such screening programs can easily do more harm than good, needlessly devastating dozens of lives for every case of infection detected.

The Army has been testing military recruits, a low-risk group, for two years. Its chief tester, Col. Donald Burke, believes that the rate of false positives is less than one in 100,000 people tested. At a recent Congressional hearing, Colonel Burke urged mass screening to identify almost every infected person in America.

But the Army is able to insist on unusually rigorous standards from its testing laboratories. States and local authorities setting up mass screening programs would reap many more false positives. Not only is the Western blot test for AIDS antibodies very difficult to perform, but there is not yet a generally agreed way to interpret its results. The slightest inaccuracy or sloppiness — a notorious problem with medical laboratories — quickly leads to more false diagnoses than true.

❋❋❋

Commercial laboratories recently given negative samples to test by the College of American Pathologists reported nearly 2 percent as positive by the Elisa test and 5 percent as positive by the Western blot. This joint error rate, according to the Office of Technology Assessment, means that in screening a low-risk population, up to 90 percent of people confirmed by the two tests as infected will not be.

People infected with the AIDS virus risk loss of jobs, insurance and housing. What responsible government could assume the burden of falsely telling nine people they were infected for each true infection identified? The cost of screening low-risk populations could be over $50,000 for each true positive detected. In states that seek to reach infected individuals for counseling, there is an innocuous and cheaper alternative — tracing the sexual and needle contacts of those already diagnosed.

Several members of the President's AIDS commission have indicated a predilection for testing various groups at low risk for AIDS. One, Cory Servaas, pressed the American Medical Association last week to say why it wasn't urging doctors to test all their patients. If the commission advocates widespread screening without insisting on far more accurate testing than is now available, it will create a program for shattering more lives than it saves.

APPENDIX VII

Refugees have fled from across the world to America in an effort to escape the tyranny imposed by oppressive socialist governments. Refugees have come from behind the Iron Curtain, Vietnam, Mainland China, Nicaragua, Central America and from Mexico — people from all over the world have fled to America and its promise of freedom — recognizing that liberty and limited government are synonymous, just as tyranny and total government are synonymous. How many people have died in small boats trying to escape from socialist Cuba or socialist Vietnam? How many more have made the long and arduous sea voyage to our shores, hoping that here they can at last be free?

Tragically, many Americans have come to take freedom for granted, not realizing that there are forces in our land which are intent upon imposing a socialist-type dictatorship in the United States. Tragically, those forces have powerful allies in many of our state governments and certainly in Washington, D. C.

Today we are moving towards a federal government that will provide for the individual from the cradle to the grave, which will take from the people according to their ability and give to others according to their need and regulate the means of production and distribution of goods throughout our nation. These programs are the basic tenets of Marxism.

To once again regain our freedom, the American public must become involved. We cannot depend upon our present leaders or hope that some man on a white horse will ride forth to lead us away from tyranny. Freedom is never free. It was purchased in past generations by the sacrifices and suffering of those who came before. It can only be maintained by our own personal sacrifice and commitment.

How can we accomplish this? What can be done? Some say it is too late, others say the job is overwhelming and nothing can be done to restrict the power of government, a government which is intent upon controlling us from the cradle to the grave. I do not believe that.

I would challenge you to become involved. You must not try to do everything, but to do what you can do. For it has been said:

I cannot do everything, but I can do something.

And that which I can do I will do.

You can target one group of people. You can target your precinct, your church or a club to which you belong. If you and a few thousand others who read my book can convince the people in your precinct, your church or your club of the problems that our nation faces — then we can begin to make inroads and begin to turn around the juggernaut which is intent upon stifling all freedom and using this epidemic to justify draconian controls over our nation. For indeed, this epidemic will destroy our nation just as surely as a nuclear attack.

There are three things you must convince people of.

1. They cannot believe what they read in the newspapers, for there are a few people working within our news media who are effectively censoring the news.

2. They must understand America is a unique nation and that our freedoms are derived from our Constitution which was drawn up by men who believed in God. Our freedoms came from God, not from government.

3. They must decide to convince others to become involved in the education and political process. The political process does not occur every two years when you go to the polls — it is something Americans must work at every day of the week.

How then will you gain the information needed to educate others? You can contact my office: 618 Frederick Street, Santa Cruz, CA 95062. I have studied the forces at work within our society — both political and spiritual — for over 25 years. I will be glad to send you a packet which will tell you how to go about educating your fellow Americans. For a nominal fee, I will provide you with audiotapes on:

1. The Judeo-Christian History of America

2. Thought Control in America

3. Political Control in America

With those three tapes, you will have more knowledge than most citizens, politicians and political scientists.

We can begin to utilize the miraculous electronic techniques available. We can communicate instantaneously by fax and by computers. I can teach you how to begin to utilize the local media to get the facts out, how to establish your own newsletters and your own newspapers with relatively little expense and effort.

The time is late. The illness of HIV disease, the illness of dependence on government, the illness of indifference and apathy are on the rise. Now is the time for a counterattack. You must always remember, "All that is necessary for evil to triumph is that good people do nothing" and "The price that good people pay for their apathy and indifference to public affairs is they are ruled by evil men."

What is at stake is our future, our freedom and our families. What is at stake is the preservation of this nation — under God — which has been the beacon of hope for people throughout the world for 200 years. If this nation falls then all will be lost and life will have no meaning.

I hope that you will join with me in this crusade to try to save this nation. Time is running out. The biological clock ticks towards the point of no return as the ever-widening ripples of disease spread silently across our tragic land.

— Stanley K. Monteith, M.D.

APPENDIX VIII

Publisher's note: This document has been typeset rather than photographically reproduced in the interest of readability.

CMA NEWS, August 6, 1982
CMA seeks immediate enactment of remedial legislation on AB 3480

CMA will seek immediate "trailer" legislation to remedy provisions of AB 3480, the bill to allow insurance companies to contract directly with hospitals and physicians at discount rates and to establish closed panels of "preferred providers." Meeting Friday in special session, Council voted to pursue amendments to AB 3480 that would protect both patients and physicians. As News has reported, AB 3480 has two major provisions: it lets insurance companies contract with physicians and hospitals at discount rates, and it allows insurance companies to limit payments to contracting providers only.

CMA's legislation does not preclude insurance company contracting. However, it prohibits insurers from controlling the practice of medicine; precludes conditioning of hospital staff membership privileges upon a physician's agreement to so contract; regulates the solicitation of providers; clarifies that the Knox-Keene Act (which regulates health care service plans) must govern any contracting arrangements if the contract deals with anything other than fees; and requires the insurer to maintain information that identifies providers and outlines contractual arrangements.

CMA's Proposal and Arguments in Support
(Received from CMA on September 7, 1982)

Section 1343.1 is added to the Health and Safety Code to read: (new) An insurer or hospital service plan operating pursuant to a certificate issued by the Insurance Commissioner which negotiates and enters into contracts for alternative rates of payment with institutional or professional providers and offers the benefit of such alternative rates to insureds who select such providers is not subject to this chapter, so long as no limitation is placed upon the right of insureds to select any hospital or physician, and so long as said contracts are limited to alternative rates charged by contracting providers, imposing no further condition or requirement upon the provider or the insured.

Explanation and argument:
This section exempts insurance contracting for "discount rates" from Knox-Keene regulation, so long as the contracts are limited to rates. If insurers contract in any way that may impact on access or quality of health care, such contracts must be regulated by Knox-Keene. This is intended to prevent the reoccurrence of the PHP scandals. CMA CAN ACCEPT HAVING PHYSICIANS CONTRACT TO ACCEPT A LESSER REIMBURSEMENT FOR HEALTH CARE. CMA IS NOT WILLING TO REDUCE THE QUALITY OF CARE OR THE AC-CESS TO CARE.

For additional copies of this book
send $14.95 plus $2.00 postage and handling (for each copy) to

AIDS Book
618 Frederick Street
Santa Cruz, CA 95062

Book Dealers write for discount information.